The Manual of Allergy and Clinical Immunology

The Manual of Allergy and Clinical Immunology

Edited by

Abeer Feteih, MD, FRCPC
Assistant Professor of Medicine
Clinical Immunologist and Allergist
Department of Internal Medicine, Faculty of Medicine in Rabigh
King Abdulaziz University
Jeddah, Saudi Arabia

Michael Fein, MD, FRCPC
Assistant Professor of Medicine
Division of Clinical Immunology and Allergy
McGill University Health Centre
Montréal, Québec, Canada

Natacha Tardio, MD, FRCPC
Assistant Professor of Medicine
Residency Training Program Director
Division of Clinical Immunology and Allergy
McGill University Health Centre
Montréal, Québec, Canada

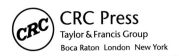

CRC Press
Taylor & Francis Group
Boca Raton London New York

CRC Press is an imprint of the
Taylor & Francis Group, an **informa** business

First edition published 2022
by CRC Press
6000 Broken Sound Parkway NW, Suite 300, Boca Raton, FL 33487-2742

and by CRC Press
2 Park Square, Milton Park, Abingdon, Oxon, OX14 4RN

Library of Congress Cataloging-in-Publication Data

Names: Feteih, Abeer, editor. | Fein, Michael (Michael N.), editor. | Tardio, Natacha, editor.
Title: The manual of allergy and clinical immunology / edited by Abeer Feteih, Michael Fein, Natacha Tardio.
Other titles: Manual of allergy and clinical immunology (Feteih)
Description: First edition. | Boca Raton, FL : CRC Press, 2022. | Includes bibliographical references and index. | Summary: "This pocketbook provides brief clinical summaries of complex and emerging major topics encountered in the field of Allergy and Immunology. As knowledge in the specialty is rapidly evolving, it condenses this material while maintaining an evidence-based approach to the practice. It is a practical and informative guide for students and clinicians"–Provided by publisher.
Identifiers: LCCN 2021045214 (print) | LCCN 2021045215 (ebook) | ISBN 9781032004464 (hardback) | ISBN 9781032004457 (paperback) | ISBN 9781003174202 (ebook)
Subjects: MESH: Immune System Diseases | Hypersensitivity | Immunotherapy | Handbook
Classification: LCC RC582 (print) | LCC RC582 (ebook) | NLM QW 539 | DDC 616.07/9–dc23
LC record available at https://lccn.loc.gov/2021045214
LC ebook record available at https://lccn.loc.gov/2021045215

ISBN: 9781032004464 (hbk)
ISBN: 9781032004457 (pbk)
ISBN: 9781003174202 (ebk)

DOI: 10.1201/9781003174202

Typeset in Minion Pro
by KnowledgeWorks Global Ltd.

Dedications

To my beloved supportive husband Mohammed, my precious son Yousef, my parents (Maha and Nizar), and my dear siblings for all your love and care.

– Abeer Feteih

To my wonderful family for all of their love and support.

– Michael Fein

To my beautiful children Mia and Noah, and wonderful husband Pierre for your inspiration, encouragement and unconditional love.

– Natacha Tardio

Contents

Preface   ix

Editors   xi

Contributors   xiii

PART 1   RHINOCONJUNCTIVITIS

1 Allergic Rhinitis   3
Abeer Feteih, Hoang Pham, Michael Fein, Geneviève Genest, and Jaime Del Carpio

2 Rhinosinusitis   13
Abeer Feteih, Hoang Pham, Michael Fein, Geneviève Genest, and Jaime Del Carpio

3 Ocular Allergy   23
Fatemah Al-Yaqout and Abeer Feteih

4 Allergen Immunotherapy   31
Abeer Feteih, Walaa Almasri, Geneviève Genest, Hoang Pham, and Phil Gold

PART 2   RESPIRATORY DISORDERS

5 Asthma and Allergic Bronchopulmonary Aspergillosis (ABPA)   41
Hoang Pham, Abeer Feteih, Geneviève Genest, and Jaime Del Carpio

6 Approach to Chronic Cough   57
Hoang Pham and Maxime Cormier

PART 3   CUTANEOUS DISORDERS

7 Atopic Dermatitis (AD)   67
Fatemah Al-Yaqout, Abeer Feteih, Walaa Almasri, Hoang Pham, and Reza Alizadehfar

8 Contact Dermatitis   75
Geneviève Bouvette, Walaa Almasri, Hoang Pham, and Abeer Feteih

9 Urticaria   81
*Abeer Feteih, Farida Almarzooqi, Michael Fein, Geneviève Genest, Hoang Pham, and
Moshe Ben-Shoshan*

10 Angioedema   91
*Abeer Feteih, Farida Almarzooqi, Michael Fein, Geneviève Genest, Hoang Pham, and
Moshe Ben-Shoshan*

PART 4   MAST CELL-RELATED DISORDERS/ANAPHYLAXIS (SYSTEMIC ILLNESSES)

11 Mastocytosis and Mast Cell Activation Syndromes   103
*Abeer Feteih, Farida Almarzooqi, Geneviève Genest, Michael Fein, Hoang Pham, and
Moshe Ben-Shoshan*

12 Anaphylaxis   115
Abeer Feteih, Michael Fein, Natacha Tardio, Geneviève Genest, Lydia Zhang, Hoang Pham, and Moshe Ben-Shoshan

13 Exercise-Induced Anaphylaxis (EIA) and Food-Dependent EIA (FDEIA)   123
Abeer Feteih, Lydia Zhang, Natacha Tardio, and Michael Fein

14 Stinging Insect Hypersensitivity   127
Abeer Feteih, Hoang Pham, Walaa Almasri, and Geneviève Genest

15 Eosinophilia and Hypereosinophilic Syndrome (HES)   135
Abeer Feteih, Hoang Pham, Geneviève Genest, and Natacha Tardio

PART 5   FOOD ALLERGY

16 Food Allergy   145
Abeer Feteih, Lydia Zhang, Natacha Tardio, Hoang Pham, and Moshe Ben-Shoshan

17 Eosinophilic Esophagitis (EoE)   153
Abeer Feteih, Hoang Pham, Michael Fein, Serge Mayrand, and Natacha Tardio

18 Celiac Disease and Non-Celiac Gluten Sensitivity   159
Stephen Tsoukas, Natacha Tardio, and Waqqas Afif

PART 6   DRUG ALLERGY

19 Drug Allergy   167
Abeer Feteih, Hoang Pham, and Ghislaine Annie Clarisse Isabwe

20 Adverse Reactions to Nonsteroidal Anti-Inflammatory Drugs and Aspirin   177
Abeer Feteih, Lydia Zhang, Geneviève Genest, and Ghislaine Annie Clarisse Isabwe

21 Adverse Reactions to Vaccines   183
Abeer Feteih, Lydia Zhang, and Geneviève Genest

PART 7   CLINICAL IMMUNOLOGY

22 General Approach to Primary Immunodeficiency (PID) in Adults   191
Abeer Feteih, Lydia Zhang, Reza Alizadehfar, and Christos Tsoukas

23 Immunoglobulin Replacement Therapy   199
Abeer Feteih, Farida Almarzooqi, Reza Alizadehfar, and Christos Tsoukas

Index   203

Preface

Allergy and Immunology is a rapidly evolving field with an abundance of growth in medical knowledge. Significant advances have been made in the diagnosis and treatment of a wide array of allergic and immunologic conditions including respiratory, cutaneous, and systemic allergic disorders. This manual was created as a practical tool for medical professionals, residents, and students to quickly access current and concise information on the main pathologies seen in this discipline. Chapters are organized so that material is easy to grasp and apply in both clinical and non-clinical settings.

Starting off as a collection of study notes from teaching faculty and senior residents in the Division of Clinical Immunology and Allergy at McGill University (Montréal, Québec), this work has significantly expanded over the last 5 years to include the contributions of various experts at the McGill University Health Centre. This includes a collaborative effort among several specialties including allergy, immunology, respirology, gastroenterology, dermatology, and pathology. Medical education, research, clinical innovation, and patient advocacy are common objectives of our teaching faculty.

We would like to sincerely thank all the authors as well as the publisher for their help in creating this manual. We hope that it encourages students, scientists, clinicians, and inquisitive minds to pursue scholarly work in this fascinating field and to contribute to its advancement.

Editors

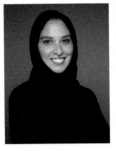

Dr. Abeer Feteih completed medical school and received her medical degree from the Faculty of Medicine at King Abdulaziz University, Jeddah, Saudi Arabia. She then completed her postgraduate medical education and training at McGill University in Montréal, Canada, which included 3 years of residency training in Internal Medicine, followed by 2 years of fellowship training in Clinical Immunology and Allergy. She received certifications from the Royal College of Physicians and Surgeons of Canada in both Internal Medicine and Clinical Immunology and Allergy. Currently, Dr. Feteih is an Assistant Professor in the Department of Internal Medicine, Faculty of Medicine in Rabigh at King Abdulaziz University. She practices Clinical Immunology and Allergy in private practice as well. Dr. Feteih has many interests in her field including urticaria and allergic rhinitis, as well as medical education, medical student and trainee wellness.

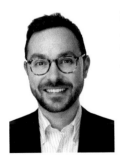

Dr. Michael Fein is an Assistant Professor of Adult Clinical Immunology and Allergy at the McGill University Health Centre. He completed a bachelor of arts in International Relations at Duke University followed by a medical doctorate at Jefferson Medical College in Philadelphia, Pennsylvania. He completed residency training in Internal Medicine and fellowship training in Clinical Immunology and Allergy at the McGill University Health Centre. He is board certified in Internal Medicine and Clinical Immunology and Allergy in both Canada and the United States. His interests include medical education and quality improvement and patient safety.

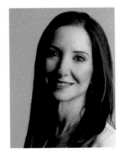

Dr. Natacha Tardio obtained her medical doctorate degree and Internal Medicine certification from Laval University in Quebec City. She then went on to complete subspecialty training in Clinical Immunology and Allergy at McGill University. She received certifications from the Royal College of Physicians and Surgeons of Canada in both Internal Medicine and Clinical Immunology and Allergy. Dr. Tardio now practices as Assistant Professor of Medicine and Residency Training Program Director in the Division of Clinical Immunology and Allergy at the McGill University Health Centre (Montréal, Québec). Her interests include medical education, eosinophilic disorders, and food allergy.

Contributors

Waqqas Afif, MD, MSc, FRCPC
Associate Professor of Medicine
Division of Gastroenterology
McGill University Health Centre
Montréal, Québec, Canada

Reza Alizadehfar, MD, FRCPC
Training Program Director
Associate Professor of Pediatrics
Division of Allergy and Clinical
    Immunology
Montréal Children's Hospital
Montréal General Hospital
McGill University Health Centre
Montréal, Québec, Canada

Farida Almarzooqi, MD
Department of Pediatrics
College of Medicine and Health Sciences,
    UAE University
Al Ain, United Arab Emirates

Walaa Almasri, MD
Division of Clinical Immunology and Allergy
McGill University Health Centre
Montréal, Québec, Canada

Fatemah Al-Yaqout, LRCP & SI, MB BCh BAO
Division of Clinical Immunology and
    Allergy
McGill University Health Centre
Montréal, Québec, Canada

Moshe Ben-Shoshan, MSc, MD
Associate Professor of Pediatrics
Montréal Children's Hospital
Department of Pediatrics
Division of Allergy Immunology and
    Dermatology
McGill University Health Centre
Montréal, Québec, Canada

Geneviève Bouvette, MD, FRCPC
Division of Clinical Immunology and Allergy
McGill University Health Centre
Montréal, Québec, Canada

Maxime Cormier, MD, FRCPC
Assistant Professor of Medicine
Department of Medicine
Division of Respiratory Medicine
McGill University Health Centre
Montréal, Québec, Canada

Jaime Del Carpio, MD, FRCPC
Associate Professor of Medicine
Division of Clinical Immunology and Allergy
McGill University Health Centre
Montréal, Québec, Canada

Michael Fein, MD, FRCPC
Assistant Professor of Medicine
Division of Clinical Immunology and Allergy
McGill University Health Centre
Montréal, Québec, Canada

Abeer Feteih, MD, FRCPC
Assistant Professor of Medicine
Clinical Immunologist and Allergist
Department of Internal Medicine
Faculty of Medicine in Rabigh
King Abdulaziz University
Jeddah, Saudi Arabia

Geneviève Genest, BSc, MD, FRCPC
Founder, McGill Reproductive Immunology
    Clinic
Director, McGill Fellowship Program,
    Reproductive Immunology
Assistant Professor of Medicine
Division of Clinical Allergy and Immunology
McGill University Health Centre
Montréal, Québec, Canada

Phil Gold, CC, GOQ, MD, PhD, FRSC, DSc (Hon) MACP, FRCP(C)
Douglas G. Cameron Professor of Medicine
Professor of Physiology and Oncology
Division of Physiology and Oncology
McGill University Health Centre
Montréal, Québec, Canada

Ghislaine Annie Clarisse Isabwe, MD, FRCPC
Division of Clinical Immunology and Allergy
McGill University Health Centre
Montréal, Québec, Canada

Serge Mayrand, MD, FRCPC
Associate Professor of Medicine
Division of Gastroenterology
McGill University Health Centre
Montréal, Québec, Canada

Hoang (Tano) Pham, MD, FRCPC
Division of Clinical Immunology and Allergy
McGill University Health Centre
Montréal, Québec, Canada

Natacha Tardio, MD, FRCPC
Residency Training Program Director
Assistant Professor of Medicine
Division of Clinical Immunology and Allergy
McGill University Health Centre
Montréal, Québec, Canada

Christos Tsoukas, CM, MD, MSc, FRCP(C), FACP, FCAHS
Professor of Medicine and Experimental Medicine
Director, Division of Clinical Immunology and Allergy
McGill University Health Centre
Montréal, Québec, Canada

Stephen Tsoukas, MD, FRCPC
Assistant Professor of Medicine
Division of Gastroenterology and Hepatology
St. Mary's Hospital
McGill University Health Centre
Montréal, Québec, Canada

Lydia Zhang, MD, FRCPC
Division of Clinical Immunology and Allergy
McGill University Health Centre
Montréal, Québec, Canada

RHINOCONJUNCTIVITIS

1 Allergic Rhinitis   3
Abeer Feteih, Hoang Pham, Michael Fein, Geneviève Genest, and Jaime Del Carpio

2 Rhinosinusitis   13
Abeer Feteih, Hoang Pham, Michael Fein, Geneviève Genest, and Jaime Del Carpio

3 Ocular Allergy   23
Fatemah Al-Yaqout and Abeer Feteih

4 Allergen Immunotherapy   31
Abeer Feteih, Walaa Almasri, Geneviève Genest, Hoang Pham, and Phil Gold

Allergic Rhinitis

ABEER FETEIH, HOANG PHAM, MICHAEL FEIN,
GENEVIÈVE GENEST, AND JAIME DEL CARPIO

This chapter will describe the different types of rhinitis and will mainly focus on allergic rhinitis.

GENERAL BACKGROUND

- Allergic rhinitis is an IgE-mediated inflammatory disease of the nasal mucosal membranes (1).
- It is estimated to affect around 20%–25% of Canadians (2).
- Rhinitis (atopic or non-atopic) is a risk factor for developing asthma. It is more likely that the person will develop asthma when the rhinitis is more persistent and severe (2).
- Allergic rhinitis in childhood is more frequent in boys, but in adults, it is more frequent in women (3).

- Symptoms of seasonal allergic rhinitis (SAR) usually do not develop until 2–7 years of age (3).
- Despite the high prevalence and negative impact on quality of life and productivity, rhinitis is often overlooked and remains undertreated (1, 3–5).

OTHER COMMON CAUSES OF RHINITIS

Rhinitis is a very common presentation with many potential etiologies. A focused history will guide diagnosis; aeroallergen skin testing, or specific IgE testing is required to evaluate for an allergic component (see Table 1.1).

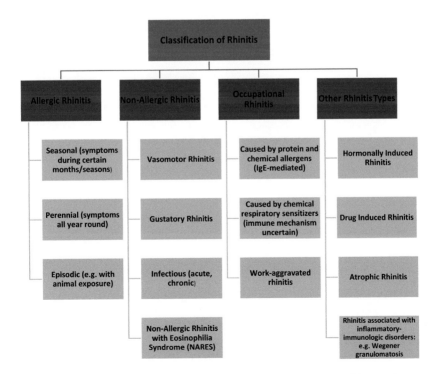

Figure 1.1 Classification of rhinitis. (Figure created with BioRender.com.) [Adapted from (3).]

DOI: 10.1201/9781003174202-2

Table 1.1 Other Causes of Rhinitis

Condition	Key suggestive features
Vasomotor Rhinitis^	Predominant rhinorrhea and nasal obstruction
	Triggered by temperature/humidity changes (e.g. cold air), irritants/strong odors (e.g. perfumes, smoke), exercise
Drug-Induced Rhinitis*	*Rhinitis Medicamentosa*—overuses topical nasal decongestants (alpha-adrenergic agonists) for more than 3 days
	Patient may be taking antihypertensive medication that disrupts sympathetic/parasympathetic vascular tone leading to nasal congestion & rhinorrhea
	NSAIDs and alcohol can cause acute rhinitis symptoms in patients with NSAID-exacerbated respiratory disease
Hormonal Rhinitis	Associated with pregnancy, menstrual cycles, menopause, and puberty, hypothyroidism and acromegaly
Non-Allergic Rhinitis with Eosinophilia Syndrome (NARES)	Prominent symptoms of perennial rhinorrhea and sneezing without other features of facial pain, nasal obstruction, nasal polyps, sinus mucosal thickening
	Marked response to intranasal steroids
	Eosinophilia in nasal tissues (research centers only)
Gustatory Rhinitis^	Clear rhinorrhea after consumption of hot and/or spicy foods
Occupational Rhinitis	Question the patient about workplace exposures such as cold dry air, dust particulate matter, vapors, smoke, chemicals, strong odors
Atrophic Rhinitis	Observed in young to middle-aged adults from dry climates; associated with nasal dryness, foul-smelling nasal crusts
Infectious Rhinitis	Acute onset of fever, nasal congestion, mucopurulent nasal discharge, headache, smell disturbance, post-nasal drip, cough
	Lacks recurrent seasonal pattern
	Lacks nasal or ocular pruritus
Local Allergic Rhinitis	Difficult to diagnose outside specialized research centres that are able to do nasal provocation tests to aeroallergens
	Frequently report watery rhinorrhea, sneezing, and itching despite negative conventional aeroallergen testing

* Other causes of drug-induced rhinitis include ACE-inhibitors (e.g. perindopril), alpha-receptor antagonists (e.g tamsulosin), and phosphodiesterase 5-selective inhibitors (e.g. sildenafil).
^Vasomotor & Gustatory rhinitis may respond to intranasal anticholinergics (e.g. ipratropium).
Adapted from (3–5).

Classification of Allergic Rhinitis [According to "Allergic Rhinitis and Its Impact on Asthma (ARIA)" (1)]

- **"Intermittent"**: Presence of symptoms <4 times a week or for <4 weeks
- **"Persistent"**: Presence of symptoms >4 days a week and for >4 weeks
- **"Mild"**: When none of the following are present:
  - Sleep disturbance
  - Impairment of daily activities, leisure, and/or sport
  - Impairment of school or work
  - Troublesome symptoms

- **"Moderate-severe"**: In the presence of ≥1 of these symptoms:
  - Sleep disturbance
  - Impairment of daily activities, leisure, and/or sport
  - Impairment of school or work
  - Troublesome symptoms

CLINICAL MANIFESTATIONS OF ALLERGIC RHINITIS [ADAPTED FROM (1, 3–5)]

Symptoms

- Nasal congestion, rhinorrhea, postnasal drip, nasal pruritus, sneezing, and itchy or watery eyes

Important Points in History Taking

- Onset/duration/chronicity of symptoms.
- Symptom pattern.
- Timing of symptoms in relation to season/month.
- Triggering factors.
- Past medical history, with particular emphasis on common comorbidities and complications of allergic rhinitis (e.g. asthma, rhinosinusitis, obstructive sleep apnea, pollen food syndrome (PFS)/oral allergy syndrome (OAS), chronic otitis media with effusion).
  - In the setting of limited access to allergy testing, a history of PFS/OAS symptoms such as local oropharyngeal pruritus upon exposure to raw stone-pitted fruits (e.g. peaches, cherries, apples) provides a major diagnostic clue to a patient's allergic status with respect to certain pollens (i.e. birch in the case of stone-pitted fruits).
- Family history (including history of atopic disease).
- Medications (e.g. trial of any anti-allergy treatments, medications that can promote rhinitis such as antihypertensives, chronic use of nasal decongestant sprays).
- History of response to previous treatment(s).
- Environmental (e.g. carpets, pets, visible mold growth/history of water damage in the home) and occupational history and exposures.
- The effect of rhinitis on quality of life (symptoms of fatigue, sleep disturbances, learning and attention issues, and absenteeism from work and/or school).

Physical Examination

- *General observations:* Frequent sniffing, mouth breathing, use of tissues, hyponasal voice, nose rubbing.
- *Allergic shiners:* Infraorbital darkening and edema due to subcutaneous venodilation, which is seen in any chronic sinonasal disorder and not specific for allergy (see Figure 1.2).
- *Dennie-Morgan lines:* Accentuated lines/folds below the lower eyelids that suggest the presence of concomitant allergic conjunctivitis (mild bilateral red conjunctival injection, chemosis, and watery discharge) (see Figure 1.2).

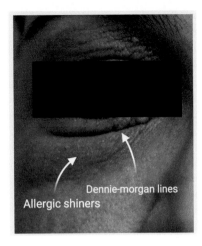

Figure 1.2 Physical exam findings in allergic rhinitis (see text). (Figure created with BioRender.com.) (Image courtesy of Dr. Dennis Sasseville.)

- *Allergic salute:* A transverse nasal crease produced by repeated rubbing and pushing the tip of the nose up with the hand.
- *Allergic facies:* Seen in children with early disease onset; it includes retracted mandible, elongated facies, high arched palate, open mouth due to mouth breathing, and dental malocclusion.
- *Nasal mucosa:* Pale bluish tint or pallor with edema of the turbinates, and anterior or posterior clear rhinorrhea; examine for nasal septum deviation and nasal polyps.
- *Posterior pharynx:* Cobblestoning, suggestive of chronic postnasal drip.
- *Tympanic membranes (TM):* Assess for retraction or accumulation of serous fluid behind the TM found in patients with swelling of the nasal mucosa and dysfunction of the eustachian tube (11).
- *Lung auscultation:* For evidence of wheezing.
- *Skin examination:* For signs of atopic dermatitis (see Chapter 7).

Differential Diagnosis of Rhinitis

1. Nasal polyps
2. Structural/mechanical factors
   - Deviated nasal septum
   - Adenoid hypertrophy
   - Trauma
   - Foreign bodies
   - Nasal tumors
   - Cleft palate
3. Ciliary dyskinesia syndrome
4. Cerebrospinal fluid (CSF) rhinorrhea

Diagnosis and Investigations of Allergic Rhinitis [Adapted from (3–6)]

- Skin prick testing for suspected environmental allergen (s).
- Size of positive skin test results (wheal) correlates with likelihood of a positive nasal provocation challenge (true allergy) and not with severity of symptoms.
- Specific IgE immunoassays may be preferred over skin testing in those with severe skin disease, in cases where antihistamines cannot be stopped, in patients who are uncooperative, or when the history suggests a high risk of anaphylaxis from skin testing (exceedingly rare with aeroallergens).
- Positive results must be correlated with history and physical examination to assess their clinical significance.

Note: Positive skin testing without symptoms has been shown to be a major risk factor for the later development of SAR (7, 8).

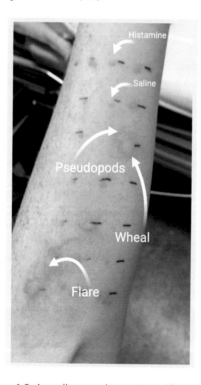

Figure 1.3 Aeroallergen skin testing. Skin testing results for aeroallergen panel with histamine (positive) and saline (negative) controls. Wheals 3 mm greater than saline control are considered positive. Flare (erythema) reactions surround wheals and pseudopods are remote wheals from site of skin test. (Figure created with BioRender.com.) (Image courtesy of Dr. Fein.)

Management of Allergic Rhinitis
Non-Pharmacologic

1. *Environmental control of indoor/outdoor allergens*
   - First-line measure to recommend, but may be difficult for the patient to achieve, especially for outdoor allergens.
   - Indoor allergen reduction interventions are most effective when done in combination.

2. *Pollen*
   - Pollen counts are usually highest on sunny, windy days with low humidity (3).
   - Advise patients to keep their windows at home closed, try to avoid going outdoors during high pollen counts, avoid drying clothes/laundry outdoors, and wash all clothes after returning back home from outside.

3. *Dust Mites [Adapted from Wilson and Platts-Mills "Home Environmental Interventions for House Dust Mite" (9)]*
   - Bedroom
     - Covering mattresses with plastic or fine woven fabric.
     - Covering pillows and comforters with fine woven fabric.
     - Washing mattress pads, sheets, and all blankets in hot water every 1–2 weeks.
     - Carpet removal if possible.
     - Decreasing upholstered furniture, drapes, and clothing.
     - Room air cleaner which is best with high-efficiency particulate air (HEPA) filter put on polished floor.
   - Whole House
     - Decreasing relative humidity to ≤45%.
     - Ventilation of the house when the humidity outside is low.
     - Choosing a house with second floor bedrooms.
     - Avoidance of concrete slabs except in the basement and avoidance of fitted carpets on a concrete slab.
   - Specific Questions beyond the Bedroom
     - Prefer area rugs over carpets; clean regularly.
     - Vacuum rugs/carpets twice weekly.
     - Reduce clutter; minimize upholstered furniture.

- Fungi
  - Face masks can reduce exposure to fungi in those who do plant/gardening work (3).
  - Eliminating sources of moisture (e.g. water intrusion, increased humidity).
  - Diluted bleach solution with detergent denatures fungal allergens and may prevent regrowth, on hard, nonporous surfaces. Porous surfaces require removal.
- Cockroach allergen (mostly found in the kitchen) (3)
  - Sealing of all sources of food.
  - Food debris removal.
  - Thorough home cleaning.
  - Using newer gel or bait pesticides (e.g. abamectin or hydramethylnon without color/odor).
  - Structural removal of harborages.
- Animals
  - It is recommended that cats and dogs be removed from the environment, if possible, or kept outside the bedroom to reduce exposure to their allergens (3, 10).
  - Cat and dog allergens were shown to produce symptoms in sensitized individuals when there is contamination of animal-free homes and schools with passive transport (e.g. clothing) (3).
  - Twenty weeks on average is needed after animal removal from the home before the allergen concentration reaches levels found in a home without an animal in it (3, 10).
  - Keeping a cat in a room without a carpet (other than bedroom) with a HEPA filter may decrease airborne allergen spreading to the rest of the house by 90% (3).
  - Some studies showed reduced airborne cat allergen by washing the animal once or twice a week (10). This recommendation is highly impractical.
- Irritants (3)
  - Nasal symptoms are related to the duration of exposure and usually resolve when the irritants, such as formaldehyde, tobacco smoke, perfume, and chlorine, are removed.

Pharmacologic Management (1, 3–5)

Many factors are to be considered when selecting pharmacotherapy options, such as type of rhinitis (allergic vs. non-allergic, intermittent vs. persistent, etc.), predominant symptoms (congestion vs. rhinorrhea, etc.), severity, impact on sleep and quality of life, comorbidities (e.g. asthma), onset of action, efficacy, adverse effects, and costs. (4). (*See Table 1.2 for specific medications and dosing.*)

- In general, most patients have likely already tried self-medicating with over-the-counter oral antihistamine options before seeking formal allergy evaluation.
  - **First-generation H1 antihistamines are *no longer* recommended as first-line options** due to adverse effects of sedation, impairment with decreased cognitive function, poor sleep quality, dry mouth, dizziness, and orthostatic hypotension (11).
- Monotherapy with one of the following three options is recommended (4):
  - **Intranasal antihistamine (INAH)** as an initial treatment option for SAR, intermittent allergic rhinitis, and non-allergic rhinitis (NAR). Alternatively, **second-generation oral antihistamines** can be considered instead of using an INAH as some patients may prefer to use oral medications.
    Note that the only single-agent INAH available in Canada is levocabastine (see Table 1.2 for dosing).
  - **Intranasal corticosteroid (INCS)** as an initial treatment option for moderate/severe SAR, perennial allergic rhinitis (PAR). Preferred monotherapy option for PAR.
  - **Combination INAH and INCS** as an initial treatment option for moderate/severe SAR. Alternatively, combination INAH and INCS is also recommended as a step-up option when moderate/severe SAR, PAR, and NAR are resistant to initial pharmacologic monotherapy.
    - Note that the only combination spray available in Canada is azelastine and fluticasone propionate (see Table 1.2 for dosing).

Table 1.2 Commonly Used Pharmacotherapy for Allergic Rhinitis in Canada

Drug	Recommended dose	Labelled indications	Special remarks (3,4)
ORAL H1-ANTIHISTAMINES			
Cetirizine	5–10 mg tab/solution OD 2–5 years: 2.5 mg OD-BID	SAR & PAR ≥ 2 years CSU ≥ 12 years	OTC
Desloratadine	5 mg tab/solution OD 2–5 years: 1.25 mg/day 6–11 years: 2.5 mg/day	SAR, PAR, CSU ≥ 2 years	OTC
Fexofenadine	60 mg tab BID or 120 mg tab OD 6–11 years: 30 mg BID	SAR, PAR, CSU ≥ 12 years	OTC
Loratadine	10 mg tab/solution OD 10 years: 10 mg OD (if ≥ 30 kg): 2–9 years: 5 mg OD	SAR, PAR, CSU ≥ 2 years	OTC
Bilastine	20 mg tab OD before meals	SAR ≥12 years CSU ≥18 years	Very low sedation profile due to novel molecular design (20) Consider if treating concomitant CSU, requiring high doses of antihistamines (11)
Rupatadine	10 mg tab/solution OD 2–11 years: 2.5 mg (if 10–25 kg) 2–11 years: 5 mg (if > 25 kg)	SAR, PAR, CSU ≥ 2 years	Has additional anti-platelet activating factor (PAF) blockade properties which may be helpful for relief of severe congestion (21)
Diphenhydramine	25–30 mg q 4–6 hours; max 150 mg/day 6–11 years: 12.5 mg q 4–6 hours 2–5 years: 6.25 mg q 4–6 hours	SAR, PAR, CSU ≥2 years	1st-generation antihistamine; use discouraged. 1st-generation antihistamines are no longer 1st-line due to significant adverse side effects; Only parenteral antihistamine available in Canada currently
INTRANASAL ANTHISTAMINES (INAHs)			
Levocabastine	50 mcg/spray; 2 sprays each nostril BID (Can increase to 2 sprays TID or QID)	AR 12 to 65 years	Only non-combination intranasal antihistamine approved in Canada Recommended as an initial therapy for SAR, NAR, and intermittent AR Recommended in combination with INCs for moderate-severe SAR, PAR, and NAR resistant to monotherapy
INTRANASAL CORTICOSTEROIDS (INCS)			
Beclomethasone	50 mcg/spray; 1–2 sprays each nostril BID or 1 spray TID-QID Max 600 mcg/day in adults; 400 mcg/day in children	SAR and PAR Nasal polyps ≥ 6 years	High bioavailability

Drug	Recommended dose	Labelled indications	Special remarks (3,4)
Triamcinolone	55 mcg/spray, 2 sprays each nostril OD 4–12 years: 1 spray each nostril OD	SAR and PAR ≥ 4 years	High bioavailability Associated with higher rate of congenital respiratory defects
Budesonide	64 mcg/spray; Max 256 mcg/day 2 sprays each nostril OD or 1 spray each nostril BID	SAR, PAR, and NAR >6 years Nasal polyps ≥ 12 years	Moderate bioavailability Safety profile in pregnancy (class B); 100 mcg spray and turbuhaler discontinued in Canada
Ciclesonide	50 mcg/spray, 2 sprays each nostril OD	SAR and PAR ≥ 12 years	Low bioavailability
Fluticasone Furoate	27.5 mcg/spray, 2 sprays each nostril OD 2–11 years: 1 spray each nostril OD	SAR and PAR ≥ 2 years	Low bioavailability New supportive safety data in pregnancy
Fluticasone Propionate	50 mcg/spray, 2 sprays each nostril OD	SAR and PAR ≥ 18 years	Low bioavailability New supportive safety data in pregnancy OTC
Mometasone	50 mcg/spray, 2 sprays each nostril OD 3–11 years: 1 spray each nostril OD May use BID for ARS (max 15 days)	SAR and PAR ≥ 3 years ARS ≥12 years Nasal polyps ≥18 years	Low bioavailability New supportive safety data in pregnancy
COMBINATION INTRANASAL CORTICOSTEROID-ANTIHISTAMINES			
Fluticasone Propionate/ Azelastine Hydrochloride	50 mcg/137 mcg; 1 spray each nostril BID	SAR >12 years	Superior to oral antihistamine; Combination may be useful for treating nasal symptoms (e.g. severe congestion) over individual components (22–23)
LEUKOTRIENE ANTAGONISTS			
Montelukast	10 mg tablet OD in the evening 6–14 years: 5 mg OD 2–5 years: 4 mg OD	Asthma ≥ 2 years EIB ≥2 years SAR ≥15 years	Counsel patients on possible serious neuropsychiatric side effects (e.g. agitation, depression, suicidal thoughts) Less effective than INCSs for rhinitis Use in select cased of concomitant asthma, exercise-induced bronchoconstriction, NERD, and/or patient preference
TOPICAL NASAL DECONGESTANTS			
Oxymetazoline	0.05%; 2–3 sprays each nostril BID for <3 days Max 2 doses/24 hours	Temporary relief ≥12 years	May be used in initial 5 days for severe mucosal edema that impairs delivery of other intranasal therapies Consider as add-on treatment to INCSs or to combination INCS-Antihistamines if persistent nasal congestion (max 4 weeks)

(Continued)

Table 1.2 Commonly Used Pharmacotherapy for Allergic Rhinitis in Canada (Continued)

Drug	Recommended dose	Labelled indications	Special remarks (3,4)
Xylometazoline	0.05–00;.1% 1–3 drops/ sprays OD-TID	Temporary relief ≥12 years	Limit to short-term & intermittent use only to avoid rebound congestion from rhinitis medicamentosa Associated with risk of reversible cerebral vasoconstriction syndrome
ORAL NASAL DECONGESTANT			
Pseudoephedrine	60 mg tablet q 4–6 hours or 120 mg ER q 12 hours; Max 240 mg/day Age 2–4: 1 mg/kg/dose q 6 hours, max 15 mg/day Age 4–5: 15 mg q 4 to 6 hours; max 60 mg/day Age 6–11: 30 mg q 4 to 6 hours; max 120 mg/day	Temporary relief ≥2 years	Consider use along with an oral antihistamine if nasal congestion is uncontrolled Caution in patients with hypertension, cardiac disease, NA-glaucoma, BPH, concomitant beta-blockers or MAOIs Other combination options are more preferred given adverse effects of pseudoephdrine; studies have shown poor efficacy
INTRANASAL ANTICHOLINERGIC			
Ipratropium	0.03%; 42 mcg/spray; 168 to 252 mcg/day 2 sprays each nostril BID-TID	Rhinorrhea in PAR and NAR ≥12 years	For symptomatic relief of rhinorrhea in patients with PAR and NAR or as add-on to INCSs for persistent rhinorrhea Commonly associated with nasal dryness and epistaxis

Note: See product monographs for individual medications.
Abbreviations: AR: Allergic rhinitis; ARS: Acute Rhinosinusitis; BID: Twice a day; BPH: Benign Prostate Hypertrophy; CSU: Chronic Spontaneous Urticaria; ER: Extended release; INCS: Intranasal Corticosteroid; MAOIs: Monoamine Oxidase Inhibitors; NAR: Non-allergic rhinitis; NA: Narrow Angle; NERD: Nonsteroidal Anti-Inflammatory Drug Exacerbated Respiratory Disease; OD: Once a day; OTC: Over the counter; PAR: Perennial allergic rhinitis; q: Every; SAR: Seasonal allergic rhinitis; TID: Thrice a day.

- If INCS is prescribed, patients should be counseled about side effects:
  - Common side effects include local nasal irritation, dryness, burning, stinging, blood-tinged secretions, and epistaxis. Risk of epistaxis can be mitigated by educating the patient about proper technique by pointing the spray away from the nasal septum. Septal perforation is extremely rare. Limited systemic absorption that varies by preparation. Consider INCS in children with reduced systemic absorption and impact on growth (e.g. fluticasone propionate and mometasone furoate) (3).

- **Leukotriene receptor antagonists (LTRAs)** (e.g. montelukast): Generally not used as first-line therapy as they are less effective than INCS but may be an option to consider if there is aversion to INCS, concerns about sedation from antihistamines, or if there is concomitant asthma/exercise-induced bronchoconstriction or NERD (4, 12, 13).
  - Patients should be counseled on possible neuropsychiatric side effects from montelukast, such as aggression, depression, suicidal thinking (rare).
- **Intranasal cromolyn:** Uncommonly used due to need for frequent dosing and delay in response.

- **Intranasal anticholinergics:** Primarily used for NAR or allergic rhinitis with predominant rhinorrhea symptoms.
- **Intranasal decongestants:** May be used in short-courses (<10 days maximum); patients should be counseled on risk of rhinitis medicamentosa (14). Rare case reports have described cerebrovascular complications, such as reversible cerebral vasoconstriction syndrome (15).
- **Allergen immunotherapy (AIT):** Refer to Chapter 4.
  - Briefly, AIT (subcutaneous or sublingual routes) may be considered through a shared decision-making process with patients who have
    (1) Moderate-severe allergic rhinitis.
    (2) Are not controlled with non-pharmacologic measures and/or pharmacotherapy.
    (3) Prefer immunotherapy as the method of treatment (e.g. due to desire to avoid adverse effects, costs, or long-term use of pharmacotherapy).
    (4) Desire the potential benefit of immunotherapy to prevent or reduce the severity of comorbid conditions like asthma.

SPECIAL POPULATIONS: PREGNANCY AND LACTATION

General Considerations
- Allergic rhinitis and rhinosinusitis are common complaints during pregnancy (16).
- Hormonal changes during pregnancy can worsen preexisting allergic rhinitis or cause new-onset rhinitis (gestational rhinitis) (16).
- Rhinitis can contribute to sleep-disordered breathing and precipitate or worsen asthma attacks during pregnancy; both of which have been linked to adverse maternal-fetal outcomes such as preeclampsia and intrauterine growth restriction (16).
- Controlling rhinitis symptoms during pregnancy improves patient quality of life and pregnancy outcomes (16).

Diagnosis
- Skin prick testing may be considered during pregnancy (expert opinion), although it is typically deferred.

- Intradermal testing is relatively contraindicated during pregnancy because of the small risk of anaphylaxis (16).

Treatment
- Most INCSs may be used during pregnancy (17, 18).
- Fluticasone furoate, mometasone, and budesonide used at recommended doses are preferred over fluticasone propionate and ciclesonide (18).
- Montelukast and zafirlukast may be continued during pregnancy if required for adequate control of rhinitis symptoms pre-conceptually; they are likely safe during breastfeeding (17–19).
- 5-Lipoxygenase inhibitors (zileuton) should be avoided during pregnancy and breastfeeding (16, 17).
- Second-generation H1 antihistamines should be considered over first-generation during pregnancy and lactation (with preference for class B agents such as loratadine and cetirizine rather than class C agents such as fexofenadine and bilastine) (16, 17).
- Oral decongestants should be avoided during the first trimester. Short course, infrequent use during the second and third trimesters can be considered (phenylpropanolamine should be avoided during the third trimester) (17).
- Short-course topical decongestant (oxymetazoline) can also be used to control symptoms (19).
- Topical decongestants could be considered for short-course, infrequent, rescue usage during pregnancy and lactation (17).
- Maintenance immunotherapy (sublingual or subcutaneous) may be continued during pregnancy but not initiated or updosed during gestation; immunotherapy may be initiated or uptitrated during breastfeeding (17, 18).

REFERENCES

1. Bousquet J et al., Allergy. (2008), PMID: 18331513/ DOI: 10.1111/j.1398-9995.2007.01620.x.
2. Keith PK et al., Allergy Asthma Clin Immunol. (2012), PMID: 22656186/DOI: 10.1186/1710-1492-8-7.
3. Wallace DV et al., J Allergy Clin Immunol. (2008), PMID: 18662584/DOI: 10.1016/j.jaci.2008.06.003.
4. Dykewicz MS et al., J Allergy Clin Immunol. (2020), PMID: 32707227/DOI: 10.1016/j.jaci.2020.07.007.
5. Corren J, Baroody FM, Togias A. Allergic and Nonallergic rhinitis. In: Burks AW, Holgate ST, O'Hehir RE, Bacharier LB, Broide DH, Hershey GK, Peebles Jr RS. Middleton's Allergy: Principles

and Practice E-Book, Ninth Edition. Amsterdam: Elsevier. Available at: https://www.clinicalkey.com/dura/browse/bookChapter/3-s2.0-C20161002419 (Accessed: August 20, 2020).

6. Bernstein IL et al., Ann Allergy Asthma Immunol. (2008), PMID: 18431959/DOI: 10.1016/s1081-1206(10)60305-5.

7. Settipane RJ et al., Allergy Proc. (1994), PMID: 8005452/DOI: 10.2500/108854194778816634.

8. Hagy GW et al., J Allergy Clin Immunol. (1971), PMID: 5285772/DOI: 10.1016/0091-6749(71)90066-2.

9. Wilson JM et al., J Allergy Clin Immunol Pract. (2018), PMID: 29310755/DOI: 10.1016/j.jaip.2017.10.003.

10. Portnoy J et al., Ann Allergy Asthma Immunol. (2012), PMID: 22469456/DOI: 10.1016/j.anai.2012.02.015.

11. Fein MN et al., Allergy, Asthma & Clin Immunology. (2019), PMID: 31582993/DOI: 10.1186/s13223-019-0375-9.

12. Weiler JM et al., J Allergy Clin Immunol. (2016), PMID: 27665489/DOI: 10.1016/j.jaci.2016.05.029.

13. Solensky R et al., Ann Allergy Asthma Immunol. (2010), PMID: 20934625/DOI: 10.1016/j.anai.2010.08.002.

14. Ducros A et al., Brain. (2007), PMID: 18025032/DOI: 10.1093/brain/awm256.

15. Pham H et al., CMAJ. (2020), PMID: 33168762/DOI: 10.1503/cmaj.201234.

16. Lal D et al., Rhinology. (2016), PMID: 26800862/DOI: 10.4193/Rhin15.228.

17. Gonzalez-Estrada A et al., Am J Med Sci. (2016), PMID: 27650241/DOI: 10.1016/j.amjms.2016.05.030.

18. Alhussien AH et al., Eur Arch Otorhinolaryngol. (2018), PMID: 29164323/DOI: 10.1007/s00405-017-4785-3.

19. Bonham CA et al., Chest. (2018), PMID: 28867295/DOI: 10.1016/j.chest.2017.08.029.

20. Church MK et al., J Eur Acad Dermatol Venereol. 2017, PMID: 28467671/DOI: 10.1111/jdv.14305.

21. Mullol J et al., Allergy. 2015, PMID: 25491409/DOI: 10.1111/all.12531.

22. Carr W et al., J Allergy Clin Immunol. 2012, PMID: 22418065/DOI: 10.1016/j.jaci.2012.01.077.

23. Dykewicz MS et al., Ann Allergy Asthma Immunol. 2017, PMID: 29103802/DOI: 10.1016/j.anai.2017.08.012.

Rhinosinusitis

ABEER FETEIH, HOANG PHAM, MICHAEL FEIN,
GENEVIÈVE GENEST, AND JAIME DEL CARPIO

GENERAL BACKGROUND

- Rhinosinusitis is the inflammation of the nasal cavities and at least one paranasal sinus.
- Acute rhinosinusitis (ARS) is common and affects 6%–15% of the general population (1).
  - Post-viral rhinosinusitis and acute bacterial rhinosinusitis (ABRS) prevalence is 17%–21% (2).
  - ABRS complicates 0.5%–2.0% of viral upper respiratory tract infections (URTIs) (3–4).
- Chronic rhinosinusitis (CRS) prevalence is 5.5%–28% (symptom-based diagnosis) but decreases to approximately 3%–6% with the addition of nasal endoscopy or computed tomography (CT) evidence (1).

DEFINITIONS AND CLASSIFICATION

There are many different definitions and classifications of rhinosinusitis. In this manual, we will discuss one that is based on the *"European Position Paper on Rhinosinusitis and Nasal Polyps (EPOS) 2020"* (1).

- *Acute Rhinosinusitis (ARS)*
  - Sudden onset of ≥2 symptoms for <12 weeks where 1 symptom must be:
    - Nasal congestion/obstruction OR nasal discharge (anterior/posterior nasal drip). PLUS
    - Facial pain/pressure and diminished/ loss of smell.
  - *Children*: Sudden onset of ≥2 symptoms for <12 weeks with nasal congestion/obstruction, discolored nasal discharge, or cough.
- *Recurrent Acute Rhinosinusitis (RARS)*
  - ≥4 episodes/year of ARS with complete resolution in between episodes.

- *Chronic Rhinosinusitis (CRS)*
  - Presence of ≥2 symptoms for ≥12 weeks where 1 symptom must be:
    - Nasal congestion/obstruction OR nasal discharge (anterior/posterior nasal drip). PLUS
    - Facial pain/pressure and diminished/ loss of smell (children may have cough as a feature).
  - There should also be abnormal findings on sinonasal endoscopy or on a CT scan of the sinuses.
  - CRS is classically sub-classified into:
    a. CRS with nasal polyps (CRSwNP)
    b. CRS without nasal polyps (CRSsNP)

Different Forms of ARS as per EPOS 2020 Conventions (1)

Acute Viral Rhinosinusitis (AVRS)

- Clinical course is similar to other viral URTIs; patients have partial or complete resolution of symptoms within 7 ± 3–4 days (particularly for nasal discharge and cough symptoms), but most symptoms resolve by day 5.
- Patients typically do not have fever. If fever is present, it is generally present early in the illness and disappears within the first 24–48 hours, with respiratory symptoms becoming more prominent after the fever has resolved.
- *The most common pathogens are rhinovirus, respiratory syncytial virus (RSV), influenza virus, coronavirus, adenovirus, enterovirus, and parainfluenza virus (5).*

Post-Viral Rhinosinusitis (Post-Viral ARS)

- Describes the phenomenon in which symptoms increase after 5 days or persist after 10 days with overall duration still <12 weeks.

Acute Bacterial Rhinosinusitis (ABRS)

- Defined as ≥3 symptoms of discolored mucus, severe local pain (often unilateral), fever>38°C, raised C-reactive protein (CRP)/erythrocyte sedimentation rate (ESR), "double" sickening (worsening illness within 10 days after an initial improvement).
- Most common bacterial organisms include *Streptococcus pneumoniae, Haemophilus influenzae,* and *Moraxella catarrhalis* (6).

Associated Symptoms

- Fever, malaise, drowsiness, dental pain, sore throat, dysphonia, cough (few complain of cough without coexisting chest disease).

Physical Examination in ABRS

- *Temperature*: Verify for fever >38.0°C.
- *Anterior Rhinoscopy*
  - Nasal secretions: Thick, yellow-green, opaque.
  - Assess for any polyps, nasal structural abnormalities.
- *Inspection and Palpation of Sinuses*: Edema and tenderness of the affected area such as the face (rare unless there is a dental origin) (1).
- Purulent exudates in the middle meatus are highly predictive of ABRS (7), but its absence does not exclude active sinus infection. Purulent drainage in the nose or posterior pharynx is the only finding of diagnostic value with a positive likelihood ratio (LR+) of 1.3 as a symptom and LR+ 0.88 on exam (8).
- Ear examination to assess for otitis media.
- Auscultation for wheezing to assess for asthma and crackles for bronchiectasis.
- Presence of clubbing (suggestive of bronchiectasis, cystic fibrosis, and primary ciliary dyskinesia).

Red Flags for Complications: Require Immediate Referral/Hospitalization

- Periorbital edema/erythema
- Displaced globe
- Double vision
- Ophthalmoplegia
- Reduced visual acuity
- Severe unilateral or bilateral frontal headache
- Frontal swelling
- Signs of meningitis
- Neurological signs
- Reduced consciousness

Complications (1)

- *Orbital complications*: Pre-septal cellulitis, orbital cellulitis, subperiosteal abscess, orbital abscess, cavernous sinus thrombosis.
- *Endocranial complications*: Epidural or subdural empyema, brain abscess, meningitis, cerebritis, and superior sagittal and cavernous sinus thrombosis.
- *Osseous complications*: Osteomyelitis (e.g. Pott's puffy tumor), subperiosteal abscess.

Differential Diagnosis of ARS (1)

- Allergic rhinitis
- Non-allergic rhinitis
- Facial pain syndromes (rare): Neuralgias, temporomandibular joint (TMJ) disorders.
- Orodontal disease/dental pain.
- Headaches (tension, migraines, cluster).
- Vasculitis (rare): Granulomatosis with polyangiitis (GPA), eosinophilic granulomatosis with polyangiitis (EGPA), or sarcoidosis.
- Acute invasive fungal rhinosinusitis: Particularly, in immunosuppressed patients and uncontrolled diabetes.
- Cerebrospinal fluid (CSF) leak.

Investigations

- Nasal endoscopy is generally not available in routine outpatient clinics and is not required for clinical diagnosis of ARS.
- CRP and ESR may correlate with CT scan changes and positive microbiological cultures (9, 10); however, they may be of limited value given their limited accuracy as individual tests (11).
- Additional investigations (e.g. imaging, microbiology) are not required for routine diagnosis of uncomplicated ARS.

Management of ABRS

- *Antibiotics*
  - *Amoxicillin-clavulanate* is recommended as first-line therapy, and doxycycline, levofloxacin, and moxifloxacin are recommended in patients allergic to penicillin (6).
  - *Dose of Amoxicillin-clavulanate (adult):* Oral 500 mg every 8 hours or 875 mg every 12 hours for 5–7 days (6).
  - *Higher Dose Amoxicillin-clavulanate:* 2 g every 12 hours or 90mg/kg/day oral twice a day for 5–7days for patients at risk for poor outcome or pneumococcal resistance (6).

- *Intranasal Saline Irrigation*: May provide symptom relief (12).
- *Intranasal Corticosteroids (INCS)*: No supportive evidence of INCS in AVRS or ABRS (13), but if there is uncertainty between ABRS or postviral ARS, consider a trial of INCS as it has been demonstrated to provide symptom relief in postviral ARS (14) and avoid unnecessary antibiotics.

Chronic Rhinosinusitis (CRS)

- *Classic classification*: Those with or without nasal polyps
- *Contemporary classification EPOS 2020* (1): Based on the functional anatomic compartments and emerging clinical relevance of pathophysiology/phenotypes/endotypes

Clinical Manifestations
CRSwNP (15)

- Hyposmia or anosmia (high-yield question often missed), nasal congestion, nasal polyps, headache, facial pressure/fullness, halitosis, fatigue, dental pain, cough, throat clearing, ear pain.
- *Comorbidities*: Inquire about asthma and nonsteroidal anti-inflammatory drug (NSAID) hypersensitivity.

CRSsNP (15)

- Nasal blockage (less prominent), anterior or posterior purulent nasal drainage are dominant, hyposmia or anosmia (less than in CRSwNP), headache, facial pressure/pain, halitosis, fatigue, dental pain, cough, throat clearing, ear pain.
- *Comorbidities*: Inquire about asthma (less common).

Important Predisposing and Concomitant Factors Associated with CRS [Adapted from (1)]

- *Environmental allergies*: Prevalence in CRS varies with phenotype; allergic fungal rhinosinusitis (AFRS) (33%), CRSwNP (31%), and CRSsNP (20.3%).
- *Asthma and other lower airway diseases*: Asthma (25%), chronic obstructive pulmonary disease (COPD), bronchiectasis.
- *NSAID-exacerbated respiratory disease* (NERD): AFRS (40%), CRSwNP (9.6%), CRSsNP (3.3%).
- *Alcohol-induced worsening of upper airway disease*: Highest prevalence in NERD and CRSwNP.

Table 2.1 Major Differences between CRSwNP and CRSsNP

Chronic rhinosinusitis WITH nasal polyps	Chronic rhinosinusitis WITHOUT nasal polyps
More anosmia	More purulent nasal discharge
More congestion/ Obstruction	More facial pain/ Pressure and headache
More Type 2 Inflammation with eosinophilia (e.g. absolute eosinophil count >300 cells/µL)	More associated with infectious processes
More risk of asthma	Humoral immunodeficiency evaluation may be more pertinent
More risk of recurrence	Less risk of recurrence

Adapted from (15, 17, 18).

- *Immunodeficiency*: IgA deficiency (sIgA), common variable immunodeficiency (CVID), specific antibody deficiency, Immunoglobulin G(IgG) subclass deficiency, X-linked agammaglobulinemia (XLA).
- *Impaired ciliary motility*: Cystic fibrosis, primary ciliary dyskinesia (including Kartagener syndrome).
- *Smoking*: Pollutant toxins are proinflammatory substances and create oxidative stress.
- *Pollution and occupational exposures*: Paper dust, cleaning agents, metal dust, animals, moisture/mold/mildew, poisonous gas, physically strenuous work, textiles work.
- *Nasal anatomic variations*: May affect progression of disease.
- *Vasculitis*: GPA, EGPA, sarcoidosis, cocaine-induced vasculitis.

Differential Diagnosis of CRS [Adapted from (1, 15)]

- Allergic rhinitis.
- Non-allergic rhinitis.
- Rhinitis medicamentosa.
- Rhinitis due to pregnancy, hypothyroidism.
- Horner syndrome.

- *Anatomic abnormalities*: Foreign body, nasal septal deviation, enlarged tonsils and adenoids.
- Migraines and facial pain syndromes.

Emerging Pathophysiologic Endotypes [Adapted from (1, 16–18)]

- *Type 2 Endotype*
  - *Presumed mechanism*
    1. Stimulation of nasal epithelial cells causes secretion of thymic stromal lymphopoietin (TSLP), interleukin-25 (IL-25), and IL-33.
    2. These induce the release of IL-4, IL-5, and IL-13 from the epithelial and mucosal mast cells.
    3. These cytokines cause class switching to IgE and IgG4 along with mast cell degranulation and eosinophil activation.
    4. Mast cell and eosinophils cause inflammation and tissue damage.
  - *Examples*: CRSwNP, NERD (a subtype of eosinophilic CRS [eCRS]), AFRS, central compartment atopic disease (CCAD).
  - *Common clinical correlates*
    - Main complaint is often smell loss or nasal blockage/congestion.
    - NSAID hypersensitivity and/or asthma, atopy.
    - Polyps and eosinophilic mucin on nasal endoscopy, tissue eosinophils >10/high-power field (hpf).
    - Elevated IgE ≥100 and peripheral eosinophilia >250 cells/μL.
    - Resistant to treatment with high recurrence rates.
- *Non-Type 2 Endotype*: Presently encompasses everything else not associated with type 2
  - Mix of type 1 and type 3 responses
    - *Proposed type 1 mechanism*: Involves epithelial response to environmental stimuli leading to a Th1 and Th17 response.
    - *Proposed type 3 mechanism*: Involves Th17 responses involved with neutrophil recruitment, activation, and proliferations as well as innate antimicrobial defenses by the airway epithelium.
  - *Examples*: CRSsNP often reflects a non-type 2 profile, non-eCRS.
  - *Common clinical correlates*
    - Main complaint is often purulent discharge/facial pain.

- Less asthma, less atopy.
- Purulence on nasal endoscopy.
- Normal IgE, no eosinophilia.

New Contemporary Classification of CRS beyond CRSsNP and CRSwNP [Adapted from (1, 16–18)]

Newly proposed classification system combines functional anatomic compartments with suspected pathophysiologic endotype mechanism.

- *Primary CRS:* Refers to CRS as a primary disorder of the "airway" or respiratory system
  - Localized/Unilateral
    - *Type 2*: AFRS
    - *Non-Type 2*: Ostiomeatal complex disease, isolated frontal sinusitis, isolated sphenoid sinusitis
  - Diffuse/Bilateral
    - *Type 2*: AFRS, CCAD, eCRS
    - *Non-Type 2*: Non-eCRS, poor corticosteroid treatment responder, older age, smokers
- *Secondary CRS:* Refers to CRS as secondary to other local or systemic causes
  - Localized/Unilateral
    - *Local pathology*: Odontogenic sinusitis, fungal ball, local neoplasm.
  - Diffuse/Bilateral
    - *Mechanical/impaired ciliary motility*: Primary ciliary dyskinesia, cystic fibrosis
    - *Inflammatory*: GPA, EGPA, sarcoidosis
    - *Immunodeficiency*: CVID, XLA, SAD, sIgA, IgG subclass deficiency

Diagnosis and Investigations

- History and physical examination including sinus/nasal exam via anterior rhinoscopy and/or nasal endoscopy.
- Aeroallergen testing (skin prick testing), sinus cultures by endoscopy, and tests for immunodeficiency/autoimmunity, cystic fibrosis, or ciliary dysfunction need to be considered (15).
  - Consider complete blood count (CBC) with differential for eosinophils, immunoglobulin levels (IgG/A/M and IgE), c-ANCA/p-ANCA.
- *Endoscopic objective evidence of rhinosinusitis* (1): Nasal polyps, mucopurulent discharge primarily from the middle meatus, and/or edema/mucosal obstruction primarily in the middle meatus.

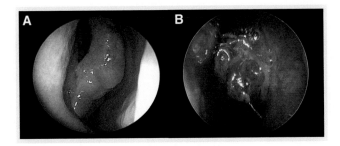

Figure 2.1 Endoscopic view of nasal inflammation in CRS. (A) Middle turbinate edema present in CCAD or IgE drive airway inflammation; (B) Middle meatus polyposis present in eCRS airway inflammation. [Reprinted with permission from Grayson et al., © The Author(s). 2019 Open Access This article is distributed under the terms of the Creative Commons Attribution 4.0 International License (http://creativecommons.org/licenses/by/4.0/), which permits unrestricted use, distribution, and reproduction in any medium, provided you give appropriate credit to the original author(s) and the source, provide a link to the Creative Commons license, and indicate if changes were made. The Creative Commons Public Domain Dedication waiver (http://creativecommons.org/publicdomain/zero/1.0/) applies to the data made available in this article, unless otherwise stated. (32).]

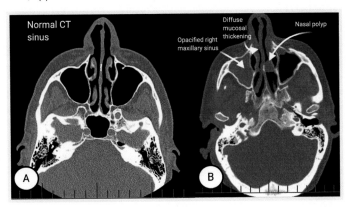

Figure 2.2 Normal and abnormal CT sinus imaging. CT imaging of paranasal sinuses is an important diagnostic tool for chronic rhinosinusitis to clarify extent of disease, presence of nasal polyps, septal deviation or other anatomic abnormalities obstructing mucous/airflow. Normal CT sinus (A) shows well-aerated maxillary and sphenoid sinuses, normal turbinates and nasal septum. CRSwNP seen in (B) demonstrates diffuse inflammatory mucosal thickening, completely opacified right maxillary sinus and presence of nasal polyps. (Figure created with BioRender.com.) (Images courtesy of Dr. Fein.)

- *CT scan for objective evidence of rhinosinusitis* (1): Mucosal changes within the ostiomeatal complex and/or sinuses.

Management Options in Adult CRS

- *Nasal Irrigation with Saline:* Use isotonic saline (or Ringer's lactate with or without xylitol, sodium hyaluronate, and/or xyloglucan). Baby shampoo and hypertonic saline solutions are *not* recommended due to side effects (1).
- *INCS:* High-quality evidence that long-term use is effective and safe for CRS (1); no difference between different nasal corticosteroids; no direct comparisons between doses and delivery methods, but some methods seem to have a larger effect on symptoms (e.g. nasal rinse with budesonide); INCS post-operatively prevents polyp recurrence; does not affect intraocular pressure or lens opacity (1).
- *Oral Glucocorticoids*
  - Short courses (7–21 days, e.g. prednisone 50 mg for 14 days) with or without INCS result in significant reduction in total symptom score and nasal polyp score (1, 19).
  - One to two courses per year can be a useful addition to INCS in patients with partially or uncontrolled disease.
  - Systemic corticosteroids (even short term) carry significant side effects such as sepsis, heart failure, gastrointestinal (GI) bleeding, venous thromboembolism, and fractures (20, 21).

- **Oral Antibiotics:** Controversial topic
  - May consider short courses of oral antibiotics for acute exacerbations of CRS, but counsel patient about GI side effects.
  - Prolonged courses of antibiotics for CRS remain controversial; doxycycline and macrolides have been described for their possible anti-inflammatory benefits in select populations, which need to be weighed against adverse effects (e.g. microbial resistance, GI upset, and QTc prolongation with macrolides) (17, 18).
- **Leukotriene Inhibitors** (e.g. montelukast)
  - A trial may be considered, especially in the presence of concomitant conditions where there is a benefit, such as allergic rhinitis (22), asthma (23), exercise-induced bronchoconstriction (24), and NSAID hypersensitivity (25).
  - Patients need to be counseled about the increased risk of serious neuropsychiatric adverse effects (e.g. sleep disturbance, nightmares, depression, anxiety, psychosis, aggression, irritability, suicidal thoughts and behavior) (22).
- **Biologics**
  - Indications (1): Presence of bilateral polyps in a patient who had endoscopic sinus surgery + at least three of the following criteria:
    - *Evidence of type 2 inflammation:* Tissue eosinophils >10/hpf, peripheral blood eosinophils >250 cells/μL, total IgE >100
    - *Need for systemic corticosteroids or contraindication to systemic steroids:* ≥2 courses per year or long-term (>3 months) low-dose steroids
    - *Significantly impaired quality of life:* Sinonasal outcome test (SNOT)-22 ≥40
    - *Significant loss of smell:* Anosmic on smell test (score depending on test)
    - *Diagnosis of comorbid asthma:* Asthma needing regular inhaled steroids
  - Defining treatment response (1): Excellent (5 criteria), Moderate (3–4 criteria), Poor (1–2- criteria), None (0 criteria)
    - *Based on five criteria:* ↓Polyp size, ↓Systemic corticosteroids, ↑Quality of life, ↑Smell, ↓Impact of comorbidities
    - Evaluate after 16 weeks: Stop if no response
    - Evaluate after 1 year: Stop if no response

  - *Approved agents:* Both improved symptoms, polyp size, smell sense, quality of life, systemic steroids, and need for sinus surgery
    - *Dupilumab* (anti-IL-4α) (26): **Adverse events** – 2 EGPA in the dupilumab group and 1 in placebo; 7 conjunctivitis in dupilumab group and 1 in placebo
    - *Omalizumab* (anti-IgE) (27): **Adverse events** – headache, injection site reaction, arthralgias; no anaphylaxis
  - Potential future agent
    - *Mepolizumab* (anti-Il-5) (28): Phase 3 endpoints achieved in press release similar results likely to follow with Benralizumab
- Management of the underlying secondary cause if present (e.g. immunodeficiency, vasculitis, uncontrolled diabetes)

Indications for Referral to Specialists (e.g. Ear, Nose, and Throat; Allergy)

- Before referral optimize patient education and adherence, initiate adequate trial of first-line medical management (e.g. saline irrigation, INCS, antibiotics if indicated), and evaluate for improvement in 6–12 weeks.
- Refer for specialist care if:
  - There is no improvement in 6–12 weeks despite adequate initial measures
  - Alarming symptoms present suggestive of complications
  - >3 episodes of ABRS in last year
  - Need for objective evidence of rhinosinusitis with nasal endoscopy
  - Need for additional workup to clarify endotype (type 2 vs. non-type 2) or differential diagnosis/concomitant conditions
    - e.g. inhalant allergy evaluation (e.g. skin prick tests), CT scans
  - Need for additional therapy
    - e.g. sinus surgery, aspirin desensitization, biologics

SPECIFIC CRS PHENOTYPES OF SPECIAL NOTE

AFRS [Adapted from (1, 15)]

- **Major Diagnostic Criteria:** Ideally all five major criteria by Bent-Kuhn should be met:

- Nasal polyposis
- Fungi elements on staining
- Eosinophilic mucin without fungal invasion into sinus tissues
- Type I hypersensitivity to fungi
- Classic radiologic findings with soft tissue differential densities on CT scan (hyperattenuation) and unilaterality or anatomically discrete sinus involvement
- **Minor Diagnostic Criteria:** Bony erosion, Charcot Leyden crystals, unilateral disease, peripheral eosinophilia, positive fungal culture, absence of immunodeficiency or diabetes.
- **Clinical Features:** Young, female > male, allergic rhinitis/atopic, warm humid climate, nasal congestion, thick "peanut buttery discharge," asthma, total IgE >500 IU/mL.
- **Common Causative Fungi:** *Bipolaris, Curvularia, Aspergillus,* and *Drechslera* species.
- **Management**
  - *Surgery*: Mainstay.
  - Systemic and/or topical corticosteroids (pre- and post-operative benefit).
    - *Pre-operatively*: Likely to reduce mucosal inflammation and radiologic scores.
    - *Post-operatively*: Improve short-term outcomes and likely reduce long-term recurrence.
  - *Antifungals (oral and topical)*: Fluconazole and itraconazole may be beneficial.
  - *Immunotherapy*: Fungal immunotherapy may be considered; treating concomitant non-fungal allergic rhinitis with immunotherapy may be effective in this population.
  - *Leukotriene receptor antagonist*: One case report; may reduce symptoms (29).
  - *Omalizumab*: Two small case series; may improve outcomes in AFRS (30, 31).

eCRS and NERD (1, 16, 32)

- *Type 2 endotype*: Tissue eosinophilia with evidence of eosinophilic activation, blood eosinophilia.
- *Clinical features*: Mid-life "adult" onset (30–50 years), adult-onset eosinophilic asthma, nasal polyposis, severe olfactory dysfunction, symptoms are responsive to corticosteroids, worsening of upper and lower respiratory symptoms with NSAIDs or alcohol.
- *Endoscopy*: Polyps from the middle meatus, thick eosinophilic mucin, secondary purulence.
- *CT scans*: Pan-sinusitis, neo-osteogenesis.
- *Treatment*: Topical corticosteroid irrigations with intermittent bursts of oral corticosteroids if severe

(limit to 2–3 times per year), endoscopic sinus surgery; consider dupilumab.
- NERD: Montelukast, aspirin desensitization

Non-eCRS (1, 16, 32)

- *Non-type 2 endotype*: Also lacking atopic sensitization.
- *Clinical features*: Older age (>50 years), female, obese, cough, poor corticosteroid response, may have asthma that is non-responsive to inhaled corticosteroids.
- *Endoscopy*: May have polyps or polypoid edema, purulent secretions, lack eosinophilic mucin.
- *CT scans*: Pan-sinusitis (similar appearance to eCRS).
- *Treatment*: Saline or corticosteroid irrigations, endoscopic sinus surgery, consider macrolide therapy trial (clarithromycin 250 mg daily for 3 months and then continue 3×/week for 12 months if responder).

Central Compartment Atopic Disease (CCAD) (1, 16, 32)

- New phenotype where sinus dysfunction is driven mainly by postobstructive mucus trapping.
- *Type 2 endotype*: Associated with IgE-mediated sensitization to inhalant allergens without eosinophilic activation in tissue or blood eosinophilia.
- *Clinical features*: Young onset (teens to 20s), classic allergic rhinitis (usually dust mite, perennial allergens, monosensitized), early-onset allergic asthma, eczema.
- *Endoscopy*: Middle turbinate edema, *polypoid* changes from turbinates and septum.
- *CT scans*: Specific central thickening of the turbinates and septum with superior and lateral sparing of the sinus cavities, normal anterolateral sinus mucosa sometimes called a "black halo sign".
- *Treatment*: Endoscopic sinus surgery, topical corticosteroids, allergen immunotherapy; omalizumab (might consider in difficult to control disease).

SPECIAL POPULATIONS: PREGNANCY

Medical Management Considerations

- Penicillins, monobactams, and cephalosporins are safest during pregnancy. Ceftriaxone should be used with precaution (risk of kernicterus). Carbapenems can be used if medically required (33).

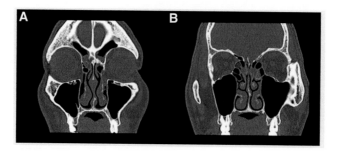

Figure 2.3 CT Sinus Imaging of CCAD. (A) Radiographic evidence of CCAD with central disease (prominent nasal turbinate and septal thickening) and peripheral clearing; (B) "black halo" sign seen in CCAD. [Reprinted with permission from Grayson et al., © The Author(s). 2019 Open Access This article is distributed under the terms of the Creative Commons Attribution 4.0 International License (http://creativecommons.org/licenses/by/4.0/), which permits unrestricted use, distribution, and reproduction in any medium, provided you give appropriate credit to the original author(s) and the source, provide a link to the Creative Commons license, and indicate if changes were made. The Creative Commons Public Domain Dedication waiver (http://creativecommons.org/publicdomain/zero/1.0/) applies to the data made available in this article, unless otherwise stated. (32).]

- Amoxicillin clavulanate may be associated with an increased risk of necrotizing enterocolitis when used in the third trimester (34) but short-course use and use during the first and second trimester is likely safe (34, 35).
- Short-course aminoglycosides may be used during pregnancy with appropriate monitoring if benefit surpasses risk. Streptomycin should be avoided (33).
- Tetracyclines have been associated with congenital malformations including neural tube defects and cleft palate as well as dental staining in offspring of mothers using tetracyclines during pregnancy (36). They should be avoided during pregnancy (36).
- Doxycycline has not been associated with these effects and may be used as a short course during pregnancy in penicillin-allergic patients (36).
- For macrolides, azithromycin is an acceptable alternative in penicillin-allergic patients; short courses are preferred over long-term usage. Erythromycin and clarithromycin should only be used if no other alternatives are available (36).
- Fluoroquinolones should be avoided in pregnancy unless no other alternatives are available (36).
- Quinolones have not been associated with unfavorable pregnancy outcomes in small case series. However, further studies are required to determine their innocuity during pregnancy. Quinolones should not be used as a first-line agent during pregnancy and should be used with caution in short courses when no other options are available (37).

- Intranasal saline and INCS are safe and well tolerated during pregnancy (see Chapter 1).
- Leukotriene inhibitors may be continued during pregnancy, 5-lipoxygenase inhibitors should be discontinued during pregnancy (see Chapter 1).
- Anti-IgE therapy (omalizumab) has not shown any adverse pregnancy outcomes and can be continued throughout pregnancy if favorable response pre-pregnancy. Omalizumab should not be initiated during pregnancy because of the risk of anaphylaxis (expert opinion). Other biologics (mepolizumab, benralizumab, and dupilumab) can be considered under expert guidance if benefits clearly surpass risk in pregnancy; otherwise, they must be discontinued at diagnosis of pregnancy (expert opinion).
- Oral glucocorticoids can be used if absolutely required. Maternal and fetal risks must be discussed with patient (see Chapter 11).

REFERENCES

1. Fokkens WJ et al., Rhinology. (2020), PMID: 32077450/DOI:10.4193/Rhin20.600.
2. Hoffmans R et al., PLOS ONE. (2018), PMID: 29401486/DOI:10.1371/journal.pone.0192330.
3. Dingle JH et al. (1974), Illness in the home: a study of 25,000 illness in a group of Cleveland families. p. 347. Cleveland, Ohio: the Press of Western Reserve University.
4. Berg O et al., Rhinology. (1986), PMID: 3775189.
5. Gwaltney JM, Jr., Clin Infect Dis. (1996), PMID: 8953061/DOI:10.1093/clinids/23.6.1209.
6. Chow AW et al., Clin Infect Dis. (2012), PMID: 22438350/DOI:10.1093/cid/cir1043.

7. Lacroix JS et al., Acta Otolaryngol. (2002), PMID: 11936912/DOI:10.1080/00016480252814216.

8. Ebell MH et al., Ann Fam Med (2019), PMID: 30858261/DOI:10.1370/afm.2354.

9. Hansen JG et al., APMIS. (2011), PMID: 21143525/DOI: 10.1111/j.1600-0463.2010.02690.x.

10. Hansen JG et al., APMIS. (2009), PMID: 19775340/DOI:10.1111/j.1600-0463.2009.02526.x.

11. Ebell MH et al., Br J Gen Pract. (2016), PMID: 27481857/DOI:10.3399/bjgp16X686581.

12. King D et al., Cochrane Database Syst Rev. (2015), PMID: 25892369/DOI:10.1002/14651858.CD006821.pub3.

13. Hayward G et al., Cochrane Database Syst Rev. (2015), PMID: 26461493/DOI:10.1002/14651858.CD008116.pub3

14. Keith et al., Prim Care Respir J. (2012), PMID: 22614920/DOI: 10.4104/pcrj.2012.00039.

15. Peters AT et al., Ann Allergy Asthma Immunol. (2014), PMID: 25256029/DOI:10.1016/j.anai.2014.07.025.

16. Grayson JW et al., JAMA Otolaryngol Head Neck Surg. (2020), PMID: 32644117/DOI: 10.1001/jamaoto.2020.1453.

17. Bachert C et al., J Allergy Clin Immunol. (2018), PMID: 29731100/DOI:10.1016/j.jaci.2018.03.004.

18. Bachert C et al., J Allergy Clin Immunol Pract. (2016), PMID: 27393777/DOI:10.1016/j.jaip.2016.05.004.

19. Hissaria P et al., J Allergy Clin Immunol. (2006), PMID: 16815148/DOI:10.1016/j.jaci.2006.03.012.

20. Yao TC et al., Ann Intern Med. (2020), PMID: 32628532/DOI: 10.7326/M20-0432.

21. Waljee AK et al., BMJ. (2017), PMID: 28404617/DOI: 10.1136/bmj.j1415.

22. Dykewicz MS et al., J Allergy Clin Immunol. (2020), PMID: 32707227/DOI:10.1016/j.jaci.2020.07.007.

23. Global Initiative for Asthma (GINA). Global Strategy for Asthma Management and Prevention (2020 Update). https://ginasthma.org/wp-content/uploads/2020/06/GINA-2020-report_20_06_04-1-wms.pdf. Accessed on 17, August 2020.1–48.

24. Weiler JM et al., J Allergy Clin Immunol. (2016), PMID: 27665489/DOI:10.1016/j.jaci.2016.05.029.

25. Joint Task Force on Practice Parameters et al., Ann Allergy Asthma Immunol. (2010), PMID: 20934625/DOI: 10.1016/j.anai.2010.08.002.

26. Bachert C et al., Lancet. (2019), PMID: 31543428/DOI:10.1016/S0140-6736(19)31881-1.

27. Gevaert P et al., J Allergy Clin Immunol. (2020), PMID: 32524991/DOI:10.1016/j.jaci.2020.05.032.

28. GlaxoSmithKline. Nucala (mepolizumab) is the first anti-IL5 biologic to report positive phase 3 results in patients with nasal polyps. April 3, 2020 [cited 2021 Feb 02]. https://www.gsk.com/en-gb/media/press-releases/nucala-mepolizumab-is-the-first-anti-il5-biologic-to-report-positive-phase-3-results-in-patients-with-nasal-polyps/#:~:text=03%20April%202020-,Nucala%20(mepolizumab)%20is%20the%20first%20anti%2DIL5%20biologic%20to,in%20patients%20with%20nasal%20polyps&text=GlaxoSmithKline%20plc%20(GSK)%20today%20announced,with%20nasal%20polyps%20(CRSwNP).

29. Schubert MS, J Allergy Clin Immunol. (2001), PMID: 11544470/DOI:10.1067/mai.2001.117592.

30. Evans MO, 2nd et al., Allergy Rhinol (Providence). (2014), PMID: 25565055/DOI: 10.2500/ar.2014.5.0098.

31. Gan EC et al., Am J Otolaryngol. (2015), PMID: 26117492/DOI:10.1016/j.amjoto.2015.05.008.

32. Grayson JW et al., J Otolaryngol Head Neck Surg. (2019), PMID: 31142355/DOI: 10.1186/s40463-019-0350-y.

33. Bookstaver PB et al., Pharmacotherapy. (2015), PMID: 26598097/DOI: 10.1002/phar.1649.

34. Clavulin product monograph, GSK, January 2020

35. Schmitz T et al., Eur J Obstet Gynecol Reprod Biol. (2019), PMID: 30870741/DOI:10.1016/j.ejogrb.2019.02.021.

36. Cross R et al., Expert Opin Drug Saf. 2016;15(3):367–82. PMID: 26680308/DOI: 10.1517/14740338.2016.1133584.

37. Yefet E et al., BJOG. (2018), PMID: 29319210/DOI:10.1111/1471-0528.15119.

Ocular Allergy

FATEMAH AL-YAQOUT AND ABEER FETEIH

GENERAL BACKGROUND

- Ocular allergies affect up to 40% of the general population (1).
- They often go untreated and are a challenge to diagnose (1, 2).
- The eye has no mechanical barrier to prevent the impact of allergens on its surface (3).
- Ocular allergy can occur in isolation, but it frequently occurs along with allergic rhinitis, asthma, and atopic dermatitis (4, 5).
- A multidisciplinary approach is often utilized for managing patients with ocular allergy (4, 6).

TYPES OF OCULAR ALLERGY

There are four major types of allergic inflammatory disorders of the ocular surface that can involve the conjunctiva, eyelids, and in severe disease the cornea (1, 4).

1. Allergic conjunctivitis (AC)
   a. Seasonal allergic conjunctivitis (SAC)
   b. Perennial allergic conjunctivitis (PAC)
2. Keratoconjunctivitis
   a. Atopic keratoconjunctivitis (AKC)
   b. Vernal keratoconjunctivitis (VKC)
3. Giant papillary conjunctivitis (GPC)
4. Contact Dermatoconjunctivitis (CDC)

CLINICAL PRESENTATIONS

- The most common symptoms and signs of the four ocular allergy subtypes are summarized in Table 3.1.

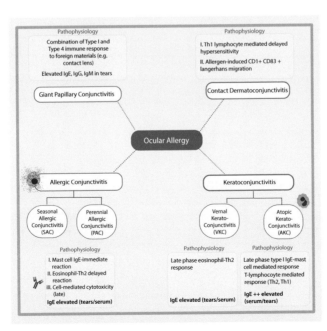

Figure 3.1 Types of ocular allergy and summarized pathophysiology. (Figure created with BioRender.com.) [Adapted from (3, 7, 8).]

DOI: 10.1201/9781003174202-4

Table 3.1 Clinical Presentations of Ocular Allergy Subtypes

	Demographics / Associations	Symptoms	Signs
AC (10)	• Inflammation of the conjunctiva • 60% of patients with AR also have evidence of AC • Most common is SAC • PAC: Year-round symptoms • PAC: Indoor, smaller allergens • No threat to sight	• Ocular itching • Watery eyes • Sensitivity to light • SAR/PAR • Symptoms of other atopic disease	• Ocular redness (hyperaemia) • Palpebral edema • Conjunctival hyperemia and chemosis • Allergic Shiners • Signs of AR • Cornea not affected
AKC (4, 11)	• M > F • Age: 20–50 years • Assoc. with AD of eyelids • Personal and FH of atopy • Perennial with worsening in winter • Loss of vision if not treated	• Severe ocular and eyelid itching • Watery eyes or mucus discharge • Burning • Dry eyes • Symptoms worsen around pets • Blurry vision and photophobia • Ocular pain (= cornea affected)	• Injection and chemosis of conjunctiva • Periocular skin eczema • Lateral canthal ulceration and lash loss • Cicatricial ectropion • Lagophthalmos • Limbus: Horner-Trantas dots • Corneal erosions and scarring • Cataracts • Keratoconus (in severe cases and untreated disease)
VKC (5, 11, 12)	• M:F (3:1 ratio) • Age: 3–25 years of age • Assoc. with other atopic diseases in 50% • FH of atopy present • Palpebral and limbal • Can lead to loss of vision if not treated	• Severe ocular itching • Tearing and mucous discharge • Thick stringy discharge • Dry eyes • Severe photophobia • Ocular pain (= cornea affected)	• Scleral injection • Giant papillae (cobblestone papillae) • Limbus: Horner-Trantass dots • Superficial punctate keratitis • Corneal plaques (shield ulcer) • Epithelial plaques • Ptosis • Keratoconus

	Demographics / Associations	Symptoms	Signs
GPC (7, 13, 14)	• M = F • Immune/mechanical process • Assoc. with CL use • In 1%–5 % of CL users • Soft hydrogel CL > rigid CL • No threat to sight	• Ocular itching after CL removal • Foreign body sensation • Burning sensation • Photophobia • Usual CL cause discomfort • Blurred vision	• Giant papilla (≥1 mm in size; superior tarsus) • Conjunctival injection and Chemosis • Conjunctival opacification • Cornea affected rarely
CDC (11, 15)	• Due to direct or indirect exposure by irritant or allergen • Due to atopic CD in > 50% • Common allergens: Gold (8.2%); Fragrance mix (7.1%) Balsam of Peru (6.3%), topical drugs; formaldehyde resins; and preservatives in eye drops or lens solution (thimerosal)	• Ocular itching • Tearing • Rash on eyelids • Sensation of fullness in the eye • Eyelid swelling • Burning sensation	• Thickened eyelids with redness • Ulcerated eyelids • Reactive papillae • Chemosis

Original content; Adapted from (1, 2, 4, 15).

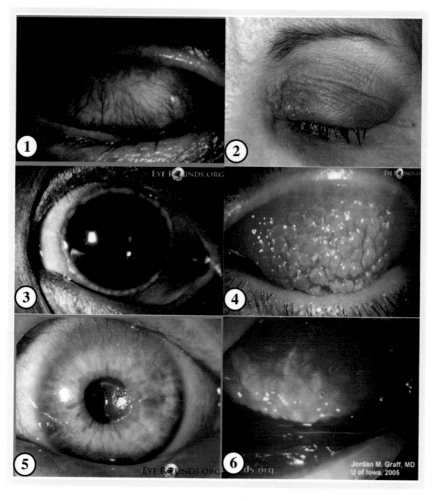

Figure 3.2 Ocular allergy (OA). (1) Mild hyperemia and edema in upper palpebra in Allergic Conjunctivitis; (2) Eczematous plaque and lid chemosis, a specific sign for AKC; (3) showing Limbal VKC with Horner's Trantas dots; (4) showing giant papillae in VKC; (5) showing corneal ulceration in a patient with VKC; (6) showing superior tarsal giant papillae in GPC. [(1) Reprinted with permission from Miyazaki, D et al., Allergology Int. (2020) (2) Reprinted with permission from La Rosa, M et al. (8) © by (Creative Commons license); (3–6) Courtesy of "EyeRounds.org University of Iowa."] (*Abbreviations:* AKC: Atopic Keratoconjunctivitis; GPC: Giant Papillary Conjunctivitis; VKC: Vernal Keratoconjunctivitis.) (Figure created with BioRender.com.)

- Ocular pruritus is the most common symptom of ocular allergy (ranging from uncomfortable to debilitating) (1, 4, 16).

DEFINITIONS [ADAPTED FROM (11)]

- Allergic shiners: Periorbital darkening due to local pigmentation and decrease in venous return.
- Cicatricial ectropion: Turning of the lid due to scarring.
- Lagophthalmos: Incomplete closure of eyelids.

- Horner-Trantas dots: Accumulated white/gray inflammatory infiltrates at the gelatinous limbus (Figure 3.2).

Diagnosis

- Recognizing the symptoms and signs (summarized in Table 3.1) that suggest ocular allergy is the first step in diagnosis.
- Symptoms and signs that are **not** suggestive [Adapted from (1, 4)]
  - Unilateral disease
  - Purulent discharge (consider infectious conjunctivitis)

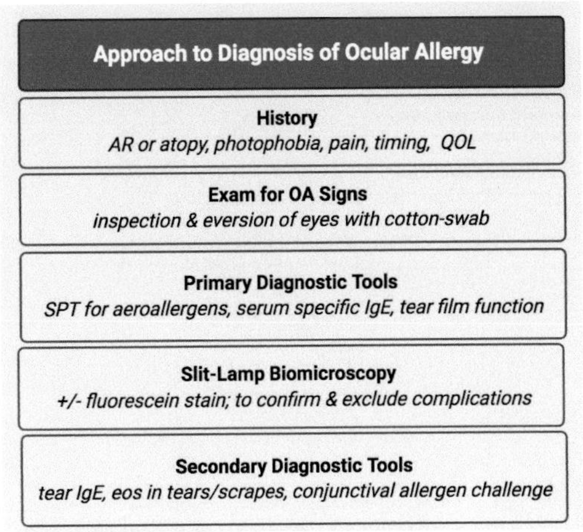

Approach to Diagnosis of Ocular Allergy

History
AR or atopy, photophobia, pain, timing, QOL

Exam for OA Signs
inspection & eversion of eyes with cotton-swab

Primary Diagnostic Tools
SPT for aeroallergens, serum specific IgE, tear film function

Slit-Lamp Biomicroscopy
+/- fluorescein stain; to confirm & exclude complications

Secondary Diagnostic Tools
tear IgE, eos in tears/scrapes, conjunctival allergen challenge

Figure 3.3 Approach to diagnosis of ocular allergy (OA). The diagnosis of OA often requires collaboration between allergists, ophthalmologists, and dermatologists. (Figure created with BioRender.com.) [Adapted from (1, 4).]

- Pain (usually only seen in severe AKC/VKC)
- Localized hyperemia (consider: subconjunctival hemorrhage or episcleritis)
- Lid margin disease (consider: blepharitis)
- Fixed pupil
- Patch testing is necessary for the diagnosis of CDC.
- Conjunctival allergen challenge is not usually done in clinical practice but can be used to aid diagnosis (4, 16).
- Total IgE in tears is <3 ng/mL (AC if >3 ng/mL) (1).

Differential Diagnosis [Adapted from (1, 16)]

- Hypo-secretive dry eye
- Mechanical conjunctivitis
- Toxic conjunctivitis
- Autoimmune conjunctivitis (such as ocular cicatricial pemphigoid with eyelid involvement)

Management of Ocular Allergy

- A multidisciplinary approach is often utilized (1, 2)
- Referral to ophthalmology if severe symptoms, ocular pain, and if vision affected (4)
- Management is divided into:
  1. **Non-pharmacological** (summarized in Figure 3.4)
  2. **Pharmacological options** for AC can be applied to other subtypes of ocular allergy (6) (Figure 3.5).

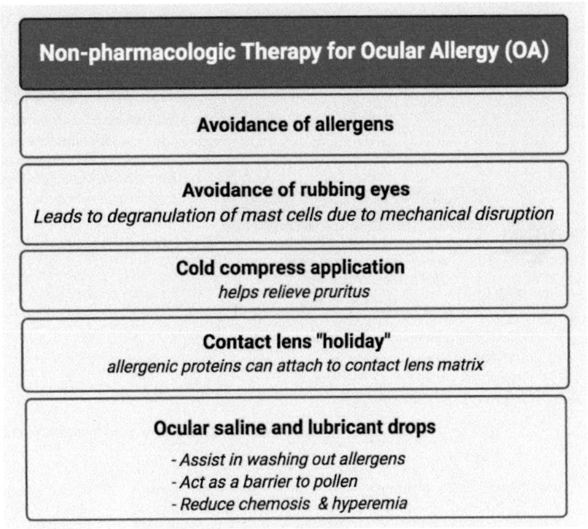

Non-pharmacologic Therapy for Ocular Allergy (OA)

Avoidance of allergens

Avoidance of rubbing eyes
Leads to degranulation of mast cells due to mechanical disruption

Cold compress application
helps relieve pruritus

Contact lens "holiday"
allergenic proteins can attach to contact lens matrix

Ocular saline and lubricant drops
- Assist in washing out allergens
- Act as a barrier to pollen
- Reduce chemosis & hyperemia

Figure 3.4 Approach to non-pharmacologic therapy in OA. (Figure created with BioRender.com.) [Adapted from (1, 6, 19).]

3. **Specific treatments** (summarized in Figure 3.6)
   - Nonsteroidal anti-inflammatory drugs (NSAIDs) reduce symptoms of ocular itching, injection, tearing (2, 6) but can cause systemic adverse effects.
   - Avoid topical decongestants due to paradoxical effect (1).
   - Topical calcineurin inhibitors do not cause intraocular pressure (IOP) increase and are steroid-sparing (6, 18, 21).
   - Systemic cyclosporine or tacrolimus therapy is effective for refractory VKC or AKC (6, 20, 22).

ABBREVIATIONS

>	More than
&	And
+	Positive
AC	Allergic conjunctivitis
AD	Atopic dermatitis
AKC	Atopic keratoconjunctivitis
AR	Allergic rhinitis
Assoc.	Associated
BID	Twice daily
B/L	Bilateral
CDC	Contact dermatoconjunctivitis
CL	Contact lens
d	Days
FH	Family history
GPC	Giant papillary conjunctivitis

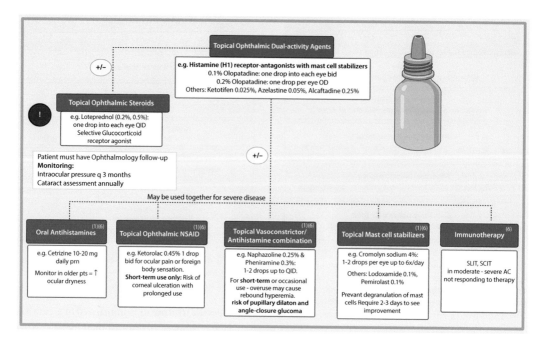

Figure 3.5 Pharmacotherapy options for treatment of ocular allergy. (Figure created with BioRender.com.) [Adapted from (1, 2, 6, 9, 16).]

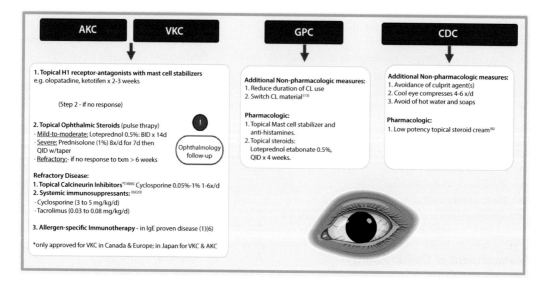

Figure 3.6 Treatment approach to specific subtypes of OA. Strongly consider ophthalmology co-management in refractory or complicated disease. (Figure created with BioRender.com.) [Adapted from (1, 6, 17–22).]

IgE	Immunoglobulin E	PAR	Perennial allergic rhinitis
IL	Interleukin	QoL	Quality of life
IOP	Intraocular pressure	QID	Four times a day
NSAIDs	Nonsteroidal anti-inflammatory drugs	SAC	Seasonal allergic conjunctivitis
PAC	Perennial allergic conjunctivitis	SAR	Seasonal allergic rhinitis

SCIT	Subcutaneous immunotherapy
SLIT	Sublingual immunotherapy
TID	Three times a day
txm	Treatment
VKC	Vernal keratoconjunctivitis

REFERENCES

1. Bielory L et al., Ann Allergy Asthma Immunol. (2020), PMID: 31759180/DOI: 10.1016/j.anai.2019.11.014.

2. Dupuis P et al., Allergy Asthma Clin Immunol. (2020), PMID: 31993069/DOI: 10.1186/s13223-020-0403-9.

3. Bielory L. J Allergy Clin Immunol. (2000), PMID: 11080700/DOI: 10.1067/mai.2000.111029.

4. Leonardi A et al., Allergy. (2017), PMID: 28387947/DOI: 10.1111/all.13178.

5. Bonini S et al., Ophthalmology. (2000), PMID: 10857837/DOI: 10.1016/s0161-6420(00)00092-0.

6. Leonardi A et al., Allergy. (2019), PMID: 30887530/DOI: 10.1111/all.13786.

7. Elhers W H et al., Curr Opin Allergy Clin Immunol. (2008), PMID: 18769199/DOI: 10.1097/ACI.0b013e32830e6af0.

8. La Rosa M et al., Ital J Pediatr. (2013), PMID: 23497516/DOI: 10.1186/1824-7288-39-18.

9. Bielory L et al., Immunol Allergy Clin North Am. (2008), PMID: 18282545/DOI:10.1016/j.iac.2007.12.005.

10. Leonardi A et al., Curr Opin Allergy Clin Immunol. (2015), PMID: 26258920/DOI: 10.1097/ACI.0000000000000204.

11. Barney NP. (2020) Allergic and Immunologic Diseases of the Eye. In: Middleton E. Middleton's Allergy: Principles and Practice, Ninth Edition, 38, 606–623.e1, Elsevier. https://www.clinicalkey.com/#!/content/book/3-s2.0-B9780323544245000393.

12. Bonini S et al., Eye. (2004), PMID: 15069427/DOI: 10.1038/sj.eye.6700675.

13. Hayes V et al., Cont Lens Anterior Eye. (2012), PMID: 16303503/DOI: 10.1016/S1367-0484(03)00019-5.

14. Donshik P et al., Trans Am Ophthalmol Soc. (1994), PMID: 10703125.

15. Rodrigues J et al., Ann Allergy Asthma Immunol. (2020), PMID: 33276116/DOI:10.1016/j.anai.2020.11.016.

16. Prokopich CL et al., Can J Optom. (2018), DOI:10.15353/cjo.80.257.

17. Vichyanond P et al., J Allergy Clin Immunol. (2004), PMID: 14767456/DOI: 10.1016/j.jaci.2003.10.065

18. Pucci N et al., Ann Allergy Asthma Immunol. (2002), PMID:12269651/DOI:10.1016/S1081-1206(10)61958-8.

19. Bilkhu P et al., Cont Lens Anterior Eye. (2012), PMID: 21925924/DOI: 10.1016/j.clae.2011.08.009.

20. Avunduk AM et al., Ophthalmologica. (2001), PMID: 11399937/DOI: 10.1159/000050876.

21. Abud TB et al., Ophthalmology. (2016), PMID: 27086024/DOI: 10.1016/j.ophtha.2016.02.044.

22. Stumpf T et al., Cornea. (2006), PMID: 17172887/DOI:10.1097/01.ico.0000240091.11854.14.

23. 23. Miyazaki, D et al., Allergology Int. (2020). DOI: 10.1016/j.alit.2020.03.005.

Allergen Immunotherapy

ABEER FETEIH, WALAA ALMASRI, GENEVIÈVE GENEST,
HOANG PHAM, AND PHIL GOLD

GENERAL BACKGROUND

- Allergen immunotherapy (AIT)
  - In IgE-mediated conditions, therapy involves repeated administration of a specific allergen with the objective of protection from allergic symptoms and inflammatory reactions associated with exposure to the allergen (1).
- Mechanism of AIT
  - Induces complex changes in different arms of the immune system including the innate, cellular, and humoral immune responses to the allergen leading to a decrease in the early and late immune responses of many organs, including the conjunctiva, skin, nasal mucosa, and respiratory bronchi (see Table 4.1) (1).
- AIT for aeroallergen and venom desensitization is approved by Health Canada by:
  - Subcutaneous immunotherapy: Aeroallergens, venom.
  - Sublingual (tablet) immunotherapy: Aeroallergens.

SUBCUTANEOUS IMMUNOTHERAPY (SCIT) [ADAPTED FROM (1, 3)]

A Brief Note on SCIT Dose and Scheduling

- Involves the gradual increase in allergen extract concentration until maintenance dose is achieved.
- Maintenance dose is considered the effective therapeutic dose, which is continued for a prolonged period at regular intervals to provide long-lasting immune response.
- Usual starting dose is 1:1000 vol/vol (4 dilutions) or rarely, 1:10,000 vol/vol (5 dilutions) in high-risk patients.

- Maintenance dose is typically 0.5 mL/injection; however, not all patients will tolerate this dose, and effectiveness may be achieved with lower maintenance dosing.
- Dosing schedules
  - Conventional:
    - Maintenance dose reached in 3–4 months; typically used for aeroallergens.
  - Cluster or rush:
    - Maintenance dose reached in days to weeks; typically used for venom immunotherapy.

Adverse Effects of SCIT

- Adverse effects range from mild/common to rare and life-threatening (see Table 4.4).
- Patients should be counseled about all possible adverse events and written informed consent is obtained prior to starting therapy.

Reduction of Immunotherapy Risks/Adverse Effects

- Assess the patient's medical condition at the time of injection (e.g. asthma control) and delay injection if indicated.
- Consider peak expiratory flow (PEF) for those with asthma before injections.
- Avoid errors (verify patient ID, dose, and technique of injection).
- Educate patients on how to recognize and treat allergic reactions.
- Instruct the patient to remain in the physician's office for at least 30 minutes after injection or longer if previous reactions, regardless of how long they have been receiving AIT.
- *When to reduce the dose*
  - If anaphylaxis occurs and immunotherapy is continued, reduce the dose by at least 50% and consider further reduction for moderate-severe reactions.

DOI: 10.1201/9781003174202-5

Table 4.1 Immune Responses after Starting Immunotherapy

Early response	Late response
• ↑ Regulatory T lymphocytes (Treg) that produce Interleukin (IL-10) and transforming growth factor beta (TGF-β) • Initial ↑ in specific immunoglobulin E (IgE)	• Change from T- helper 2 cell (Th2) to a T- helper 1 (Th1) response of cytokines to the allergen • Progressive ↓ in specific IgE • ↑ in specific IgGl, IgG4 and IgA (blocking antibodies)

Adapted from (1, 2).

- When there has been a newly prepared allergen extract/new vial.
- Any significant interruptions in the treatment schedule.
- Use of a more diluted initial AIT extract in those with an elevated sensitivity based on history or by specific IgE testing.
- Prescription of an epinephrine auto-injector to patients at higher risk for adverse effects and for those with a history of systemic reactions secondary to immunotherapy.

Table 4.2 Indications and Contraindications for Starting AIT

Indications

• Allergic rhinitis (see Chapter 1) • Allergic conjunctivitis • Allergic asthma	After clinical correlation and demonstration of specific IgE antibodies to relevant allergens, AIT may be considered through a shared-decision making process with patients who have moderate-severe allergic rhinitis/rhinoconjunctivitis and (1, 3–5) 1. Are not controlled with non-pharmacologic measures and/or pharmacotherapy 2. Prefer immunotherapy as the method of treatment (e.g. due to desire to avoid adverse effects, costs, or long-term use of pharmacotherapy) 3. Desire the potential benefit of immunotherapy to prevent or reduce the severity of comorbid conditions like allergic asthma
• Atopic dermatitis	• Many studies suggest that immunotherapy could be effective in those with coexistent aeroallergen sensitivity (dust mites) (6)
• Hymenoptera insect stinging hypersensitivity	• Refer to Chapter 14 on Stinging Insect Hypersensitivity

Contraindications (1, 3)

- Uncontrolled or severe asthma
- Major comorbidities such as cardiovascular disease
- Beta-blockers (relative contraindication with venom immunotherapy)
- Build-up phase in pregnancy

Special populations: Immunotherapy can be considered (1)

- Immunodeficiency disorders
- Autoimmune disorders

Allergen Immunotherapy is a disease modifying treatment for allergic rhinitis, allergic conjunctivitis, atopic dermatitis, and venom allergy. AIT is the most effective treatment in allergic rhinoconjunctivitis, however patient selection is important through a shared-decision making process with consideration of risks versus benefit and ability/willingness to adhere to this therapy.

Adapted from (1, 3–6).

Table 4.3 Major Allergens and Effective Doses in AIT

Allergen	Major allergenic component	Dose per ml, presuming 0.5 ml/dose, as per CSACI (3)	Effective dose range (per dose), as per 2011 practice parameter (1)
Dermatophagoides pteronyssinus	Der p 1	2000 AU	500–2000 AU/dose
Dermatophagoides farinae	Der f 1	2000 AU	500–2000 AU/dose
Dust Mite Mix		1000 AU each	
Cat (hair or pelt)	Fel d 1	2000 BAU	1000–4000 BAU
Grass (timothy)	Phl p 5	5000 BAU	1000–4000 BAU
Short Ragweed	Amb a 1	5000 PNU	1000–4000 AU 6–12 mcg
Fungi/mold (non-standardized) e.g. Altemaria or Cladosporium*		5000 PNU	Highest tolerated dose
Other Pollen (non-standardized) e.g. Tree mix		5000 PNU	0.5 ml of 1:100 or 1:200 wt/vol
Birch	Bet v 1	5000 PNU	
Dog	Can f 1	5000 PNU	15 mcg of Can f 1
Hymenoptera	(Refer to Chapter 14)	100 mcg/ml (1 ml dose)	50–200 mcg of each venom
Fire Ant	(Refer to Chapter 14)		0.5 ml of 1:100 wt/vol up to 0.5 ml of 1:10 wt/vol

* Allergens may be mixed in different combinations which may vary but molds should not be mixed with other non-mold extracts due to high protease activity.
Note: Maintenance dose is typically 0.5mL/injection.
Abbreviations: AU: Arbitrary units, BAU: Bioequivalent Allergy Units, PNU: Protein Nitrogen Unit.
Adapted from (1, 3).

Risk Factors for Anaphylaxis during Immunotherapy

1. **Patient factors**
   - Poorly controlled asthma
   - Persistent airflow limitation (FEV_1 <70%)
   - Active wheezing on day of immunotherapy
   - Current use of beta-blockers or angiotensin-converting enzyme (ACE)-inhibitors
   - History of anaphylaxis associated with AIT
2. **Administration factors**
   - Changes in potency associated from starting a new maintenance vial
   - Intravenous injections
   - Errors in dosing (wrong vial, dose, or patient)

Follow-Up of Patients on Immunotherapy

This patient follow-up should be every 6 months for the first year and then every 6–12 months while patients are on immunotherapy for the following reasons:

- To assess efficacy of the treatment.
  - Efficacy may be seen after reaching the maintenance dose, and should be seen by 1 year.
- To implement and reinforce its safe administration and to monitor for adverse reactions.
- Evaluating compliance to treatment.
- To determine an end date for successful immunotherapy.
- Assessing the need for dosing schedule or allergen content modifications.
  - Dosing frequency may be extended under extreme circumstances such as shortages of extract supply or during pandemics.

Duration of Treatment

Generally it is 3–5 years. Treatment is individualized according to patient response and preferences. Some cases such as with mast cell disorders with anaphylaxis to Hymenoptera require life-long treatment (refer to Chapter 14).

Table 4.4 Adverse Reactions to SCIT and Their Management

Types of reactions	Characteristics	Prevalence	Management
Local	• Redness, swelling and pruritus at injection site • Does not seem to predict subsequent systemic reactions although a higher frequency of large local reactions (LLR) might be at an increased risk for future systemic reactions • LLR defined as >25 mm	• Very common • Occurs between 26%–82% of patients and 0.7%–4% of injections (7–9)	• Cold compresses/ice • Antihistamines • Topical corticosteroids • Leukotriene antagonists (e.g. in a rush protocol immunotherapy) • Consider splitting the dose between each arm if local reactions intolerable
Systemic	• Majority occurs within 30 minutes after the injection (10) • Refer to Chapter 12	• < 1% of those treated with conventional immunotherapy and > 34% of patients in some studies who receive rush immunotherapy (11–14)	• Epinephrine is the first line treatment • Refer to Anaphylaxis chapter for complete management • Systemic cutaneous reactions (urticaria) occurring during the 30 min observation period should be preemptively treated with epinephrine as reactions may quickly progress to anaphylaxis
Delayed Systemic	• Typically less severe than immediate systemic • Occur 30 minutes or more after injection	• Up to 50% may occur after 30 min wait period (15)	• High-risk patients should carry an epi-pen throughout the day of their injection.
Fatal	• Extremely rare, but do occur • Major risk factors include uncontrolled asthma, dosing errors and administration during susceptible pollen season	• 1/2,500,000 (16) to 1/8,000,000 injections (17–18)	

Adapted from (1, 7–9, 11–15, 17, 18).

Sublingual Immunotherapy (SLIT)

Although subcutaneous immunotherapy (SCIT) has been used for over 100 years, SLIT became an accepted alternative to SCIT in 1998 (19).

The immunologic principles behind SLIT are the same as SCIT, with the major differences in the route, frequency, and location of administration.

General Information [Adapted from (3, 20–23)]

- **Route:** One tablet is placed sublingual (under the tongue) and should remain there until it dissolves completely.
- **Frequency:** One tablet daily.

- **Instructions on tablet administration:** The patient should be instructed not to take the tablet with any food or beverage, not to swallow for at least 1 minute, and to avoid food or drink for 5 minutes after taking the tablet.
- **First dose:** Should be given at the physician's office/medical health care setting with experience and supervision.
- **Observation period:** Patient observation for 30 minutes after the first dose to monitor for any adverse effects (local or systemic), and if the first dose is well tolerated, the subsequent doses are taken by the patient at home.
- **Initiation and length of treatment**
  - Pollen SLIT is given pre-/co-seasonally (see Table 4.5) but may be given year-round.
  - Dust mite SLIT is given year-round.
  - Treatment duration is 3–5 years.
  - Re-initiation of years 2–5 for pollen SLIT should be observed again in the physician's office.
- There are not enough data on the safety of SLIT during pregnancy or breastfeeding (24).

Side Effects of SLIT
Local Symptoms [Adapted from (3)]

- ~40% of patients.
- Oral pruritus, throat and ear discomfort.
- Reactions are usually transient and mostly during the first week of treatment.
- Pretreatment with antihistamines (non-sedating) may be helpful.

Systemic Allergic Reactions [Adapted from (3)]

- Very small risk (<1:500 over 3 years, less than the risk with SCIT)

Development of Eosinophilic Esophagitis (EoE)

- Potential risk while taking SLIT (24)

Contraindications to SLIT [Adapted from (24) Based on the U.S. Food and Drug Administration (FDA)-Approved SLIT Tablet-Prescribing Information]

- History of any severe local reaction to SLIT
- Any history of a severe systemic reaction to any form of immunotherapy
- Severe, unstable, or uncontrolled asthma
- History of EoE
- History of hypersensitivity to any of the inactive ingredients of the preparation
- Patients with serious medical conditions that may decrease their capability of surviving a significant systemic reaction or increasing the risk of adverse reactions post epinephrine (some examples include recent myocardial infarction, unstable angina, and hypertension that is uncontrolled) (24)

Patient Instructions at Home

- Inform patients about the need to temporarily stop SLIT if they develop mouth lesions (e.g. mouth ulcers, thrush, oral lichen planus), and post oral surgery/dental extraction (20, 21, 23).
- If one dose is missed, the next dose can be taken in the next scheduled time but should not be doubled. If the dose is missed for more than 7 days, the dose needs to be readministrated with supervision by the treating allergist (24).

Table 4.5 Health Canada Approved Sublingual Immunotherapy Tablets

SLIT	Extract composition	Age Indication (years)	Dose initiation	Timing of initiation before pollen season	Daily dose
Itulatek®	White birch	18–65	Full dose	At least 16 weeks	12 SQ-Bet
Oralair®	5 grass-mix	5–50	3-day escalation	~16 weeks	300IR
Grastek®	Timothy grass	5–65	Full dose	At least 8 weeks	2800 BAU
Ragwitek®	Short ragweed	18–65	Full dose	At least 12 weeks	12 Amb a 1-U
Acarizax®	D. farinae and D. pteronyssinus	18–65	Full dose	Not applicable/Start any time	12 SQ-HDM

Adapted from (19–21, 23).

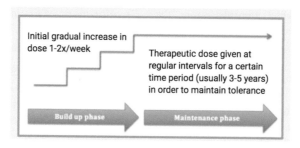

Figure 4.1 Dosing of AIT. Several dosing protocols are utilized for AIT, however the general principle includes a build-up phase of increasing dose followed by maintenance therapy over a prolonged time period. [Adapted from (1, 3).]

Choosing SCIT versus SLIT (25)

- SCIT and SLIT both have proven efficacy in seasonal and perennial allergic rhinitis.
- Choice of the AIT route largely depends on patient preference and availability of particular allergen extracts for treatment (e.g. cat allergen only available in SCIT).
- Shared decision making is important in AIT to ensure success of chosen therapy.
- Educate patients on risks of each therapy, efficacy, visits required, and cost.
- Re-evaluate choice of therapy periodically and change as needed.

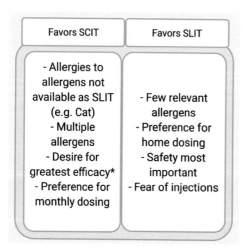

Figure 4.2 Choosing SCIT versus SLIT. After presented with both options for AIT patients will typically have a clear preference based on above characteristics. (Figure created with BioRender.com.) [Adapted from (25).]

*There are no head-to-head studies of SCIT versus SLIT, however, anecdotally SCIT may be slightly more effective.

SPECIAL POPULATIONS: PREGNANCY

- Immunotherapy is not started during pregnancy usually due to potential adverse effects of systemic reactions and its consequent treatment on the mother and her fetus or the two of them (some examples include spontaneous abortion or fetal hypoxia) (26).
- The initiation of immunotherapy in pregnant women may be considered only if the clinical indication for it is a medical condition with an elevated risk (e.g. Hymenoptera hypersensitivity causing anaphylaxis) (1).
- If in the buildup phase of immunotherapy and pregnancy occurs while the patient is obtaining a dose that is unlikely therapeutic, stopping treatment needs to be considered (1).
- Maintenance doses can be continued throughout the pregnancy period.
- Immunotherapy doses in pregnant women are generally not increased (1).
- The continuation of maintenance AIT during pregnancy appears safe. Furthermore, few data available suggest that the initiation of AIT during pregnancy might also be safe; however, more data are required for a definitive conclusion. Last, available studies do not show a convincing reduction in the development of atopy in offspring from the administration of AIT during pregnancy (27).

REFERENCES

1. Cox L et al., J Allergy Clin Immunol. (2011), PMID: 21122901/DOI: 10.1016/j.jaci.2010.09.034.
2. Kucuksezer UC et al., Allergol Int. (2020), PMID: 32900655/DOI: 10.1016/j.alit.2020.08.002.

3. Kim H et al., Immunotherapy Manual 2016. Canadian Society of Clinical Allergy & Immunology. https://csaci.ca/wp-content/uploads/2017/12/IT-Manual-2016-5-July-2017-rev.pdf. Accessed on June 15, 2019.

4. Dykewicz MS et al., J Allergy Clin Immunol. (2020), PMID: 32707227/DOI: 10.1016/j.jaci.2020.07.007.

5. Global Initiative for Asthma (GINA). Global Strategy for Asthma Management and Prevention (2020 Update). https://ginasthma.org/wp-content/uploads/2020/06/GINA-2020-report_20_06_04-1-wms.pdf. Accessed on 17, August 2020.1-48.

6. Bussmann C et al., J Allergy Clin Immunol. (2006), PMID: 17157659/DOI: 10.1016/j.jaci.2006.07.054.

7. Nelson BL et al., Ann Allergy. (1986), PMID: 3963525.

8. Prigal SJ, Ann Allergy. (1972), PMID: 5056915.

9. Tankersley MS et al., J Allergy Clin Immunol. (2000), PMID: 11080704/DOI: 10.1067/mai.2000.110468.

10. Cox LS et al., J Allergy Clin Immunol Pract. (2017), PMID: 28065342/DOI: 10.1016/j.jaip.2016.11.009.

11. Bousquet J et al., J Allergy Clin Immunol. (1989), PMID:2708740/DOI:10.1016/0091-6749(89)90017-1.

12. Windom HH et al., Curr Opin Allergy Clin Immunol. (2008) PMID: 18978474/DOI: 10.1097/ACI.0b013e32831845fb.

13. Bernstein DI et al., Ann Allergy Asthma Immunol. (2010), PMID: 20568387/DOI: 10.1016/j.anai.2010.04.008.

14. Portnoy J et al., Ann Allergy. (1994), PMID: 7978533.

15. Daveiga S et al., J Allergy Clin Immunol. (2008), DOI:10.1016/j.jaci.2007.12.495

16. Bernstein DI et al., J Allergy Clin Immunol. (2004), PMID: 15208595/DOI: 10.1016/j.jaci.2004.02.006.

17. Cox L et al., J Allergy Clin Immunol. (2010), PMID: 20144472/DOI: 10.1016/j.jaci.2009.10.060.

18. Epstein T G et al., Ann Allergy Asthma Immunol. (2013), PMID: 23535092/DOI: 10.1016/j.anai.2013.01.015.

19. Quirt J et al., Allergy Asthma Clin Immunol. (2018), PMID: 29339956/DOI: 10.1186/s13223-017-0225-6.

20. GRASTEK® (Timothy Grass Pollen Allergen Extract). https://www.grastek.com/app/uploads/sites/3/2017/11/USPI_US_GRX_20170818.pdf. Accessed June 14, 2019.

21. RAGWITEK® (Short Ragweed Pollen Allergen Extract) Tablet for Sublingual Use Prescribing Information. https://ragwitek.com/app/uploads/sites/4/2017/11/USPI_US_RGW_20170818.pdf. Accessed on June 15, 2019.

22. ACARIZAX™ Standardized Allergen Extract, House Dust Mites (*D. farinae and D. pteronyssinus*) Tablet for Sublingual Use Prescribing Information. https://pdf.hres.ca/dpd_pm/00039166.PDF. Accessed on June, 17 2019.

23. Oralair® (Sweet Vernal O, Perennial Rye, Timothy, and Kentucky Blue Grass Mixed Pollens Allergen Extract) Tablet For Single Use Prescribing Information. https://www.oralair.com/assets/pdf/ORALAIR-Prescribing-Information_Medication-Guide-2018.pdf. Accessed on June, 15 2019.

24. Greenhawt M et al., Ann Allergy Asthma Immunol. (2017), PMID: 28284533/DOI: 10.1016/j.anai.2016.12.009.

25. Roberts G et al., Allergy. (2018), PMID: 28940458/DOI: 10.1111/all.13317.

26. Metzger WJ et al., J Allergy Clin Immunol. (1978), PMID: 632475/DOI: 10.1016/0091-6749(78)90202-6.

27. Oykhman P et al., Allergy Asthma Clin Immunol. (2015), PMID: 26561490/DOI: 10.1186/s13223-015-0096-7.

RESPIRATORY DISORDERS

5 Asthma and Allergic Bronchopulmonary Aspergillosis (ABPA)   41
   Hoang Pham, Abeer Feteih, Geneviève Genest, and Jaime Del Carpio
6 Approach to Chronic Cough   57
   Hoang Pham and Maxime Cormier

Asthma and Allergic Bronchopulmonary Aspergillosis (ABPA)

HOANG PHAM, ABEER FETEIH, GENEVIÈVE GENEST, AND JAIME DEL CARPIO

This chapter will discuss asthma mainly in adults with a focus on long-term management and new treatment options.

GENERAL BACKGROUND

- Asthma is a heterogeneous, chronic inflammatory disease of the airways presenting with cough, wheeze, dyspnea, and/or chest tightness. These symptoms are caused by variable expiratory airflow limitation, ranging from mild to severe, and may lead to exacerbations requiring emergency treatments (1).
- Asthma is a common worldwide health problem that affects children and adults. In Canada, the point prevalence of asthma from 2009 to 2010 was more than 2.4 million Canadians (8.4%) aged 12 years and up (2).
- Asthma exacerbations affect quality of life, contribute to loss of lung function over time, and have a large economic impact (3, 4).

CLASSIFICATION [ADAPTED FROM THE "GLOBAL INITIATIVE FOR ASTHMA (GINA) 2020 UPDATE" (1)]

- Asthma severity is classified according to symptoms and the amount of medication required to control symptoms. Exacerbations and FEV_1 are also taken into account.
- Below is a simplified way to characterize asthma severity based on presenting symptoms, as severity is usually assessed retrospectively from the level of treatment required to control symptoms

and prevent exacerbations (see Figure 5.3 to understand the approximate level of treatment required for each step):

- **Mild Asthma: Step 1 or 2**
  - *GINA Step 1:* Symptoms <2×/month (no risk factors for exacerbations).
  - *GINA Step 2:* Symptoms twice a month or more, but less than daily.
- **Moderate Asthma: Step 3**
  - *GINA Step 3:* Symptoms most days or waking up with asthma once a week or more.
- **Severe Asthma: Steps 4–5**
  - *GINA Step 4:* Symptoms most days or waking with asthma once a week or more, or low lung function.
  - *GINA Step 5:* Severe uncontrolled asthma.
  - *Severe versus difficult-to-control asthma:* Difficult-to-control asthma becomes classified as severe asthma if it requires step 4–5 treatments to prevent loss of control or remains uncontrolled, even after optimizing other factors such as adherence, inhaler technique, and comorbidities.

Asthma Pathophysiology, Endotypes, and Phenotypes [Adapted from (1, 5–7)]

- Asthma is a markedly heterogeneous disease.
- *Endotype:* Refers to cellular/molecular mechanistic pathways.
  - *T2-high endotype mechanism:* Observed in ~50% of asthmatics
    - Stimulation of a dysregulated airway epithelial barrier by allergens, pollution, and/or viruses promotes the

DOI: 10.1201/9781003174202-7

release of alarmins called thymic stromal lymphopoietin (TSLP), interleukin-33 (IL-33), and IL-25.

- These alarmins act through T-helper subset 2 (Th2) cells and group 2 innate lymphoid cells (ILC2) to generate type 2 cytokines (IL-4, IL-5, and IL-13).
- These type 2 cytokines promote the recruitment, activation, proliferation, and survival of several inflammatory cells including mast cells, eosinophils, basophils, and B cells.
- These cells release inflammatory mediators, including histamine, prostaglandin D2 (PGD2), cysteinyl leukotrienes, and immunoglobulin E (IgE), which cause airway hyperresponsiveness, smooth muscle hypertrophy, and airway remodeling.
- *Associated biomarkers*
  - *Sputum eosinophils* >3% – available in specialized centers only.
  - *Peripheral blood eosinophils* >150 to 400 cells/μL – variable cutoffs used to predict response to anti-IL-5 biologics; exacerbation rates increased progressively, particularly starting when absolute eosinophil counts (AECs) are >300 cells/μL (8); easy to measure but values fluctuate depending on many factors such as degree of asthma control, medication adherence, OCS usage and unexplained physiologic fluctuations butin general true eosinophilic asthmatics keep PBE above 300 cells/uL, corticosteroid therapy.
  - *Total IgE* – associated with atopy; elevated levels crudely correlate with asthma severity, probability of wheeze, and reduced lung function; used to predict response to anti-IgE therapy, but not useful for monitoring response.
  - *Allergen sensitization tests* – skin prick tests (SPTs) or serum-specific IgE (sIgE) are used to assess degree of allergic sensitization, which correlates with asthma symptoms in early onset asthma.

  - *Fractional excretion of nitric oxide* (FeNO) >50 ppb (>35 in children) – correlates with IL-4 and IL-13 activity, airway hyperresponsiveness, and uncontrolled asthma.
- *T2-low endotype mechanism* (9): Relatively under investigated; sometimes called "non-T2."
  - *Non-T2 inflammation (neutrophilic):* Airway neutrophilia, possibly linked to dysregulated type 1 (T1) inflammation mediated through interferon-γ or type 3 (T3) inflammation mediated through IL-17.
  - *Non-inflammatory (paucigranulocytic):* Hypothesized to be driven by a "primary" smooth muscle dysfunction.
  - *Systemic inflammation:* Associated with IL-6, obesity, and metabolic dysfunction.
  - Some T2-low asthma may be T2-high asthma masked by oral corticosteroids (OCS).
  - *Associated "biomarkers"*
    - Absence of T2 markers.
    - Neutrophilic subtype: Sputum neutrophilia >40%–60%.
    - Paucigranulocytic ("non-inflammatory") subtype: Normal sputum eosinophils and neutrophils.
    - Lack of corticosteroid responsiveness.
- *Phenotype:* Refers to clinical presentation
  - Key discriminating factors between various common phenotypes are age of onset (early vs. late), atopic status, eosinophilia, and lung function.
  - Many of these "phenotypes" overlap, in particular, the allergic eosinophilic phenotypes, especially if AEC >150 cells/μL is adopted as the cutoff for eosinophilic asthma.
    - Furthermore, a possible T2-associated phenotype exists with mixed granulocytic (eosinophilic and neutrophilic) inflammation.
- *T2-high associated phenotypes*
  - Early-onset allergic asthma.
  - Late-onset eosinophilic asthma.
  - Nonsteroidal anti-inflammatory drug-exacerbated respiratory disease (NERD).

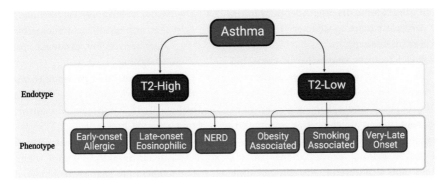

Figure 5.1 Classification of asthma by endotype and phenotype. Asthma is a heterogenous disease and phenotyping is important for treatment options and prognosis. (*Abbreviations:* T2: type 2; NERD: NSAID exacerbated respiratory disease.) (Figure created with BioRender.com.) [Adapted from (1, 5–7).]

- *T2-low associated phenotypes*
  - Obesity-associated asthma.
  - Smoking-associated asthma.
  - "Very"-late-onset non-allergic non-eosinophilic asthma.

Clinical Manifestations (All Vary in Intensity over Time)

- Cough
- Wheezing
- Shortness of breath (SOB)
- Chest tightness

QUESTIONS ON HISTORY (1)

- Age of asthma onset/diagnosis
  - Practical tip: Ask when the patient started using inhalers as a rough approximation
- Symptom pattern and control: Frequency of daytime symptoms, frequency of waking up with asthma, frequency of short-acting beta agonist (SABA) reliever use, any activity limitation due to asthma
  - Does pattern of symptoms vary with season?
- Trigger(s): Exercise, cold air, irritants (e.g. perfumes, cigarette smoke), aeroallergens, viral infections
- Environmental history: Type and age of residence (e.g. basement apartment), carpets, animals, molds/dampness/water damage, cockroaches, rodents
- Response to treatment(s): Symptomatic improvement with reliever medications, inhaled corticosteroids (ICS), leukotriene antagonist (LTRA), OCS

- Past medical history of allergic rhinitis, eczema, food allergies, chronic sinusitis with or without nasal polyps, gastroesophageal reflux disease (GERD), obstructive sleep apnea (OSA), depression/anxiety
- Past history of nasal sinus surgery
- Always ask about sense of smell, since severe hyposmia in an asthmatic frecuently indicates the presence of nasal polyposis
- Medication-adverse reactions including acetylsalicylic acid (ASA), NSAIDs, alcohol; Beta-blocker intolerance
- Medication adherence should be established by direct questioning: "How many times a day, a week, a month, a year do you use your fluticasone?"
- Social history: Occupation, occupational exposures, private health care coverage
- Smoking history: Pack-per-year history
- Family history of atopic disease
- Questionnaires available such as the Asthma Control Questionnaire (ACQ) and Asthma Control Test (ACT)

Physical Examination

- **Normal exam** (especially if mild intermittent asthma outside of an exacerbation).
- **Anthropomorphics:** Weight, height, and body mass index.
- **Nasal examination:** With otoscope or endoscope if available to observe nasal mucosal edema, status of the middle meatus, and possible presence of nasal polyps.
- **Respiratory examination:** Wheezing with prolonged expiratory phase on auscultation, check for clubbing (which should prompt additional evaluation, such as for cystic fibrosis).

- **Signs of other atopic disease:** Allergic rhinitis, atopic dermatitis (refer to Chapters 1 and 7 for physical exam findings).
- **Craniofacial features suggestive of comorbid OSA** (10): Obesity, wide neck circumference, nasal septal deviation, turbinate hypertrophy, crowding of posterior oropharynx (e.g. tonsillar enlargement, soft palate elongation, macroglossia, dental malocclusion), retrognathia.
- **Acute severe asthma exacerbation:** Patients may have signs of respiratory distress including severe SOB, use of accessory muscles, tachypnea, tachycardia, inability to complete full sentences, tripod position, and hypoxia (late finding).

Major Differential Diagnoses (Selected) (1): Varies Considerably with Age and Depends on Predominant Symptom

- *Vocal cord dysfunction (VCD):* Asthma mimic (42%), but also can be an asthma comorbidity (33%) (11)
  - *Symptoms:* Dyspnea (typically exertional), wheeze, stridor, cough, chest tightness, throat tightness, hoarseness/voice change; seen more in females, adolescents, or young adults (12, 13)
  - *Triggers* [Adapted from (13, 14)]
    - Exercise: Stridor at peak exercise that resolves rapidly within minutes of activity cessation
    - Irritants: Fragrances, cigarette smoke, fumes, vapor, mist, dust
    - Emotional stress
  - *Pittsburgh VCD Index:* A validated screening tool to help differentiate VCD versus asthma using key features (15)
    - Throat Tightness (4 pts), Sensitivity to Odors (3 pts), Dysphonia (2 pts), Absence of Wheezing (2 pts)
    - Positive screen if score >4 pts, sensitivity 83%, specificity 95%
  - *Treatment*
    - Sometimes a diagnostic clue is their lack of responsiveness to SABA and ICS
    - May respond to speech-language pathology, cognitive behavioral therapy, low-dose amitriptyline, and supraglottic surgical intervention in exceptional cases (12)

- *Dysfunctional breathing/hyperventilation:* It can exist as an asthma mimic or a comorbidity
  - Characterized by dizziness, paresthesias, and sighing
- *Cough hypersensitivity syndrome (CHS):* Consider this entity, which may be superimposed on asthma, if cough is the predominant or sole symptom (refer to Chapter 6)
  - Characterized by allotussia (16): Cough triggered by innocuous stimuli such as ambient temperature changes (cold air), deep inspiration, laughing, singing, voice projection, exposure to aerosols, perfumes, bleaches
- *Angiotensin-converting enzyme (ACE)-inhibitor cough:* Medication review
- *Chronic obstructive pulmonary disease (COPD):* Can be challenging to distinguish and may overlap
  - Elicit history: Symptom pattern (variable versus persistent symptoms), history of asthma (childhood vs current), and exposure history (smoking, etc.).
  - Spirometry (see section Diagnosis and Investigations): Assess for obstruction (post-bronchodilator FEV_1/FVC <0.70 required to diagnose COPD) and bronchodilator reversibility (marked reversibility >400 mL is more probable of asthma and unusual for COPD).
  - Treat cautiously:
    - High-dose ICS should be avoided due to risk of pneumonia in COPD (1, 17).
    - However, ICS therapy (with long-acting bronchodilator therapy) for COPD may be added if there is history/features of asthma, hospitalizations, ≥2 exacerbations/year requiring OCS, and AEC >300 cells/μL (1, 17–19).
- *Bronchiectasis:* Consider lung imaging workup if history suspicious for lung parenchymal diseases.
- *Other small airway diseases*
  - Allergic bronchopulmonary aspergillosis (ABPA): See section Allergic Bronchopulmonary Aspergillosis (ABPA) below
  - Eosinophilic granulomatosis with polyangiitis (EGPA)
- *Other large airways diseases*
  - Tracheobronchomalacia and excessive dynamic airway collapse.
    - Patients may also report wheeze.
  - Consider pulmonary consultation for bronchoscopy for these less common conditions.

- *Congestive heart failure (CHF):* SOB, orthopnea, paroxysmal nocturnal dyspnea, lower leg edema
  - A good reminder to consider non-pulmonary causes of respiratory symptoms

Diagnosis and Investigations

The following clinical features and investigations are employed to establish a diagnosis of asthma (1):

1. **History of typical respiratory symptoms** (see above)
2. **Spirometry**
   - Decreased FEV_1/FVC ratio: In practical terms, <0.70 in adults and <0.85 in children and adolescents. Normal subjects have FEV_1/FVC >0.75–0.80 in adults and >0.90 in children.
   - Decreased FEV_1 (it can be normal).
   - FEV_1 reversibility: After 400 mcg of salbutamol >12% and > 200 mL improvement in FEV_1.
3. **Methacholine provocation test (if symptoms are suggestive and spirometry results are non-diagnostic):** Conventionally, a fall in FEV_1 by >20% with a methacholine concentration (PC20) of <4 mg/mL is considered positive for airway hyperresponsiveness (4–16 mg/mL is a borderline result, which may be considered relevant if patient is taking ICS).
4. **Full pulmonary function tests including lung volumes and diffusing capacity for carbon monoxide (DLCO):** Not needed for initial or routine evaluation.
5. **Aeroallergen SPT**
   - Essential for establishing the phenotype of early-onset allergic asthma.
   - The 2007 National Heart, Lung, and Blood Institute (NHLBI) EPR-3 Guidelines recommend allergy SPT in all persistent asthmatics (20).
   - Casale et al. outlines a pragmatic approach for aeroallergen testing indications (21):
     - Persistent asthmatics, patients needing OCS or high-dose ICS, preschool children with repeated wheeze, patients seeking to understand their disease and/get guidance on pets, and evaluate candidate for allergen immunotherapy and biologicals (namely, anti-IgE)

6. **Complete blood count (CBC) with differential (eosinophil count)**
   - To screen for evidence of eosinophilic inflammation, which also serves as a biomarker of severity (see type 2 (T2)-high biomarkers above)

Other Tests

- Sputum eosinophils
  - Chronic airway inflammation (elevated sputum eosinophils>3%) is also an important component of the GINA asthma definition, which may help establish an asthma diagnosis and guide management.
  - However, this test is not widely available and often not performed routinely.
- FeNO is an indirect evaluation of eosinophilic airway inflammation.
  - More widely available (can be performed in clinic) and also an indirect measure of ICS compliance.

Features Indicating Increased Risk of Asthma-Related Death

- If the patient required asthma care in an emergency room or hospitalization in the last year
- If the patient is not using an ICS
- Adherence to ICS is poor
- Previous near-fatal asthma history needing intubation and ventilation
- If the patient is now on or stopped using OCS
- Overusing SABA (especially >1 canister/month)
- Psychosocial issues or psychiatric condition
- No written asthma action plan
- Food allergy (confirmed)

Management [Adapted from Global Initiative for Asthma (GINA), Global Strategy for Asthma Management and Prevention (2020 Update): A "Stepwise Approach for Adjusting Treatment for Individual Patient Needs" (1)]

Note: This chapter will not discuss the management of acute asthma exacerbations.

Non-Pharmacologic

- Education on asthma diagnosis and treatment plan
- Review inhaler technique
- Asthma action plan
- Discuss pneumococcal and seasonal influenza vaccination

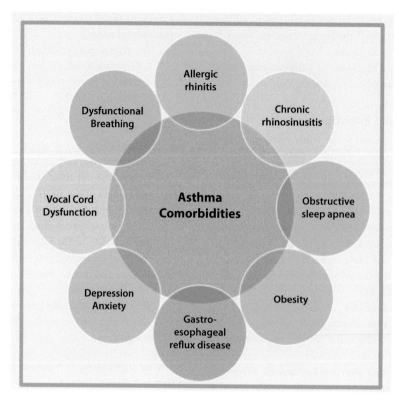

Figure 5.2 Asthma comorbidities. Addressing and treating comorbid conditions in asthma is important for achieving good asthma control. (Figure created with BioRender.com.)

- Smoking cessation
- Identification and elimination of triggers (e.g. allergens, irritants)
- Regular physical activity encouragement
- Patient should avoid NSAIDs and aspirin if intolerant
- Treatment of comorbidities (see Figure 5.2)
- ***Before stepping up asthma treatment, evaluate for common problems first***
  - Inhaler technique, adherence, persistent allergen exposures, control of comorbidities (e.g. obesity, GERD, OSA, anxiety/depression, rhinosinusitis)

Pharmacologic

- *Anti-inflammatory reliever (AIR): Therapy with as-needed formoterol-ICS*
  - New treatment approach developed to address the issue of low medication adherence to anti-inflammatory therapy and overuse of SABAs in mild asthma (22–25).
  - *Evidence:* Derived from four randomized controlled trials: SYGMA 1/2 (22, 23), Novel START (24), and PRACTICAL (25).

- Budesonide-formoterol Turbuhaler dry powder inhaler (DPI) combination (200/6 μg) on demand was superior to on-demand salbutamol (24, 25) or terbutaline (22, 23) and non-inferior (22–24) or superior (25) to maintenance budesonide DPI (200 μg) for preventing asthma exacerbations and lower overall ICS exposure.
  - *Select key exclusion criteria (23):* History of life-threatening asthma exacerbation including intubation and intensive care admission, any systemic glucocorticoid in last 30 days.
- *Single inhaler maintenance and reliever therapy (SMART)*
  - Budesonide-formoterol combination inhaler used as maintenance and reliever therapy is superior to salbutamol or formoterol as reliever therapy and maintenance budesonide for exacerbation reduction (26).
  - Budesonide-formoterol combination inhaler used as maintenance and reliever therapy is superior to fixed-dose ICS/long-acting

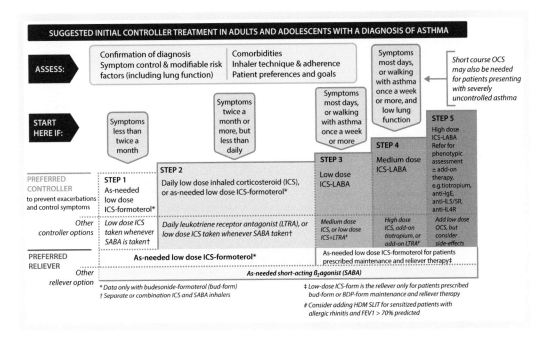

Figure 5.3 Suggested initial controller treatment in adults and adolescents with a diagnosis of asthma. Asthma therapy is targeted toward symptom frequency, as well as history/risk of exacerbations. Severity of asthma correlates with GINA "step" required to control symptoms with step 4–5 considered severe asthma. (©2020 Global Initiative for Asthma, reprinted with permission. Available from www.ginasthma.org.)

beta agonist (LABA) with SABA reliever for exacerbation reduction and overall ICS exposure (27).

Salient Features of the GINA Guidelines Since 2019

- **Salbutamol as monotherapy is eliminated.**
- As-needed (PRN) salbutamol is now PRN salbutamol + ICS, in other words, every time salbutamol is used ICS should be used at the same time.
- ICS-formoterol is now accepted as a reliever and as a controller medication, "Anti-Inflammatory Reliever Strategy" (see above).
- Sublingual Immunotherapy (SLIT) for house dust mites is recommended in GINA steps 3 and step 4.

Comments on ICS-LABA Combinations in Canada

1. **Budesonide and formoterol** (Symbicort™) – formoterol is both a LABA and a fast-acting beta agonist (FABA).
2. **Mometasone furoate and formoterol** (Zenhale™) – not officially approved for as-needed use.

3. **Fluticasone propionate and salmeterol** (Advair™) – although salmeterol is a LABA, **it is not a FABA and inappropriate for PRN use.**
4. **Fluticasone furoate and vilanterol** (Breo Ellipta™) – vilanterol is the only 24-hour-acting LABA available in asthma treatment, making it suitable for once-daily dosing.

Other Advanced Add-On Treatment Considerations in Severe Asthma: Important to Consider in Severe Non-Type 2 (Non-Allergic, Non-Eosinophilic) Asthma

1. **Tiotropium respimat** 2.5 mcg 2 puffs once daily
2. **Chronic azithromycin** 500 mg PO 3×/week (decreases exacerbations regardless of eosinophilia (28))
3. **Bronchial thermoplasty** – select centers in Canada only; considered in the setting of severe asthma with a non-inflammatory/paucigranulocytic "endotype" where smooth muscle dysfunction and airway hyperresponsiveness are hypothesized to be driving pathogenic factors (29)

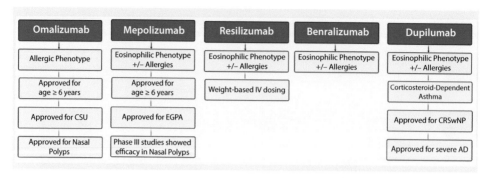

Figure 5.4 Asthma biologics and associated special features. (*Abbreviations:* AD: Atopic Dermatitis; CRSwNP: Chronic Rhinosinusitis with Nasal Polyps; CSU: Chronic Spontaneous Urticaria; EGPA: Eosinophilic Granulomatosis with Polyangiitis.) (Figure created with BioRender.com.) [Adapted from (30–34).]

Approved Biologics in Asthma

Refer to the product monographs for details, indications, and contraindications

1. **Anti-IgE monoclonal antibody**
   - Omalizumab (XOLAIR™) (30)
2. **Anti-IL-5 monoclonal antibodies**
   - Mepolizumab (NUCALA) (31)
   - Reslizumab (CINQAIR) (32)
3. **Anti-IL-5 receptor monoclonal antibody**
   - Benralizumab (FASENRA) (33)
4. **Anti-IL-4 receptor alpha monoclonal antibody**
   - Dupilumab (DUPIXENT) (34)

How to Choose between Biologics

- No absolute directives since allergic eosinophilic asthma populations frequently overlap.
- Allergic comorbidities such as allergic rhinitis, food allergies, early onset of asthma favors omalizumab.
- Anti-IL-5 in eosinophilic populations with or without allergies.
- Comorbidities such as atopic dermatitis favor dupilumab.
- Nasal polyposis: Dupilumab and omalizumab are approved for this indication. Beneficial effects have also been demonstrated with anti-IL5; however, it is not approved for this indication alone.

Follow-Up and Reviewing the Response to Treatment and Medication Adjustment (1)

- Patient follow-up
  - 1–3 months after starting treatment.

- Verify the response to the treatment.
- Not all patients respond equally to the same medication.
  - Eosinophilic allergic asthmatics respond better to ICS.
- Thereafter, review the patient every 3–12 months to decide the need for step-up or step-down therapy
- In pregnancy: Every 4–6 weeks
- Post asthma exacerbation: Patient should be seen within 1 week afterward
- Monitor for adverse effects to corticosteroids, especially if on OCS and suggested by the history:
  - Osteoporosis, diabetes mellitus

Allergic Bronchopulmonary Aspergillosis (ABPA)

- ABPA is a complex, progressive disease caused by a hypersensitivity reaction (type I and III) to *Aspergillus fumigatus*, typically affecting patients with underlying asthma or cystic fibrosis (35).
  - Affected asthmatics usually have severe asthma with a T2-high phenotype.
  - Suspect ABPA in patients with asthma and frequent exacerbations despite maximal medical therapy and good adherence.
  - Allergic bronchopulmonary mycosis (ABPM): Similar to ABPA caused by other fungi including *Penicillium* and *Schizophyllum commune*.
- *Clinical features:* Wheezing, productive cough with brown mucous plugs, occasional malaise/weight loss/hemoptysis, fleeting pulmonary opacities, central bronchiectasis (1, 35–37).

- *Diagnostic workup:* Many different criteria developed, but a recently validated criteria set has been proposed with a sensitivity of 89.9% and specificity of 96% for ABPM without cystic fibrosis (35).
  - Patients require >6 criteria to be diagnosed with ABPM:
    - Current or previous history of asthma or asthmatic symptoms
    - AEC >500 cells/µL
    - Elevated total IgE >417 IU/mL (>1000 µg/L)
    - SPT or sIgE for filamentous fungi
    - Specific IgG or precipitins for filamentous fungi
    - Filamentous fungal growth in sputum cultures or bronchial lavage fluid
    - Presence of fungal hyphae in bronchial mucous plugs
    - Central bronchiectasis on computed tomography (CT)
    - Presence of mucous plugs in central bronchi on CT/bronchoscopy or mucous plug expectoration history
    - High-attenuation mucus in bronchi on CT
- *Management*
  - OCS are the mainstay of treatment with suggested long courses (6–12 months) of prednisone 0.75 mg/kg/day × 6 weeks then 0.5 mg/kg/day × 6 weeks then taper by 5 mg/day every 6 weeks with disease activity monitored by symptoms, total IgE, and spirometry (36, 37).
  - Azole antifungals have been shown to have efficacy in steroid-dependent ABPA, but this may be due to cytochrome P450-dependent CYP3A4 enzyme inhibition, enhancing the bioavailable dose of corticosteroids (36).
  - Anti-IgE therapy with omalizumab 750 mg monthly significantly reduced exacerbation rates in patients within 4 months (37).

SPECIAL POPULATIONS: PREGNANCY

General Considerations (38, 39)

- Normal physiological respiratory changes during pregnancy include increased minute ventilation, compensated respiratory alkalosis, and decreased chest wall compliance/decreased functional residual capacity (with preservation of FEV_1, FVC, and the FEV_1/FVC ratio) as pregnancy progresses.
- Dyspnea is a common symptom during pregnancy and can present as early as several weeks after conception.
- Asthma is common during pregnancy, occurring in 5%–8% of pregnant women.
- Although most asthmatic pregnant women have preexisting asthma, asthma can first present during pregnancy.
- Pregnancy can lead to more frequent/severe asthma exacerbations in patients with preexisting asthma.
- Uncontrolled asthma has a significant impact on pregnancy/neonatal outcomes and is associated with increased risk for placenta-related complications, unplanned C-section, preterm labor/delivery, and small-for-gestational age infants.
- With certain exceptions, the risk of uncontrolled asthma surpasses potential side effects of asthma medications on the fetus.
- Appropriate asthma control during pregnancy improves maternal and fetal pregnancy outcomes.

Management (38, 39)

- Patients with asthma considering pregnancy benefit from a pre-conceptual visit to review medications and to assess fitness for pregnancy.
- Management of related comorbidities must be considered:
  - Allergen avoidance
  - Treatment of coexistent rhinitis (reviewed in Chapter 1)
  - Control of gastroesophageal reflux (H2 antihistamine; consider proton pump inhibitors if H2 antihistamine ineffective)
- Pregnant women with asthma should be assessed frequently during pregnancy, at least once a trimester or more often if asthma is uncontrolled.
- Compliance to treatment and control of exacerbating factors must be reviewed at each visit.
- Patients with moderate-severe asthma should be followed in a high-risk obstetrical unit, intermittent fetal monitoring should be considered after 32 weeks.
- Patients should receive yearly inactivated influenza vaccine.

Table 5.1 Commonly Used Asthma Inhaler Therapies in Canada (40–58)

Drug (approximate ICS dose equivalents)	Recommended dose (use lowest effective dose to control symptoms)	Labelled indications	Special remarks
	SHORT-ACTING BETA-2-AGONIST (SABA)		
Salbutamol 100 mcg/dose (MDI) 200 mcg/dose (DISKUS)	Recommended dose range: • 100 mcg 1–2 inhalations every 4–6 hours as needed • 200 mcg 1 inhalations every 4–6 hours as needed Max dose: 800 mcg/day (max 400 mcg/day ages 4–11)	Symptomatic relief of bronchospasm in asthma, EIB, COPD for ages > 4 years	• MDI can be used with spacer device • Some patients may demonstrate more proficiency with a particular device
Terbutaline 0.5 mg/dose (Turbuhaler)	Recommended dose range: • 0.5 mg every 4–6 hours as needed Max dose: 3 mg/day	Symptomatic relief of bronchospasm in asthma, bronchitis and emphysema for ages > 6 years	• Some patients may prefer to have all their inhalers be of the same type (e.g., Terbutaline and Pulmicort both come as Turbuhalers) • Dose counter present
	INHALED CORTICOSTEROIDS (ICS)		
Beclomethasone Dipropionate 50, 100 mcg/dose (MDI) Low <200 mcg/day (<200 mcg/day in children) Med 201–500 mcg/day (201–400 mcg/day in children) High >500 mcg/day (>400 mcg/day in children)	Recommended dose range: • 50–400 mcg twice daily (ages > 12) • 50–100 mcg twice daily (ages 5–11) Max dose: 800 mcg/day (200 mcg/day ages 5–11)	Maintenance therapy of asthma ages > 5 years old	• Daily doses >200 mcg/day is not approved for use in children in Canada

Drug (approximate ICS dose equivalents)	Recommended dose (use lowest effective dose to control symptoms)	Labelled indications	Special remarks
Budesonide 100, 200, 400 mcg/dose (Turbuhaler) Low <400 mcg/day Med 401–800 mcg/day High >800 mcg/day (same in children)	Recommended dose range: • 100–2600 mcg 2 to 4 times daily (ages >12) • 100–200 mcg twice daily (ages 6–12) Max dose: 2400 mcg/day (400 mcg/day ages 6–12)	Maintenance therapy of asthma ages > 6 years old	• Licensed for once daily dosing in Canada (generally up to 400 mcg on a single occasion may be considered in ages >12) • Turbuhaler device may reduce need for hand-breath coordination • Dose counter present
Ciclesonide 100, 200 mcg/dose (MDI) Low <200 mcg/day Med 201–400 mcg/day High >400 mcg/day (same in children)	Recommended dose range: • 100–400 mcg once or twice daily (ages >12) • 100–200 mcg once daily (ages 6–11) Max dose: 800 mcg/day (max 200 mcg/day ages 6–11)	Maintenance therapy of asthma ages > 6 years old	• Licensed for once daily dosing in Canada • Prodrug and is hydrolyzed to its pharmacologically active metabolite by esterase enzymes primarily in the lungs
Fluticasone Furoate 100, 200 mcg/dose (Ellipta) Low 100 mcg/day High 200 mcg/day	Recommended dose range: • 100 or 200 mcg once daily Max dose: 200 mcg/day	Maintenance therapy of asthma ages >12 years old	• Licensed for once daily dosing in Canada • High ICS dose achieved with only 1 inhalation/day (may facilitate easier adherence) • Ellipta device may reduce need for hand-breath coordination • Dose counter present
Fluticasone Propionate 50, 125, 250 mcg/dose (MDI) 100, 250, 500 mcg/dose (Diskus) Low < 250 mcg/day (<200 mcg/day in children) Med 251–500 mcg/day (201–400 mcg/day in children) High >500 mcg/day (>400 mcg/day in children)	Recommended dose range: • 100–1000 mcg twice daily(ages>16) • 100–200 mcg twice daily(ages 4-16) • 100 mcg twice daily (ages 12months to 4 years, MDI only with pediatric space device) Max dose: 2000 mcg/day (400 mcg/day ages 4–16; 200 mcg/day 12 months–4 years)	Maintenance therapy of asthma ages >12 months old (MDI), >4 years old (DISKUS)	• Licensed as young as 12 months of age • MDI can be used with spacer device

(Continued)

Table 5.1 Commonly Used Asthma Inhaler Therapies in Canada (40–58) (Continued)

Drug (approximate ICS dose equivalents)	Recommended dose (use lowest effective dose to control symptoms)	Labelled indications	Special remarks
Fluticasone Propionate 55, 113, 232 mcg/dose (Respiclick) Low 110 mcg/day Med 226 mcg/day High 464 mcg/day	Recommended dose range: • 55, 113, or 232 mcg twice daily Max dose: 464 mcg/day	Maintenance therapy of asthma ages >12 years old	• Novel inhalation device with one step for opening and loading the dose • Dose counter present • Respiclick device may reduce need for hand-breath coordination
Mometasone Furoate 100, 200, 400 mcg/dose (Twisthaler) Low 100–200 mcg/day (100 mcg/day in children) Med >200–400 mcg/day (>200–<400 mcg/day in children) High >400 mcg/day (>400 mcg/day in children)	Recommended dose range: • 100–400 mcg once or twice daily Max dose: 800 mcg day (100 mcg/day ages 4–11)	Maintenance therapy of asthma ages >4 years old	• Licensed for once daily dosing in Canada • Twisthaler device may reduce need for hand-breath coordination

COMBINATION INHALED CORTICOSTEROID LONG-ACTING BETA-2-AGONIST (ICS-LABA)

Drug (approximate ICS dose equivalents)	Recommended dose (use lowest effective dose to control symptoms)	Labelled indications	Special remarks
Budesonide-Formoterol 100/6, 200/6 (Turbuhaler) Low <400 mcg/day Med 401–800 mcg/day High >800 mcg/day	Recommended dose range: 100/6 or 200/6 mcg 1–2 inhalations once or twice daily Max dose: • Not more than 6 inhalations on a single occasion • Max 1600 mcg/day of budesonide — max 48 mcg/day of formoterol — 100/6 or 200/6 mcg 4 inhalations twice daily (8 inhalations/day) • Essentially, patients have an additional 4 puffs for anti-inflammatory reliever therapy daily as needed if their maintenance dose is 2 inhalations twice daily.	For ages >12 years old a. Anti-inflammatory reliever therapy as needed for acute relief using 200/6 mcg device b. Anti-inflammatory reliever therapy plus maintenance therapy using 100/6 or 200/6 mcg device as daily maintenance and as needed c. Maintenance therapy with separate SABA for acute relief d. Moderate-to-severe COPD if combination appropriate	• Contains fasting-acting beta-agonist, formoterol, enabling as-needed relief (option a and b) • Turbuhaler device may reduce need for hand-breath coordination • Approved for both asthma and COPD which may be useful in overlap cases • Having one inhaler for both maintenance and acute relief may be preferable for the patient (option b)

Drug (approximate ICS dose equivalents)	Recommended dose (use lowest effective dose to control symptoms)	Labelled indications	Special remarks
Mometasone-Formoterol 100/5, 200/5 mcg (MDI) Low 100–200 mcg/day (100 mcg/day in children) Med >200–400 mcg/day (>200–<400 mcg/day in children) High >400 mcg/day (>400 mcg/day in children)	Recommended dose range: • 100/5 or 200/5 mcg 2 inhalations twice daily Max dose: 800/20 mcg day	For ages >12 years old for maintenance therapy of asthma	• Although it contains formoterol, it is not officially approved by Health Canada for acute relief • MDI can be used with spacer device
Fluticasone Propionate-Salmeterol 125/25, 250/25 mcg (MDI) 100/50, 250/50, 500/50 (Diskus) Low <250 mcg/day (<200 mcg/day in children) Med 251–500 mcg/day (201–400 mcg/day in children) High >500 mcg/day (>400 mcg/day in children)	Recommended dose range: • 125/25 or 250/25 mcg 2 inhalations twice daily • 100/50, 250/50, or 500/50 1 inhalation twice daily Max dose: 1000/100 mcg/day	For ages > 4 years old a. For maintenance therapy of asthma b. For maintenance therapy of COPD if combination appropriate	• Approved for both asthma and COPD which may be useful in overlap cases • Salmeterol is a long-acting beta agonist but not a fast-acting beta agonist (thus, should not be used for acute relief) • MDI can be used with spacer device
Fluticasone Furoate-Vilanterol 100/25, 200/25 mcg (Ellipta) Low 100 mcg/day High 200 mcg/day	Recommended dose range: • 100/25 or 200/25 1 inhalation once daily Max dose: 100–200/25 mcg/day	For ages > 18 years old a. For maintenance therapy of asthma b. For maintenance therapy of COPD if combination appropriate (only 100/25 mcg device)	• Approved for both asthma and COPD which may be useful in overlap cases • Vilanterol is an ultra-long acting beta agonist which enables once daily dosing (may be easier to adhere)

Abbreviations: COPD: chronic obstructive pulmonary disease; EIB: exercise-induced bronchoconstriction; MDI: metered dose inhaler.

- Asthma management during pregnancy is similar to the non-pregnant state and should be adjusted to the severity of asthma at each visit.
- **Patients should be maintained on the same pre-pregnancy inhaler regiment if asthma is well controlled pre-conception.**
- Theophylline can be continued during pregnancy, but serum theophylline levels should be monitored more frequently; theophylline can also increase formoterol toxicity.
- LTRA can be continued throughout pregnancy.
- 5-Lipoxygenase inhibitors should be discontinued prior to conception.
- Omalizumab can be continued throughout pregnancy (but should only be started during pregnancy if benefit clearly surpasses the risk of anaphylaxis associated with initiation).
- There is no current data on anti-IL5 biologic use during pregnancy; however, observational studies are ongoing. A patient with previously severe eosinophilic asthma well controlled with anti-IL-5 therapy should be maintained on it throughout pregnancy (expert opinion).
- There is no existing safety data concerning tiotropium usage during pregnancy. The decision to do so should be done on an individualized basis after a proper risk assessment.
- Treatment of acute exacerbations during pregnancy is similar to the non-pregnant state; fetal monitoring should be considered if >24 weeks gestation.
- Keep in mind that a normal pregnant woman has a compensated respiratory alkalosis. A normal PCO_2/acidemia can signal impending/imminent respiratory failure and warrants intensive care unit (ICU) admission and fetal monitoring.

REFERENCES

1. Global Initiative for Asthma (GINA). Global Strategy for Asthma Management and Prevention (2020 Update). https://ginasthma.org/wp-content/uploads/2020/06/GINA-2020-report_20_06_04-1-wms.pdf. Accessed on 17, August 2020. 1–48.
2. Government of Canada. Fast Facts about Asthma: Data compiled from the 2011 Survey on Living with Chronic Diseases in Canada. http://www.phac-aspc.gc.ca/cd-mc/crd-mrc/asthma_fs_asthme-eng.php. Accessed August 17, 2020.
3. Bai TR et al., Eur Respir J. (2007), PMID: 17537763/DOI:10.1183/09031936.00165106.
4. Castillo JR et al., J Allergy Clin Immunol Pract. (2017), PMID: 28689842/DOI:10.1016/j.jaip.2017.05.001.
5. Kaur R et al., J Allergy Clin Immunol. (2019), PMID: 31277742/DOI: 10.1016/j.jaci.2019.05.031.
6. Moore WC et al., Am J Respir Crit Care Med. (2010), PMID: 19892860/DOI: 10.1164/rccm.200906-0896OC.
7. Kuruvilla ME et al., Clin Rev Allergy Immunol. (2019), PMID: 30206782/DOI:10.1007/s12016-018-8712-1.
8. Price DB et al., Lancet Respir Med. (2015), PMID: 26493938/DOI:10.1016/S2213-2600(15)00367-7.
9. Fitzpatrick AM et al., J Allergy Clin Immunol Pract. (2020), PMID: 32037109/DOI:10.1016/j.jaip.2019.11.006.
10. Laratta CR et al., CMAJ. (2017), PMID: 29203617/DOI:10.1503/cmaj.170296.
11. Traister RS et al., Allergy Asthma Proc. (2013), PMID: 23883599/DOI:10.2500/aap.2013.34.3673.
12. Morris MJ et al., Chest. (2010), PMID: 21051397/DOI:10.1378/chest.09-2944.
13. Halvorsen T et al., Eur Respir J. (2017), PMID: 28889105/DOI:10.1183/13993003.02221-2016.
14. Marcinow AM et al., Otolaryngol Head Neck Surg. (2015), PMID: 26307573/DOI:10.1177/0194599815600144.
15. Traister RS et al., J Allergy Clin Immunol Pract. (2014), PMID: 24565771/DOI:10.1016/j.jaip.2013.09.002.
16. Song WJ et al., Allergy Asthma Immunol Res. (2017), PMID: 28677352/DOI:10.4168/aair.2017.9.5.394.
17. Global Initiative for Chronic Obstructive Pulmonary Disease (GOLD). Global Strategy for Prevention, Diagnosis, and Management of COPD 2021 Report. https://goldcopd.org/2021-gold-reports/. Accessed on 17, August 2020.1-48.
18. Gershon AS et al., JAMA. (2014), PMID: 25226477/DOI:10.1001/jama.2014.11432.
19. Kendzerska T et al., Ann Am Thorac Soc. (2019), PMID: 31298938/DOI: 10.1513/AnnalsATS.201902-126OC.
20. National Asthma Education and Prevention Program. J Allergy Clin Immunol. (2007), PMID: 17983880/DOI: 10.1016/j.jaci.2007.09.043.
21. Casale TB et al., J Allergy Clin Immunol Pract. (2020), PMID: 32687905/DOI:10.1016/j.jaip.2020.07.004.
22. O'Byrne PM et al., N Engl J Med. (2018), PMID: 29768149/DOI: 10.1056/NEJMoa1715274.
23. Bateman ED et al., N Engl J Med. (2018), PMID: 29768147/DOI:10.1056/NEJMoa1715275.
24. Beasley R et al., N Engl J Med. (2019), PMID: 31112386/DOI: 10.1056/NEJMoa1901963.
25. Hardy J et al., Lancet. (2019), PMID: 31451207/DOI:10.1016/S0140-6736(19)31948-8.
26. Rabe KF et al., Lancet. (2006), PMID: 16935685/DOI:10.1016/S0140-6736(06)69284-2.
27. Buhl R et al., Respir Res. (2012), PMID: 22816878/DOI: 10.1186/1465-9921-13-59.

28. Gibson PG et al., Lancet. (2017), PMID: 28687413/ DOI:10.1016/S0140-6736(17)31281-3.

29. Svenningsen S et al., Front Med (Lausanne). (2017), PMID: 29018800/DOI: 10.3389/fmed.2017.00158.

30. XOLAIR® (omalizumab) Injection for Subcutaneous Use. https://www.gene.com/download/pdf/xolair_prescribing.pdf. Accessed on 21, June 2019.

31. NUCALA (mepolizumab) for Injection. Interleukin-5 (IL-5) inhibitor. https://ca.gsk.com/media/1209435/nucala.pdf. Accessed on 21, June 2019.

32. Cinqair® (Reslizumab) injection 100mg/10ml. https://www.cinqair.com/globalassets/cinqair/prescribinginformation.pdf. Accessed on 21, June 2019.

33. Fasenra™ (benralizumab) Injection for Subcutaneous Use. https://www.azpicentral.com/fasenra/fasenra.pdf - page=1. Accessed on 21, June 2019.

34. Dupixent® (dupilumab) Injection for Subcutaneous Use. Interleukin-4 Receptor Alpha Antagonist. https://d1egnxy4jx1q3f.cloudfront.net/Regeneron/Dupixent_FPI.pdf. Accessed on 21, June 2019.

35. Asano K et al., J Allergy Clin Immunol. (2020), PMID: 32920094/DOI:10.1016/j.jaci.2020.08.029.

36. Hew M, Douglass JA, Tay TR, O'Hehir RE. Allergic Bronchopulmonary Aspergillosis, Hypersensitivity Pneumonitis, and Epidemic Thunderstorm Asthma. In: Burks AW, Holgate ST, O'Hehir RE, Bacharier LB, Broide DH, Hershey GK, Peebles Jr RS. Middleton's Allergy: Principles and Practice E-Book, Ninth Edition. Amsterdam: Elsevier. Available at: https://www.clinicalkey.com/dura/browse/bookChapter/3-s2.0-C20161002419 (Accessed: Feb 03, 2021).

37. Voskamp AL et al., J Allergy Clin Immunol Pract. (2015), PMID: 25640470/DOI:10.1016/j.jaip.2014.12.008.

38. Bonham CA et al., Chest. (2018), PMID: 28867295/ DOI:10.1016/j.chest.2017.08.029.

39. Namazy JA et al., Semin Respir Crit Care Med. (2018), PMID: 29427983/DOI:10.1055/s-0037-1606216.

6

Approach to Chronic Cough

HOANG PHAM AND MAXIME CORMIER

BACKGROUND

Cough represents a disruption of normal breathing patterns and can be conceptualized as a triphasic event (1, 2).

1. **Inspiratory phase:** Inspiratory effort.
2. **Compressive phase:** Expiratory effort against a closed glottis.
3. **Expulsive phase:** Opening of the glottis and a rapid expiratory airflow.

CLASSIFICATION

The most common and useful classification of cough is based on duration (1).

- **Chronic cough:** Cough lasting more than 8 weeks in adults, more than 4 weeks in children (2).

- **Subacute cough:** Cough lasting for 3 to 8 weeks.
- **Acute cough:** Cough lasting for less than 3 weeks.

DEFINITIONS

Chronic cough research has evolved and academics, societies, and researchers groups have adopted the following definitions (1):

- **Refractory chronic cough (RCC):** Cough that persists despite optimal treatment for the presumed associated condition(s).
- **Unexplained chronic cough (UCC) or idiopathic chronic cough (ICC):** No diagnosable cause for cough has been found (despite extensive assessment for both common and uncommon causes).
- **Cough hypersensitivity syndrome (CHS):** A syndrome, first proposed by the European Respiratory Society (ERS) Task Force,

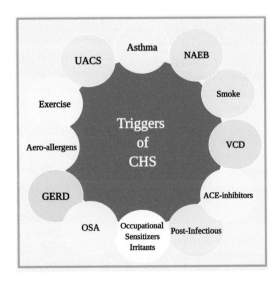

Figure 6.1 Triggers of cough hypersensitivity syndrome. (*Abbreviations:* CHS: Cough hypersensitivity Syndrome, UACS: Upper airway cough syndrome, NAEB: Non-asthmatic eosinophilic bronchitis, OSA: Obstructive sleep apnea, GERD: Gastroesophageal reflux disease, VCD: Vocal cord dysfunction.) (Figure created with BioRender.com.) [Adapted from 1–3, 5).]

characterized by allotussia, hypertussia, and laryngeal paresthesia (2). It's analogous to chronic pain syndromes with heightened perception of pain to relatively innocuous or mildly irritating stimuli. CHS can result from the summation of multiple different trigger exposures and hypersensitivities from different etiologies (3).

– *Allotussia:* Cough triggered by low-intensity-level thermal, mechanical, or chemical exposures, which usually does *not* produce cough in healthy subjects (e.g. ambient temperature changes, deep inspiration, laughing, prolonged phonation, exposure to aerosols and perfumes, and eating dry food textures).
– *Hypertussia:* Excessive cough response to known noxious stimuli that normally induce cough.
– *Laryngeal paresthesia:* Sensation of airway irritation that is not alleviated by cough.
  • *Urge to cough:* An alternative phrase used to describe laryngeal paresthesia

Epidemiology (2)

• *Prevalence:* 5%–10% of the adults
• *Potential complications of severe chronic cough:* Incontinence, cough syncope, and social isolation
• Regardless of the underlying disease or exposure leading to chronic cough, all patients presenting with chronic cough, as their predominant symptom, share a *common clinical presentation, now conceptualized as CHS:*
  – Marked sensitivity to environmental irritants such as perfumes, bleaches, cold air, exercise, stress, singing, talking/voice projection
  – Sensations of tickling/irritation in the throat with an urge to cough
  – Two-thirds are females
  – Peak prevalence in fifties and sixties
  – Commonly associated conditions include irritable bowel syndrome, obesity, and a variety of neuropathic syndromes

Pathophysiology (3, 4)

Cough is a protective vagal reflex to prevent aspiration into the lungs and expel excess mucus and debris in the lungs

• Peripherally, coughing is stimulated by vagal sensory nerves in the larynx and airways upon activation by various stimuli like irritants and excess mucus through *chemo*sensitive C fibers and Aδ fiber *mechano*receptors.
• Centrally, these peripheral fibers synapse at the brainstem and then form complex neural networks in the cerebral cortex, which then coordinates an efferent cough response.
• In broad terms, there are two putative mechanisms of chronic cough:
  1. Increased exposure of sensory nerve terminal to irritants or excess mucus with upregulation of cough receptors (e.g. P2X3, TRPV1), thereby decreasing the threshold for neuronal excitability to these triggers
  2. Changes in the excitability of the neuronal pathways that may affect airway sensory nerve and/or their central nervous system (CNS) connections, "central sensitization of the cough reflex"
     – Increased activation in certain midbrain areas may alter central cough control.
     – Decreased activation in other cortices involved with cough inhibition.
• In short, a chronic cough phenotype (CHS) likely represents the summation of an underlying disease ("intrinsic factor") + trigger exposure ("external factor") + a component of cough hypersensitivity.

Diagnostic Evaluation of Chronic Cough Using the Framework of CHS

1. Focus on identifying the **two components of CHS** (5)Possible trigger exposures (external factors) and/or underlying diseases (intrinsic factors)
2. Cough/laryngeal hypersensitivity ("irritable larynx")

Note: This diagnostic approach generally applies to ages 14 and up.

• *Step 1:* **Classify the duration of the cough**
  – *Acute:* **<3 weeks**
    • *Most probable diagnoses:* Upper respiratory tract infection, exacerbation of asthma or chronic obstructive pulmonary disease (COPD), pneumonia
  – *Subacute:* **3–8 weeks**
    • *Most probable diagnoses:* Postinfectious cough syndrome, asthma or COPD exacerbation, eosinophilic bronchitis, upper airway cough syndrome (UACS)

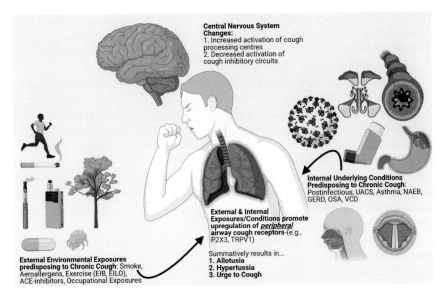

Figure 6.2 Pathophysiologic components of chronic cough and cough hypersensitivity syndrome. (*Abbreviations:* EIB: Exercise-induced bronchoconstriction; EILO: Exercise-induced laryngeal obstruction; GERD: Gastroesophageal reflux disease; NAEB: Non-asthmatic eosinophilic bronchitis; OSA: Obstructive sleep apnea; P2X3: Purinergic receptor P2X ligand-gated ion channel subunit 3; TRPV1: Transient receptor potential vanilloid type 1; UACS: Upper airway cough syndrome; VCD: Vocal cord dysfunction.) (Figure created with BioRender.com.)

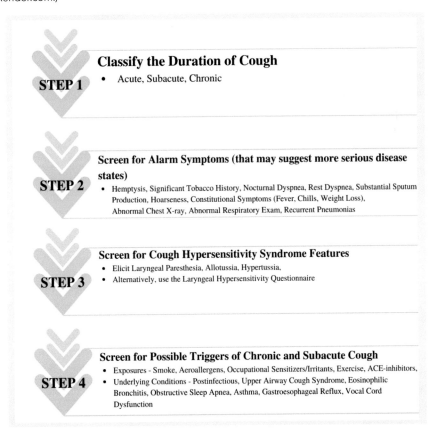

Figure 6.3 Diagnostic evaluation flowchart of chronic cough. (Figure created using BioRender.com.)

- *Note:* Postinfectious cough syndrome may last up to ~6 months.
  - **Chronic: > 8 weeks**
    - *Most probable diagnoses:* UACS, cough-variant asthma, gastroesophageal reflux disease (GERD), angiotensin-converting enzyme (ACE) inhibitor-induced cough, and eosinophilic bronchitis, postinfectious cough syndrome
- **Step 2: Screen for alarm symptoms (6)**
  - *Key red flags:* Smoking history, spontaneous cough that is not preceded by an urge or tickle, waking up due to cough, objective sputum production, hemoptysis, persistent non-episodic voice change, abnormal chest exam, abnormal chest imaging
  - *Do not miss diagnoses:* Malignancy, parenchymal lung disease, infection, cardiac disease, foreign body, congenital airway abnormalities
  - *Take home message:* Presence of alarm symptoms suggests a pathologic/anatomical cause of chronic cough

Note: Refer to Australian Cough Guidelines for comprehensive list of alarm symptoms and significant conditions not to be missed (6)

- *Step 3:* **Screen for laryngeal hypersensitivity/ dysfunction, "irritable larynx"**
  - *Elicit laryngeal paresthesia*
    - Abnormal sensation in throat or upper airway, "tickle", itch, pain, "something is stuck in my throat", globus sensation
  - *Elicit allotussia*
    - Cough is triggered by non-tussive stimuli like cold air, perfume, voice projection, exercise
  - *Elicit hypertussia*
    - Exaggerated cough in response to expected tussive stimuli (e.g. smoke, cleaning products, fumes)
  - A positive screen suggests a neuropathic dysfunction of the sensory pathways contributing to chronic cough
- *Step 4:* **Screen for possible (external) triggers of chronic and subacute cough**
  - *Exposures*
    - *Occupational and Environmental Exposures*
      - Assess history of smoking

- Assess atopic status with respect to aeroallergens
- Assess possible occupational exposures
  - *Sensitizers:* Flour, animal proteins, wood dust, isocyanates, hair products
  - *Irritants:* Vapors, gas, dust particulates, fumes
  - Review Material Safety Data Sheets (MSDS)
  - Consult occupational medicine if needed
- *Exercise*
  - Can also trigger underlying asthma, exercise-induced bronchoconstriction, or exercise-induced laryngeal obstruction, which may need concurrent specific treatment
- *ACE-I treatment*
  - Occurs in up to ~20% of patients with up to 5% of treated patients needing to stop ACE-I because of cough.
  - Starts usually within first few weeks of treatment, but can start up to months later (7).
  - There is a higher prevalence in Asians, Blacks, and women (7).
  - This is mediated by bradykinin, which is a potent generator of cough through stimulation of vagal afferent nerve fibers
  - Stops within days to weeks after stopping ACE-I (8).
  - Can change to ARB because it is associated with much lower rates of cough (7, 8).
- *Diseases*
  - *Postinfectious cough syndrome (5, 8)*
    - *Presentation:* A dry and irritating cough following an upper respiratory tract infection (URTI) that would have been expected to last for a week, but persists for months (usually up to 8 weeks but can be longer).
      - *Bordetella pertussis* infection is the classic example, but other infections have been described to be associated

with prolonged postinfectious cough like *Mycoplasma*, respiratory viruses (influenza, respiratory syncytial virus, parainfluenza).

- *Mechanism:* Hypothesized heightened cough reflex sensitivity, postnasal drip, and/or transient vocal cord dysfunction (VCD) following URTI.
- Asthma exacerbation and eosinophilic bronchitis are important differential diagnoses to consider as well.
- *Management:* Improves with time; there is variable success with various symptom relief measures (e.g. first-generation antihistamines, inhaled steroids, nasal ipratropium, but need to caution patient of side effects).
  - First-generation antihistamines may be acting through multiple mechanisms: (a) Sedation, (b) Anticholinergic drying effects, and (c) Agonizing cough inhibition regions of the CNS (9).

- **Upper airway cough syndrome (UACS) (5, 8–11)**
  - Previously known as postnasal drip syndrome.
  - UACS is a broad term used to describe a syndrome that overlaps with postinfectious cough, but the top three causes are (1) sinusitis, (2) perennial non-allergic rhinitis, and (3) allergic rhinitis (10).
    - Less common causes include postinfectious rhinitis, vasomotor rhinitis, drug-induced rhinitis/rhinitis medicamentosa, and environmental irritant rhinitis.
    - Ask if there is regular use of over-the-counter nasal decongestants.
    - See Chapters 1 and 2 for details on rhinitis and rhinosinusitis.
    - Cough is now emphasized as a common symptom in allergic

rhinitis and non-allergic rhinitis in the 2020 Rhinitis Practice Parameter Update (11).

- *Mechanisms:* Not fully elucidated yet
  - Variable extrathoracic airway obstruction from the larynx in response to nasal inflammation/postnasal drip (increasing support)
  - Irritation of upper airway structures and **direct** stimulation of cough receptors
  - Irritation of upper airway structures and **indirect** stimulation from postnasal drip (regarded as less important mechanism currently)
- *Investigations:* Allergy testing has great utility here in identifying aeroallergen triggers that may be driving rhinosinusitis.
- *Management:* Initial trial of therapy depends on suspected underlying disorder; refer to Chapters 1 and 2 for full details.
  - *Spotlight on azelastine:* This intranasal antihistamine has demonstrated TRVP1 desensitization, which is one of the sensory cough receptors (12).

- **Eosinophilic bronchitis (5, 8)**
  - Can occur as part of asthma or without asthma
  - *Investigations (difficult to perform in routine settings):* Induced sputum with cell count analysis (only available in specialized centers), bronchoalveolar lavage with cell count analysis, or by finding an elevated fractional exhaled nitric oxide in a breath test (FeNO) (a useful non-invasive rule-in test)
  - *Management:* Medium/high-dose inhaled corticosteroid therapy (budesonide 800 mcg/day, ciclesonide 800 mcg/day, fluticasone propionate 1000 mcg/day, fluticasone furoate 200 mcg/day, mometasone 800 mcg/day), which often completely resolves the cough (10)

- *Obstructive sleep apnea (OSA)* (5)
  - *Presentation:* Classically, cough is not usually perceived to be associated with OSA; however, the prevalence of OSA in patients with chronic cough is between 33% and 68% (13).
    - Cough can be the sole presenting symptom.
    - Nocturnal cough is an important unique feature if their presentation is uncommon in a general chronic cough population.
    - Excessive daytime sleepiness is not a consistent finding in cough-OSA.
  - *Investigations:* Polysomnography.
  - *Mechanism:* Not known, but speculated to involve cough reflex hypersensitivity, laryngopharyngeal reflux, or airway inflammation.
  - *Management:* Nasal continuous positive airway pressure can significantly improve chronic cough; after 1 month, 66%–93% of patients had improvement in cough (14).
- *Asthma (or cough-variant asthma):* See full chapter on asthma (Chapter 5)
  - Usually start to respond to inhaled corticosteroid treatment by 1–3 weeks with total cessation of cough by 6–8 weeks (10).
- *GERD:* Complex relationship with chronic cough (2, 5, 8)
  - *Possible mechanisms*
    - Activation of lower esophageal sensory nerves in the distal esophagus by gastric acid.
    - Irritation and inflammation of the larynx from acid or non-acid refluxate can occur as part of proximal GERD.
    - Pulmonary aspiration of gastric contents.
    - Persistent and recurrent coughing leads to increased intraabdominal pressure as well as relaxation of the lower esophageal sphincter, promoting GERD, raising the possibility of a cycle of reflux-cough.
    - Esophageal dysmotility.
    - GERD is already quite prevalent in other conditions associated with chronic cough such as rhinitis, asthma, and OSA.
  - *Investigations:* Commonly empiric treatment of GERD in association with clear history of GERD symptoms confirms diagnosis.
  - *Management:* Proton pump inhibitors (PPIs) used *in isolation* did not improve or eliminate cough in adults with chronic cough based on a systematic review of randomized controlled trials (15).
    - However, PPI studies with concomitant diet modification and weight loss have led to better outcomes.
    - *Lifestyle measures for GERD* (15): Elevate head of bed, avoid supine position after meals, selective elimination of dietary triggers (e.g. spicy foods, caffeinated drinks, carbonated drinks, peppermint, citrus), smoking cessation.
  - If there is partial response to PPIs, one may need high-dose PPI to yield clinical benefit (e.g. pantoprazole 40 mg bid, dexlansoprazole 60 mg daily) (16).
  - Recent recognition that concomitant treatment of laryngeal hypersensitivity may also be necessary when treating cough associated with GERD (17).
  - In addition to adding lifestyle measures and considering laryngeal hypersensitivity-specific treatments, routinely screen for other dyspepsia red flags, especially PPI-refractory GERD, such as weight loss, anemia, overt gastrointestinal bleeding (hematemesis, melena), dysphagia.
  - Often need prolonged treatment with PPI in combination with concurrent treatment of associated conditions like rhinitis to yield clinical benefit.

- *VCD/inducible laryngeal obstruction* **(5, 18, 19)**

  - *Presentation:* Cough (~25%–50%), dysphonia/hoarseness/voice loss, throat tightness, chest tightness, stridor, wheeze.
  - *Triggers:* Respiratory aerosols/irritants (perfumes, smoke, vapors, dust, gas, fumes), voice projection, exercise, and intense emotional stress.
  - *Investigations:* Variable extrathoracic airflow limitation on a flow-volume curve, fiberoptic laryngoscopy, or dynamic 320-slice computed tomographic scan of the larynx.
    - VCD is highly variable in its presentation and *provocation may be required with an inhaled irritant (e.g. perfume) or exercise if normal findings at rest.*
    - A normal endoscopic examination of the vocal cords while the patient is asymptomatic does not rule-out VCD.
  - *Management:* VCD may be responsive to trigger avoidance, optimization concurrent GERD or rhinitis, speech language pathology intervention (phonation exercises), cognitive behavioral therapy, and surgery (in very limited circumstances).

Management: Addressing the Two Components of CHS

1. *Trigger management:* Specific medical therapy as detailed above
   - Avoid the relevant exposures if possible.
   - Optimize underlying conditions that may be contributing to cough – often need to concomitantly treat multiple etiologies (rhinitis, allergies, GERD, asthma) to yield clinical benefit.
2. *Cough/laryngeal hypersensitivity*
   - *Speech therapy:* Effective for chronic cough with laryngeal dysfunction/hypersensitivity (20)

- 2–4 sessions of education, cough suppression techniques, breathing exercises, and counseling
- Reduction in cough frequency, cough severity, cough-related quality of life
- May be combined with neuromodulator

- *Central neuromodulators:* Possibly effective for a *central* component of cough reflex sensitization; however, small trials often relied on subjective quality of life tools as primary outcomes, which are not reliable as these medication have mood-stabilizing properties (4) and anticholinergic side effects (21)
  - Off-label use of amitriptyline, gabapentin, pregabalin, morphine
- *Novel peripheral neuronal treatments:* Avoid CNS sedation and anticholinergic side effects
  - Current clinical trials are underway for many different targets, but only purinergic receptor P2X and ligand-gated ion channel subunit 3 (P2X3) receptor antagonists have reached phase 3 studies, namely gefapixant (not approved yet by Health Canada, only press-release data so far).
  - *P2X3:* ATP-activated ion channels on sensory nerves:
    - Each channel has three subunits – identical P2X3 subunits OR contains a single P2X2 subunit.
    - Press release data reported that adult patients (N=2044) treated with gefapixant 45 mg PO twice daily had a statistically significant 18.45% reduction compared with placebo with respect to 24-hour cough frequency at 12-weeks (COUGH-1 trial) and 14.64% reduction at 24 weeks (COUGH-2 trial). However, 58.0%–68.6% had mild-moderate taste disturbance (22).
    - Taste disturbance is hypothesized to be related to the modest selectivity for P2X3 over P2X2/3 channels; thus, more selective agents for P2X3 may cause less taste disturbance and three other products are under development (4).

REFERENCES

1. McGarvey L et al., J Allergy Clin Immunol Pract. (2019), PMID: 31002958/DOI: 10.1016/j.jaip.2019.04.012.

2. Morice AH et al., Eur Respir J. (2020), PMID: 31515408/DOI: 10.1183/13993003.01136-2019.

3. Song WJ et al., Allergy Asthma Immunol Res. (2017), PMID: 28677352/DOI: 10.4168/aair.2017.9.5.394.

4. Smith JA et al., J Allergy Clin Immunol Pract. (2019), PMID: 31279461/DOI: 10.1016/j.jaip.2019.04.027.

5. Gibson PG, J Allergy Clin Immunol Pract. (2019), PMID: 31279460/DOI: 10.1016/j.jaip.2019.03.050.

6. Gibson PG et al., Med J Aust. (2010), PMID: 20201760/DOI: 10.5694/j.1326-5377.2010.tb03504.x.

7. Joint Task Force on Practice Parameters et al., Ann Allergy Asthma Immunol. (2010), PMID: 20934625/DOI: 10.1016/j.anai.2010.08.002.

8. Chung KF, Mazzone SB. Cough. In: Murray and Nadel's Textbook of Respiratory Medicine E-Book, Sixth Edition. Philadelphia: Elsevier. Available at: https://www-clinicalkey-com.proxy3.library.mcgill.ca/#!/content/book/3-s2.0-B9781455733835000300 (Accessed: Sept 29, 2020).

9. Song WJ et al., Allergy Asthma Immunol Res. (2017), PMID: 28677352/DOI: 10.4168/aair.2017.9.5.394.

10. Madison JM, Irwin RS. Approach to the Patient with Chronic Cough. In: Burks AW, Holgate ST, O'Hehir RE, Bacharier LB, Broide DH, Hershey GK, Peebles Jr RS. Middleton's Allergy: Principles and Practice E-Book, Ninth Edition. Amsterdam: Elsevier. Available at: https://www.clinicalkey.com/dura/browse/bookChapter/3-s2.0-C20161002419 (Accessed: Oct 15, 2020).

11. Dykewicz MS et al., J Allergy Clin Immunol. (2020), PMID: 32707227/DOI: 10.1016/j.jaci.2020.07.007.

12. Singh U et al., Am J Rhinol Allergy. (2014), PMID: 24980233/DOI: 10.2500/ajra.2014.28.4059.

13. Chan K et al., Pulm Pharmacol Ther. (2015), PMID: 26068465/DOI: 10.1016/j.pupt.2015.05.008.

14. Sundar KM et al., Cough. (2013), PMID: 23845135/DOI: 10.1186/1745-9974-9-19.

15. Kahrilas PJ et al., Chest. (2016), PMID: 27614002/DOI: 10.1016/j.chest.2016.08.1458.

16. Katz PO et al., Am J Gastroenterol. (2013), PMID: 23419381/DOI: 10.1038/ajg.2012.444.

17. Fass R et al., Neurogastroenterol Motil. (2010), PMID: 19740116/DOI: 10.1111/j.1365-2982.2009.01392.x.

18. Morris MJ et al., Chest. (2010), PMID: 21051397/DOI: 10.1378/chest.09-2944.

19. Halvorsen T et al., Eur Respir J. (2017), PMID: 28889105/DOI: 10.1183/13993003.02221-2016.

20. Vertigan AE et al., J Allergy Clin Immunol Pract. (2019), PMID: 30940533/DOI: 10.1016/j.jaip.2019.03.030.

21. Ryan NM et al., Lancet. (2012), PMID: 22951084/DOI: 10.1016/S0140-6736(12)60776-4.

22. Kenilworth, NJ. Merck's Gefapixant (45 mg Twice Daily) Significantly Decreased Cough Frequency Compared to Placebo at Week 12 and 24 in Patients with Refractory or Unexplained Chronic Cough [Internet]. BUSINESS WIRE. 2020 Sep 08 [Cited Nov 1, 2020]. Available from: https://www.businesswire.com/news/home/20200908005244/en/.

PART ③

CUTANEOUS DISORDERS

7 Atopic Dermatitis (AD)   67
   Fatemah Al-Yaqout, Abeer Feteih, Walaa Almasri, Hoang Pham, and Reza Alizadehfar
8 Contact Dermatitis   75
   Geneviève Bouvette, Walaa Almasri, Hoang Pham, and Abeer Feteih
9 Urticaria   81
   *Abeer Feteih, Farida Almarzooqi, Michael Fein, Geneviève Genest, Hoang Pham, and
   Moshe Ben-Shoshan*
10 Angioedema   91
   *Abeer Feteih, Farida Almarzooqi, Michael Fein, Geneviève Genest, Hoang Pham, and
   Moshe Ben-Shoshan*

7

Atopic Dermatitis (AD)

FATEMAH AL-YAQOUT, ABEER FETEIH, WALAA ALMASRI,
HOANG PHAM, AND REZA ALIZADEHFAR

GENERAL BACKGROUND AND EPIDEMIOLOGY

- Atopic dermatitis (AD) is a common, chronic relapsing inflammatory skin disease (1).
- Can present at any age with adult-onset in ~25% of AD (2, 3).
- Affects 10%–20% of children and 1%–3% of adults (4, 5).
- The atopic march model describes a close relationship among AD, food allergy (FA), asthma, and allergic rhinitis (AR) (6, 7).
- A strong association exists between AD and allergic sensitization (8, 9).
- Uncontrolled AD can be associated with reduced health-related quality of life (QoL) and may lead to missed work/school.

IMMUNOPATHOLOGY AND GENETICS OF AD (6–8, 10, 11)

- Skin barrier defects can be genetic or acquired.
- Filaggrin (*FLG*) protein mutations occur in around 50% of patients (homozygous mutations = more severe AD).
- Studies established that the key drivers in AD are T-helper 2 cells (Th2)-specific cytokines, interleukin (IL)-4, IL-13, and IL-31.
- Clear skin in patients with AD is also evidenced to have higher numbers of immune cells with Th2 signaling and secretion of IL-4 and IL-13.
  - Cytokine profiles may vary from different clinical phenotypes (e.g. Asians with AD may have more upregulation of the Th17 axis compared with European Caucasians) (9)

Clinical Manifestations (1, 2, 7)

- Pruritus is the most common symptom, hence, the common descriptor: "the itch that rashes."
- *Acute AD:* Intensely itchy, papules on an erythematous base with excoriations, vesiculations, serous exudate.
  - *Subacute AD:* Erythematous, excoriated, scaling papules
- *Chronic AD:* Lichenification (thickened skin) and fibrotic papules
  - Acute lesions can be present.
  - Chronic relapsing pattern is common.
- *Typical distribution*
  - *Infants:* Face, scalp, extensor extremities, trunk.
    - AD usually spares the diaper area and groin; thus, diaper dermatitis may occur in the setting of a superimposed candidal infection.
  - *Older Children and adults:* Flexor folds (age >1 year), hands, neck, and feet.
- Personal or family history of atopic conditions (e.g. asthma, AR, AD, FA.)

Diagnosis and Assessment [Adapted from (1, 2, 7, 17, 18, 20, 21)]

- *Clinical diagnosis:* Based on history and physical examination consistent with symptoms and signs of AD (see Clinical Manifestations section above). No single skin finding or lab test that is solely specific for AD.
  - Criteria have been developed to assist with the diagnosis (1, 2, 16).
- Assessment and longitudinal follow-up of severity should use validated tools such as the Eczema Area Severity Index (EASI) (see below) or SCORing Atopic dermatitis (SCORAD) (2, 18–20, 28).
  - Severity is based on percentage of body surface (BS) involvement and impact on QoL.
- Laboratory investigations may reveal elevated IgE and eosinophils (not specific for AD, however).

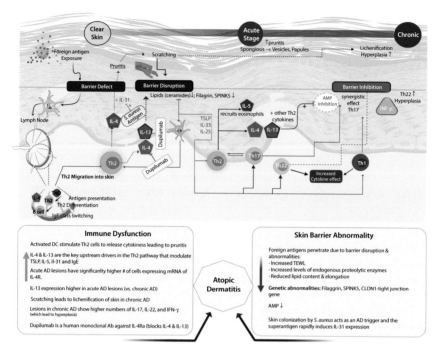

Figure 7.1 Pathophysiology of atopic dermatitis (AD). Pathophysiology of AD is complex and involves skin barrier defects, disruption, and inhibition. Immune mediated inflammation is driven primarily by Th2 cells and associated cytokines IL-4 and IL-13. (*Abbreviations:* AMP: Antimicrobial peptide; APC: Antigen presenting cell; CLDN1: Claudin-1 -tight junction gene; DC: Dendritic cells; IL-4Ra: Interleukin 4 receptor a; IL: Interleukin; IL-4: Interleukin 4; IL-13: Interleukin 13; IgE: Immunoglobulin E; IFN-γ: Interferon gamma; LC: Langerhans cells; SPNK5: Serine Protease Inhibitor; Kazal Type 5Th1: T-Helper 1 cells; Th2: T-Helper 2 cells; TEWL: Transepidermal water loss; TSLP: Thymic stromal lymphopoietin.) (Figure created with BioRender.com.) [Adapted from (8, 10–16).]

Associated Features in Establishing AD Diagnosis (1, 2, 7, 20)

- Intolerance to wool textiles
- Course influenced by emotional stress and environmental changes
- Dennie-Morgan infraorbital folds
- Keratosis pilaris
- Hyperlinear palms
- Ichthyosis

Note: Please refer to the minor criteria of Hanifin and Rajka for comprehensive list of associated features (1–2).

Differential Diagnosis of AD (Select List) (1, 2, 7, 15, 20, 21)

- *Infection:* Scabies, dermatophytosis
- *Malignancy:* Cutaneous T-cell lymphoma
- *Chronic dermatoses:* Seborrheic dermatitis, irritant or allergic contact dermatitis, psoriasis, lichen simplex chronicus

- *Immunodeficiencies:* Netherton syndrome, hyper-IgE syndromes, Wiskott-Aldrich syndrome, severe combined immunodeficiency (e.g. Omenn syndrome)
- *Autoimmune:* Dermatitis herpetiformis, dermatomyositis, prodromal bullous pemphigoid (elderly)
- *Metabolic:* Zinc deficiency, phenylketonuria

Comorbidities (2, 7, 20, 21)

- *Mental health:* Depression, anxiety, sleep disturbance
- *Eczema herpeticum (EH):*
  - More severe AD with likely history of asthma and food allergies
  - Predisposition to cutaneous infections (*Staphylococcus aureus* or *molluscum contagiosum*)
- *Eczema vaccinatum:* Risk of life-threatening complications after smallpox vaccine

- Superimposed dermatophytosis with *Malassezia sympodialis*
- *Bacterial infections:*
  - *S. aureus* skin colonization is higher in AD compared with other skin disorders.
  - *S. aureus* secretes exotoxin superantigens that in moderate to severe AD results in IgE-mediated inflammation.

Management Approach (2, 7, 20, 21)

- A simplified approach is "ABC":
  - **A**voidance of triggers and education on AD diagnosis and management plan
  - **B**arrier repair
  - **C**ontrol of inflammation & infection

- Management utilizes the therapies summarized in Table 7.1 and follows a stepwise approach based on severity of AD (see Figure 7.2).
- In addition patient-individualized management should address pruritus and sleep disruption if they exist (e.g. meditation, sleep hygiene, cognitive behavioral therapy (22).
- The available topical corticosteroid (TCS) potencies are highlighted in Figure 7.3.

Patient Education and Follow-Up [Adapted from (2, 7, 20, 21)]

- Discussions with patients should address AD disease course, management options, and the avoidance of triggering factors.

Table 7.1 Management Options in AD

Treatment	Recommendations and discussion	Reference
Non-Pharmacological		
Emollients	First-line therapy; aids in controlling pruritus	6, 7, 29, 30
	Lipid moisturizers (high in ceramide) may improve skin barrier function	
	Applying emollients immediately before or over TCS may decrease effectiveness	
Avoidance of Triggers and Aeroallergens	Avoid tight clothing and wash clothes before wearing (to remove chemicals, formaldehyde, residual detergent); avoid fabric softeners	19, 9, 27
	Avoidance of common irritants (e.g. acids, bleaches, fragrances and wool, fabric softeners)	
	Exacerbations of AD can occur with exposure to allergens (e.g. house dust mite, animal dander, pollens)	
	Limit use of non-soap or mild soap cleansers	
Limited Food Allergy Testing	Only if consistent with clinical history or if <5 years with refractory moderate-severe AD and history of food reactions	19, 22, 30
	4–6-week dietary elimination of suspected food allergen before formal allergy testing	
	If testing planned, consider testing to milk, egg, peanut, wheat, soy, fish which account for 90% of exacerbating food allergens	
Wet-Wrap Dressings	Aid in epidermal barrier recovery and penetration of TCS (they also act as a barrier to itching)	6, 9
	For refractory disease in addition to TCS; overuse can lead to chilling, maceration, secondary infections, and rarely adrenal suppression	
Patch Testing	Consider testing in presentations suspicious for ACD	23
Pharmacological		
Dilute Bleach Baths	5–15 minutes, 2x/week in recurrent skin infections; for maintenance therapy, not for acute flares (0.005% sodium hypochlorite 1 teaspoon per gallon of water)	9, 19

(Continued)

Table 7.1 Management Options in AD *(Continued)*

Treatment	Recommendations and discussion	Reference
Vitamin D	May help if levels are low	19
Phototherapy	For recalcitrant AD or after failure of first line treatment along with topical agents (narrow-band UVB preferred)	26
Tar Products	Tar shampoos useful in scalp involvement. Do not use on acute inflamed skin due to SE of skin irritation	6
Antihistamines	Can be used for sedative effects — not proven to reduce pruritus in AD (topical formulas can lead to sensitization through the skin)	19, 23
Managing Pruritus	Cyclosporine and Dupilumab effective Opioid receptor antagonists (naltrexone 50–100 mg/day) effective but SE of nausea and dizziness	21, 28
TCS	First-line when non-pharmacological approachs fail Applied on affected areas only For maintenance therapy in recurrent moderate-severe AD: • Continue low potency TCS 2x/week to previously involved areas that are clear	9, 27, 35
Topical PDE4 Inhibitors	For mild-moderate AD (e.g. Crisaborole BID)	6, 24, 35
Topical Calcineurin Inhibitors	Second line if no improvement with TCS and in patients who cannot tolerate TCS For mild-moderate AD especially on face and interiginous areas (e.g. Tacrolimus ointment 0.03% BID)	2, 6, 36
Systemic CS	Indicated for acute severe exacerbations and as bridge to other systemic treatments Caution with use as short courses can lead to atopic flares after discontinuation (taper before discontinuation)	23, 24
Antimicrobials		
a. Systemic Antibiotics	Short course of systemic antibiotics if evidence of *S. aureus*. If suspecting MRSA, culture and start antibiotic therapy (e.g. clindamycin, doxycycline, TMP/SMX)	6, 19, 26
b. Systemic Antivirals	Systemic antivirals for eczema herpiticum	
c. Systemic Antifungal	Consider fungal infection with *Malassezia* spp. in head and neck AD refractory to treatment	
Systemic Immunomodulation	For severe AD refractory to topical treatment and phototherapy E.g. cyclosporine, azathioprine, methotrexate, MMF, IFNγ	9, 24
Allergen Immunotherapy (AIT)	May be effective in patients with AD and aeroallergen sensitivity	37, 38
Biologics		
a. Omalizumab	Mast cell and basophil activation blocker (anti-IgE therapy) Literature documented benefit and resolution in severe AD (small RCTs and case reports)	9, 38, 40, 42
b. Dupilumab	Monoclonal Ab against IL-4Rα (blocks IL-4 and IL-13) FDA approved for moderate-severe AD (age >6 years) not well controlled with topical therapy Efficacy demonstrated in RCTs with a safe administrative profile	
c. Nemolizumab	Monoclonal antibody against IL-31α Potential benefit for refractory AD with ongoing studies	

Note: Table created with BioRender.com.
Adapted from (2, 7, 20–25).

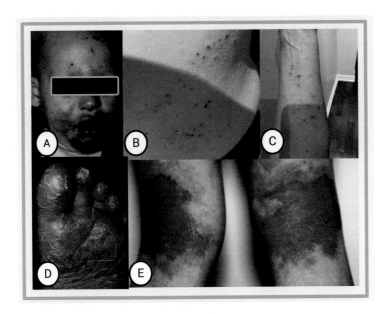

Figure 7.2 (A) Acute facial eczema in an infant with complete sparing of nasal skin known as the "headlight sign," considered pathognomonic for AD; (B and C) New diagnosis of AD in a 52-year-old female showing the flank (B) hyperkaratosis pilaris and (C) forearm shows presence of erythematous plaques. Lack of licheniflcation indicates acute AD rather than chronic AD; (D) Juvenile Plantar (Plantar AD/Winter AD); note absence of interdigital-space involvement; frequently incorrectly treated as "athlete's foot."; (E) acute/subacute AD in popliteal fossa of a young child, note erythematous, eroded and excoriated plaques. [Images courtesy of Dr. Denis Sasseville for images (A), (D), (E). Images courtesy of Dr. Fatemah Al-Yaquout for image (B) and (C).] (Figure created with BioRender.com.)

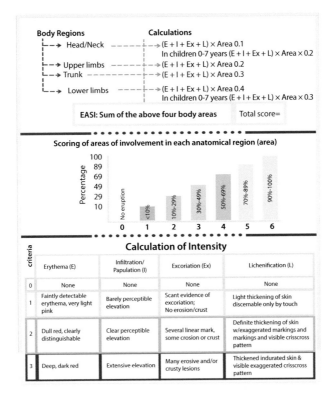

Figure 7.3 Eczema Area Severity Index. (Figure created with BioRender.com.) [Adapted from (18).]

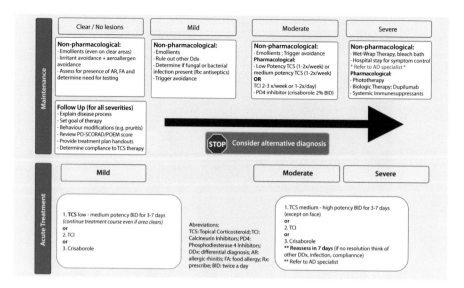

Figure 7.4 Algorithm for managing AD. (Figure created with BioRender.com.) [Adapted from (2, 7, 20–21).]

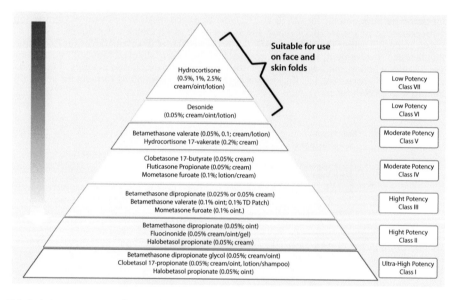

Figure 7.5 Relative potencies of topical corticosteroids (TCS). TCS are mainstays of treatment in AD. Lowest effective dose should be used. Acute treatment for 3–7 days with maintenance therapy if needed applied 2 days/week to recurrent areas of affected skin. (Figure created with BioRender.com.) [Adapted from (20, 26, 27).]

- Tools to assess the impact of AD on self-reported QoL should be utilized on follow-up (e.g. Patient-Oriented Eczema Measure [POEM] or Patient-Oriented SCORAD [PO-SCORAD]) (2, 18–20).
- Degree of pruritus and sleep quality are important follow-up questions.
- Providing written treatment plans and recommended care products (e.g. skin-care products) may improve compliance.

ABBREVIATIONS

>	More than
&	And
+	Positive
%	Percent
IL	Interleukin
Ab	Antibody

AD	Atopic dermatitis
Admin	Administration
AKC	Atopic keratoconjunctivitis
AR	Allergic rhinitis
Assoc.	Associated
B/L	Bilateral
BID	Twice daily
CBT	Cognitive behavior therapy
CS	Corticosteroids
d	Days
DDx	Differential diagnosis
e.g.	Example
EASI	Eczema Area & Severity Index
FA	Food allergy
FH	Family history
FLG	Filaggrin epidermal barrier protein
IFN-γ	Interferon gamma
IgE	Immunoglobulin E
IL-4Rα	Interleukin 4 receptor α
Max	Maximum
MC	*Molluscum contagiosum*
MMF	Mycophenolate mofetil
Mo.	Month
Mod.	Moderate
OD	Once daily
Oint	Ointment
PO-SCORAD	Patient-oriented SCORAD
POEM	Patient-oriented eczema measure
QoL	Quality of life
RCT	Randomized control trial
Rx	Prescription
S. aureus	*Staphylococcus aureus*
SCIT	Subcutaneous immunotherapy
SCORAD	SCORing atopic dermatitis
SE	Side effect
SLIT	Sublingual immunotherapy
Sp	Species
TCS	Topical corticosteroid
TD	Transdermal patch
Temp.	Temperature
Th1	T-helper 1 cells
Th2	T-helper 2 cells
TID	Three times a day
Top	Topical
Txm	Treatment

REFERENCES

1. Hanifin JM, Rajka G. Acta Derm Venereol. 1980, DOI:10.2340/0001555592447.
2. Fishbein AB et al., J Allergy Clin Immunol Pract. 2020, PMID: 31474543/DOI:10.1016/j.jaip.2019.06.044.
3. Lee HH, et al., J Am Acad Dermatol. 2019, PMID: 29864464/DOI: 10.1016/j.jaad.2018.05.1241.
4. Larsen FS, et al., Immunol Allergy Clin North Am. 2002, DOI: https://doi.org/10.1016/S0889-8561(03)00066-3.
5. Davidson WF, et al., J Allergy Clin Immunol. 2019, PMID: 30639346/DOI:10.1016/j.jaci.2019.01.003.
6. Czarnowicki T, et al., J Allergy Clin Immunol. 2017, PMID: 28583445/DOI:10.1016/j.jaci.2017.04.004.
7. Boguniewicz M, Leung DYM. Atopic Dermatitis. In: Burks AW, Holgate ST, O'Hehir RE, Bacharier LB, Broide DH, Hershey GK, Peebles Jr RS. Middleton's Allergy: Principles and Practice E-Book, Ninth Edition. Amsterdam: Elsevier. Available at: https://www.clinicalkey.com/dura/browse/bookChapter/3-s2.0-C20161002419 (Accessed: August 20, 2020).
8. Boguniewicz M, et al., J Allergy Clin Immunol. 2015, PMID: 25662304/DOI:10.1016/j.jaci.2014.12.1907.
9. Kim J, et al., Allergy Asthma Proc. 2019, PMID: 30819278/DOI:10.2500/aap.2019.40.4202.
10. de la O-Escamilla NO, et al., Pediatr Ann. 2020, PMID: 32155280/DOI:10.3928/19382359-20200217-01.
11. Czarnowicki T, et al., J Allergy Clin Immunol. 2015, PMID: 25936564/DOI:10.1016/j.jaci.2015.03.032.
12. Lee CH, et al., Br J Dermatol. 2006, PMID: 16704640/DOI: 10.1111/j.1365-2133.2006.07191.x.
13. Bowdish DM, et al., Curr Top Microbiol Immunol. 2006, PMID: 16909917/DOI: 10.1007/3-540-29916-5_2.
14. Agrawal R, et al., Curr Allergy Asthma Rep. 2014, PMID: 24633617. DOI: 10.1007/s11882-014-0433-9.
15. Schmidt E, et al., Immunol Allergy Clin North Am. 2012, PMID: 22560135/DOI: 10.1016/j.iac.2012.04.002.
16. Williams HC, et al., Br J Dermatol. 1994, PMID: 7918015. DOI: 10.1111/j.1365-2133.1994.tb08530.x.
17. Yang G, et al., Int J Mol Sci. 2020, PMID: 32326002/DOI: 10.3390/ijms21082867.
18. Hanifin JM, et al., Exp Dermatol. 2001, PMID: 11168575/DOI: 10.1034/j.1600-0625.2001.100102.x.
19. Chopra R et al., Br J Dermatol. 2017, PMID: 28485036/DOI: 10.1111/bjd.15641.
20. Schneider L et al., J Allergy Clin Immunol. 2013, PMID: 23374261/DOI: 10.1016/j.jaci.2012.12.672.
21. Langan SM et al. Lancet. 2020, PMID: 32738956/doi: 10.1016/S0140-6736(20)31286-1.

22. Eichenfield LF et al., J Allergy Clin Immunol. 2017, PMID: 28390477/DOI: 10.1016/j.jaci.2017.01.009.

23. Sidbury R et al., J Am Acad Dermatol. 2014, PMID: 24813298/DOI: 10.1016/j.jaad.2014.03.030.

24. Sidbury R et al., J Am Acad Dermatol. 2014, PMID: 25264237/DOI: 10.1016/j.jaad.2014.08.038.

25. Weisshaar E et al., Acta Derm Venereol. 2019, PMID: 30931482/DOI: 10.2340/00015555-3164.

26. Cornell RC et al., Br J Dermatol. 1981, PMID: 7259982/DOI: 10.1111/j.1365-2133.1981.tb00888.x.

27. Noda S et al., J Allergy Clin Immunol. 2015, PMID: 25541257/DOI: 10.1016/j.jaci.2014.11.015.

28. Honari G. (2017) Clinical Scoring of Atopic Dermatitis. In: Humbert P, Fanian F, Maibach H, Agache P. Agache's Measuring the Skin. Springer, Cham. https://doi.org/10.1007/978-3-319-32383-1_94.

8

Contact Dermatitis

GENEVIÈVE BOUVETTE, WALAA ALMASRI, HOANG PHAM, AND ABEER FETEIH

GENERAL BACKGROUND

- Contact dermatitis (CD): Eczematous skin disorder caused by contact with an exogenous substance that elicits an allergic and/or irritant response (1)
  - Subtypes of CD: Allergic contact dermatitis (ACD) and irritant contact dermatitis (ICD) (1)

Epidemiology

- Point prevalence: ~4.17% in the United States (2)

Pathogenesis

- ACD: A two-step process of type IV delayed hypersensitivity

1. Sensitization phase: Dermal dendritic cells present a low molecular weight allergen/hapten as an antigen to T cells, which drain to a regional lymph node.
2. Elicitation phase: Upon re-exposure, after ~72 hours, effector T cells, classically attributed to CD4+ T-helper type 1 cells (Th1), generate inflammatory mediators; interleukin (IL)-1α, IL-1β, IL-6, IL-8, and IL-13; tumor necrosis factor (TNF)-α; and granulocyte colony-stimulating factor (G-CSF), which activate mast cells and macrophages leading to dermatitis through inflammation, cell destruction, and repair (3–5).
   - More recent studies suggest that mixed Th1/Th2, Th2, Th17, Th22, and innate immune cells may play a role as immune signaling may be antigen dependent (3, 4).
- ICD: Localized, non-allergic, inflammatory response from direct cell damage to the epidermal barrier, resulting in keratinocyte cell death, releasing similar pro-inflammatory cytokines, without prior sensitization required (3, 6, 7).

Anatomic Distribution and Commonly Associated Contact Allergens (1, 4)

- Top three most common sites: Generalized, hand, and face (1)
- *Generalized:* Formaldehyde, textile dyes
  - *Generalized and intertriginous/flexural distribution:* Systemic CD after systemic exposure (e.g. ingestion, intravenous, transcutaneous)
- *Hand:* Quaternium-15, formaldehyde, Balsam of Peru (BOP), fragrance mix (FM), nickel, topical antibiotics, rubber chemicals, paraphenylenediamine (PPD)
- *Face including eyelids:* Tosylamide and/or formaldehyde resin (ectopic transfer), acrylates (ectopic transfer), botanicals, FM, BOP, nickel, preservatives, excipients
- *Neck and scalp:* Nickel, quaternium-15, FM, BOP, PPD, glyceryl thioglycolate, tosylamide and/or formaldehyde resin, acrylates, cocamidopropyl betaine (CAPB), botanicals
- *Feet:* Rubber chemicals, adhesives, leather components

High-Risk Occupations/Industries for Developing Occupational Contact Dermatitis (OCD) (1, 4, 8)

- Painting
- Cosmetic industry (e.g. hairdressers, estheticians)
- Food facility (e.g. caterers, chefs)
- Health care professionals
- Agriculture, forestry, and fishing
- Cleaning
- Construction
- Mechanics, metal working
- Electronics

Note: Routinely explore occupational history, especially if there is wet work, temperature extremes, and repeated exposures.

DOI: 10.1201/9781003174202-11

Clinical Manifestations

[Adapted from the American Academy of Allergy, Asthma & Immunology (AAAAI); the American College of Allergy, Asthma & Immunology (ACAAI); and the Joint Council of Allergy, Asthma & Immunology "Contact Dermatitis: A Practice Parameter Update 2015" (1)]

Allergens Associated with ACD (Select List) (1, 3, 4)

- Metals: Nickel, cobalt, gold, chromium
- Preservatives: Formaldehyde and formaldehyde releasers (e.g. quaternium-15), isothiazolinones (methylchloroisothiazolinone [MCI], methylisothiazolinone [MI])
- Fragrances: BOP, FM 1 and 2
- PPD in permanent hair dyes, such as in black dye and black rubber
  - Reactions to PPD: can be very severe (1)
- Topical medications:
  - Anesthetics: Benzocaine, lidocaine
  - Antibiotics: Neomycin, bacitracin
  - Corticosteroids (CS)
- Excipients: Propylene glycol
- Rubber accelerators: Thiuram, carbamates, mercaptobenzothiazole
- Adhesives: Epoxy glue, acrylates
- Botanicals: Propolis (beeswax), essential oils, tea tree oil,
  - urushiol (e.g. can be responsible for ACD to poison ivy, cashew nutshells, mango skin)

History [Adapted from (1, 3, 4)]

- Personal or family history of atopic disease (asthma, eczema, allergic rhinitis)
- Symptoms onset and duration.
- Skin disease distribution (e.g. eyelids, hands, feet, axilla).
- Response to treatments, especially topical treatments.

- Detailed history of work/occupation and environmental exposures, including:
  - Nature of the occupation
  - Duration of each activity
  - Occurrence of similar skin effects in coworkers that may aid in identifying potential causes of work-related ICD or ACD (8–10)
- Pertinent changes in work environments that result in new direct chemical exposures to the skin, including vapors and fumes.
- History of frequent handwashing and the use of cleansing agents may compromise the skin barrier and cause irritant hand dermatitis (e.g. in hospital workers) (11).
- **Material Safety Data Sheets (MSDS)** obtained from the manufacturer can be helpful because the worker may be unaware of specific chemicals to which they are exposed.
- Hobbies and non-work activities such as gardening, painting, ceramic work, and carpentry.
- History of animal/animal product exposure.
- Personal products used by the patient.
- Cosmetics and personal hygiene products that are directly applied to involved skin or ectopically transferred to uninvolved skin as potential sources of allergens, called "**ectopic ACD.**" Typical causes of ectopic ACD:
  - Nickel transferred to the eyelid by fingers.
  - Toluenesulfonamide/formaldehyde resin (TSFR) in nail polish (may cause eyelid dermatitis with sparing of the periungual skin and distal fingers).
    - Acrylate transfer from artificial nails.
  - Patients with allergy to hair products that contain CAPB, a surfactant in shampoo, can present with eyelid dermatitis without concurrent dermatitis on the scalp, neck, or ears.

Table 8.1 Clinical Manifestations of Contact Dermatitis

Clinical manifestations	Acute CD	Recurrent or persistent episodes of CD
Pruritus	✓	✓
Erythematous Papules	✓	
Vesicles	✓	
Crusted Lesions	✓	
Skin thickening/hardening/ lichenification		✓
Scaling		✓
Fissuring		✓

Adapted from (1).

Physical Examination (1)

- Total body skin exam with particular attention to specific commonly affected sites:
  - Face, eyelids, lips, oral mucosa, neck and scalp, hand, axillae, anogenital area, feet

Note: Although history and physical exam can strongly suggest a cause of ACD, self-reported nickel allergy only has a positive predictive value of 60% when verified with confirmatory patch testing. Even experienced clinicians are only able to correctly predict the sensitizer in 10%–20% (4, 12, 13).

Major Differential Diagnoses of ACD (1)

- ICD
- AD
- Seborrheic dermatitis
- Dyshidrotic eczema
- Psoriasis
- Dermatitis herpetiformis
- Mycosis fungoides and cutaneous T-cell lymphoma

Note: Each specific anatomical region has its own differential diagnosis, such as perioral dermatitis in lip dermatitis and lichen planus for oral mucosa.

Diagnosis and Investigations

- **Patch testing (PT) (1, 4, 14)**
  - Gold standard test for the diagnosis of ACD.
  - Allergens are applied to the skin (typically the back) on patches in a vehicle of either petroleum or water and left in place for 48-hours. Several standard series of allergens are available including the North American Contact Dermatitis Group (NACDG Research Group)

series (65 allergens) and the Thin-layer Rapid Use Epicutaneous Patch Test (T.R.U.E.) series (35 allergens).
  - T.R.U.E. is standardized across lot numbers and is highly reproducible; however, it is not easily modifiable or individualized. Use in isolation may be a limiting factor in identifying culprit allergen.
  - Selection of allergens for PT is more accurate when it is based on the clinical history.
  - Indications for pre-operative PT in patients with a history of metal allergy are still being developed and are currently controversial, but testing can aid in choosing which implant to use in patients with a high suspicion of metal allergy as they show improved outcomes (4, 15–18).
    - This testing is not recommended for patients without a history of metal sensitivity.
    - Post-operatively PT may be used if there is implant failure to determine whether there is any contact sensitivity after other more common causes have been evaluated (infection, mechanical failure) or if there is a new-onset eczematous or vesicular skin eruption near site of metal implantation (4).
- **PT Reading (1, 4)**
  - First reading at 48 hours: PT panels need to be removed and markings may need to be redone if faded.
  - Second reading between 3 and 7 days: this flexibility enables PT clinics to vary schedules; for example, some centers select to do

Table 8.2 Patch Test Scoring System by the International Contact Dermatitis Research Group

Reaction	Skin findings	Interpretation
No Reaction	∅	(−)
Doubtful Reaction	Faint or non-homogenous erythema only	(+/−)
Weak Positive Reaction	Non-vesicular erythema, infiltration, discrete papules	(1+)
Strong Positive Reaction	Erythema with infiltration, papules and discrete vesicles	(2+)
Extreme Positive Reaction	Intense erythema and infiltration, coalescing vesicles, bulla	(3+)
Irritant Reaction	Discrete homogenous or patchy erythema without infiltration. Rash generally appears early and tends to improve over the 96 hours (often resolved by second reading)	(IR)
Not Tested	∅	(NT)

Adapted from (21).

a reading at day 5 when the yield of positive reactions is the highest for most allergens (1, 19, 20).

- A scoring system developed by the International Contact Dermatitis Research Group is used for reading patch test reactions (see Table 8.2) (21, 32)

Factors to Consider When Performing PT

- **Do not offer PT** to patients who have an active dermatitis especially in the region of the PT.
  - Reschedule when underlying dermatitis is controlled.
- **Elements that could attenuate PT results (4):**
  - Oral CS (>20 mg/day of prednisone equivalents): wean to lowest effective dose, if possible.
  - Cyclosporine (>2–3 mg/kg/day): wean to lowest effective dose, if possible.
  - Medium-to-high potency topical CS (e.g. betamethasone dipropionate 0.05%): do not apply to PT site for 5–7 days prior.
  - Topical calcineurin inhibitors: do not apply to PT site for 5–7 days prior.
  - Excessive sun exposure and sunbed: avoid for 2–4 weeks before PT.
  - Dupilumab: mixed reports; repeat PT if ACD highly suspected if dupilumab stopped (4).
- **Antihistamines** *do not* have to be stopped before PT.
- **"Excited skin syndrome"** ("angry back syndrome"): occurs when there is a strong positive regional reaction induced by a particular tested allergen, resulting in additional positive reactions to other allergens, which are negative on subsequent testing. Excited skin syndrome occurs most frequently when testing with marginal irritants in the setting of atopic dermatitis or stasis dermatitis.

- **Recall dermatitis:** A rare phenomenon in which re-exposure to culprit sensitizer can reproduce an ectopic flare-up reaction at existing or previous sites; rare reports have described PT exposure as a trigger for these recall reactions (22).
- **Repeat open application test (ROAT):** A technique used to test products that may be irritating to the skin where the suspected sensitizer is applied twice a day for 7–14 days to an innocuous area, such as two fingerbreadths away from the antecubital fossa; may be appropriate for testing of cosmetics and personal care products (4).

Management
Non-Pharmacologic

- Patient counseling on avoidance of contact with the offending agent(s) is essential for an effective treatment of ICD and ACD.
- Substitution of a potential allergen with a different product in the workplace that is less allergenic may be effective (23).
- Rotation of job tasks could decrease irritant exposure but may not eliminate the risk of sensitization.
- Use of personal protective equipment (e.g. gloves, goggles, face shields, uniforms, and equipment to protect the skin) can help in forming a barrier against certain allergens and irritants.
- Use of cotton liners under gloves can be useful (23).
- Use of moisturizers, particularly lipid-rich moisturizers (23, 24).

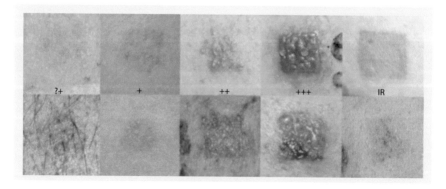

Figure 8.1 Scoring system for patch test readings. Patch test results according to the International Contact Dermatitis Research Group. (*Abbreviations:* ? /–: Doubtful; +: Weak positive, ++: Strong positive, +++: Extreme strong positive; IR: Irritant reaction; see Table 8.1 above.) [Reprinted with permission from Goyal P et al. (32).]

Pharmacologic

- **Topical CS**: Their use over prolonged periods of time should be avoided and should not be a substitute for defining the etiology of the dermatitis.

  *If symptoms worsen, the possibility of **contact sensitization to the CS itself, the vehicle, or other ingredients** in the topical CS should be considered (25–27).*

- **Topical calcineurin inhibitors:** Topical tacrolimus and pimecrolimus have been used for treating AD successfully; however, their efficacy has not been established in ACD or ICD (1).

- **Other treatments:** Cyclosporine, azathioprine, and psoralen plus ultraviolet A (UVA) have been used in steroid-resistant ACD such as chronic hand dermatitis (28–31).

REFERENCES

1. Fonacier L et al., J Allergy Clin Immunol Pract. (2015), PMID: 25965350/DOI:10.1016/j.jaip.2015.02.009.

2. Lim HW et al., J Am Acad Dermatol. (2017), PMID: 28259441/DOI: 10.1016/j.jaad.2016.12.043.

3. Brar KK, Ann Allergy Asthma Immunol. (2021), PMID: 33091591/DOI:10.1016/j.anai.2020.10.003.

4. Schmidlin K et al., J Allergy Clin Immunol Pract. (2020), PMID: 32112924/DOI:10.1016/j.jaip.2020.02.009.

5. Kalish RS, Arch Dermatol. (1991), PMID: 1929465/DOI:10.1001/archderm.1991.01680090122016.

6. Bains SN et al., Clin Rev Allergy Immunol. (2019), PMID: 30293200/DOI:10.1007/s12016-018-8713-0.

7. Smith HR et al., Clin Exp Dermatol. (2002), PMID: 11952708/DOI:10.1046/j.1365-2230.2002.00997.x.

8. Milam EC et al., J Allergy Clin Immunol Pract. (2020), PMID: 33161959/DOI:10.1016/j.jaip.2020.08.004.

9. Mirabelli MC et al., Contact Dermatitis. (2012), PMID: 22268785/DOI: 10.1111/j.1600-0536.2011.02023.x.

10. Lazzarini R et al., An Bras Dermatol. (2012), PMID: 22892770/DOI: 10.1590/s0365-05962012000400008.

11. Lan CC et al., Contact Dermatitis. (2011), PMID: 21138443/DOI:10.1111/j.1600-0536.2010.01813.x.

12. Josefson A et al., Contact Dermatitis. (2010), PMID: 20536476/DOI: 10.1111/j.1600-0536.2010.01702.x.

13. Wilkinson J, Shaw S. (1998) Contact Dermatitis. Textbook of dermatology, Sixth Edition. Oxford, UK: Blackwell Science Ltd.

14. Lachapelle JM, Maibach HI. (2012) Patch Testing and Prick Testing: A Practical Guide Official Publication of the ICDRG. Berlin, Heidelberg: Springer.

15. Atanaskova Mesinkovska N et al., Arch Dermatol. (2012), PMID: 22351785/DOI:10.1001/archdermatol.2011.2561.

16. Krecisz B et al., Int J Occup Med Environ Health. (2012), PMID: 23212287/DOI:10.2478/S13382-012-0029-3.

17. Reed KB et al., Arch Dermatol. (2008), PMID: 18711071/DOI: 10.1001/archderm.144.8.999.

18. Schalock PC et al., Contact Dermatitis. (2012), PMID: 21957996/DOI:10.1111/j.1600-0536.2011.01971.x.

19. Jonker MJ et al., Contact Dermatitis. (2000), PMID: 10871096/DOI:10.1034/j.1600-0536.2000.042006330.x.

20. Geier J et al., Contact Dermatitis. (1999), PMID: 10073438/DOI: 10.1111/j.1600-0536.1999.tb06008.x.

21. Wilkinson DS et al., Acta Derm Venereol. (1970), PMID: 4195865/DOI:102340/0001555550287292.

22. Jacob SE et al., Dermatitis. (2008), PMID: 19134429.

23. Nicholson PJ et al., Contact Dermatitis. (2010), PMID: 20831687/DOI:10.1111/j.1600-0536.2010.01763.x.

24. Saary J et al., J Am Acad Dermatol. (2005), PMID: 16243136/DOI:10.1016/j.jaad.2005.04.075.

25. Davis MD et al., J Am Acad Dermatol. (2007), PMID: 17239989/DOI: 10.1016/j.jaad.2006.11.012.

26. Dooms-Goossens A et al., Contact Dermatitis. (1992), PMID: 1505184/DOI:10.1111/j.1600-0536.1992.tb00290.x.

27. Dooms-Goossens A et al., Contact Dermatitis. (1992), PMID: 1505190/DOI:10.1111/j.1600-0536.1992.tb00304.x.

28. Bourke J et al., Br J Dermatol. (2009), PMID: 19302065/DOI:10.1111/j.1365-2133.2009.09106.x.

29. Granlund H et al., Acta Derm Venereol. (1997), PMID: 9059680/DOI:10.2340/00015555775458.

30. Rosen K et al., Acta Derm Venereol. (1987), PMID: 2436414.

31. Schram ME et al., Arch Dermatol. (2011), PMID: 21482898/DOI: 10.1001/archdermatol.2011.79.

32. Goyal P et al., J Mahatma Gandhi Univ Med Sci Tech. (2016), DOI: 10.5005/jp-journals-10057-0001.

9

Urticaria

ABEER FETEIH, FARIDA ALMARZOOQI, MICHAEL FEIN, GENEVIÈVE GENEST, HOANG PHAM, AND MOSHE BEN-SHOSHAN

GENERAL BACKGROUND AND EPIDEMIOLOGY

- Cumulative lifetime prevalence of urticaria (*all types*): ~8%–22% with a point prevalence of ~0.1% (1, 2).
- Cumulative lifetime prevalence of *acute* urticaria: 12%–24% with a point prevalence of 0.1%–0.6% (1).
  - Chronic urticaria (CU) develops in 20%–45% of individuals presenting with acute urticaria (1).
- Cumulative lifetime prevalence of *chronic* urticaria: ~1.4% with a point prevalence of ~0.7% (3).
  - Women have a slightly higher point prevalence than men (1.3% vs. 0.8%).
- Quality of life is significantly affected by uncontrolled CU, leading to interrupted sleep, lack of concentration, and missed work or school.
  - This negative impact is greater than that of most other skin conditions and similar to that of severe coronary artery disease (2).

DEFINITIONS

- **Urticaria (hives)** are transient, pruritic, erythematous papules or plaques (wheals) of variable sizes affecting the epidermal layer of the skin (4).
- **Angioedema** is a sudden onset of non-pitting swelling of the deeper dermal subcutaneous/submucosal tissues, affecting the face, neck, lips, and limbs, and generally lasts up to 72 hours (4).

Classification and Pathophysiology

1. **Acute spontaneous urticaria (ASU)** is the spontaneous occurrence of wheals, angioedema, or both within a period of *less than 6 weeks* (4).

2. **CU** is an intermittent appearance of either spontaneous or induced wheals, angioedema or both *most days of the week for more than 6 weeks* (4).
   a. **Chronic spontaneous urticaria (CSU)**
      - Majority have no specific cause identified.
      - ~50% of cases are associated with autoimmunity/autoallergy:
        - Basophil and mast cell mediator release due to *autoantibodies* (IgE or IgG) directed against:
          - Autoantigen (self-proteins), such as interleukin (IL)-24 (5); (**type 1 autoallergy, IgE-mediated**)
          - High-affinity IgE-receptor (FcεR1) or IgE (constant region); (**type IIb autoimmunity, IgG-mediated**)
   b. **Chronic inducible urticaria (CIndU)**
      - Urticaria provoked by identifiable physical triggers that are reproducible with specific testing (Table 9.1). Patients may simultaneously have several forms of CIndU or CSU and CIndU.

Clinical Manifestations

History

- Characteristics of skin lesions (pruritic, circumscribed, erythematous), duration of individual lesions (<24 hours), presence of hives (<6 weeks vs. >6 weeks), and onset (sudden).
- Review the patient's skin lesion photographs to aid in diagnosis.
- **Urticarial vasculitis features should be ruled out:** Longer lasting hives (>24 hours) and non-blanching, painful lesions, can be accompanied by residual hyperpigmentation/purpura, and associated systemic symptoms (e.g. fever and joint pain).

DOI: 10.1201/9781003174202-12

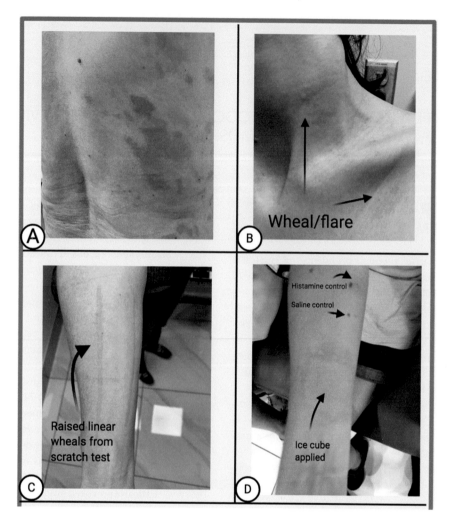

Figure 9.1 Spontaneous and physical urticarias. (A) Chronic spontaneous urticaria; (B) *Aquagenic urticaria* provoked by 35 degree water towel test applied to patient's neck/chest; (C) Dermatographism on volar aspect of forearm; (D) Positive ice cube test with large wheal and flare reaction in a patient with cold urticaria. (Figure created with BioRender.com.) (Images courtesy of Dr. Michael Fein.)

- **Physical triggers:** Exposure to pressure, heat, cold, water, vibration, sweat, and sun exposure (5).
- **Exacerbating factors:** Drugs such as nonsteroidal anti-inflammatory drugs (NSAIDs; e.g. aspirin), angiotensin-converting enzyme (ACE)-inhibitors, and hormones (oral contraceptives), as urticaria may occur with menstrual cycle and result from *autoimmune progesterone dermatitis* (rare) (6).
- **Associated features (with urticaria related to systemic disorders):** Fever, weight loss, and arthralgias.
- **Quality of life:** Interference with work, sleep, hobbies, and social life.

- **Response to treatment:** What treatments have been tried including dose, duration, and side effects (if any).

Physical Examination [Adapted from (6)]

- **Urticarial lesions:** Raised, erythematous plaques that may have a pale center. *Look for ecchymosis/purpura, which may suggest urticarial vasculitis.*
- **Shape:** Round, oval, serpiginous, and numerous lesions, which may become confluent.
- **Size:** Range is between less than 1 cm and several centimeters.

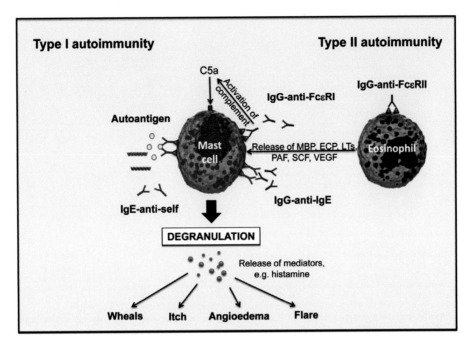

Figure 9.2 Mechanisms of mast cell activation in patients with chronic spontaneous autoimmune urticaria. Type I autoimmunity: Type I autoantigens ("autoallergens") can activate mast cells and basophils by crosslinking IgE-AAbs. Type II autoimmunity: IgG-AAbs can do the same by binding to IgE or to FcεRI, which might involve complement C5a and the CD88/C5aR receptor. IgG-AAbs against the low-affinity IgE receptor (FcεRII) might activate eosinophils and induce subsequent mast cell degranulation. (*Abbreviations:* ECP: Eosinophil cationic protein; LTs: Leukotrienes; MBP: Major basic protein; PAF: Platelet-activating factor; SCF: Stem cell factor; VEGF: Vascular endothelial growth factor.) (Figure created with BioRender.com.) [Reprinted from *J Allergy Clin Immunol*, 139 (58), Kolhkir et al. Autoimmune chronic spontaneous urticaria: What we know and what we do not know, 1772–8, (2017), with permission from Elsevier.]

- **Angioedema:** Of the face, tongue, lips, extremities, or genitals can occur with hives or can occur alone.
  - Angioedema without urticaria should be investigated for other causes of angioedema (e.g. hereditary angioedema; see Chapter 10).
- In cases when the lesion(s) time course recall is a challenge for the patient, skin marking with a pen is useful to document resolution time.

Differential Diagnosis [Adapted from (6)]

- Acute urticaria is a very common manifestation of IgE-mediated allergic disease (foods, aeroallergens, medications, etc.) and a thorough history can usually identify particular triggers.
- Urticaria in different forms is associated with many systemic diseases which should be considered according to the clinical history (Figure 9.3).
- Infections:
  - Bacterial and viral infections often provoke acute urticaria (especially in children).

  - Screening for chronic viral and bacterial infections (e.g. *Helicobacter pylori*) is not indicated in workup of CU unless there is a clinical suspicion.
  - Parasitic infections: Several parasitic infections have been reported in association with CSU.
    - Screening for parasitic infection is only suggested if there are symptoms, travel to endemic areas, and/or peripheral eosinophilia.

Diagnosis and Investigations

1. **Acute urticaria:** Investigations rarely required. Test only for **relevant** allergens on history.
2. **CU:** Investigations not usually required unless an underlying medical condition is suspected. According to the European Academy of Allergology and Clinical Immunology/Global Allergy and Asthma European Network/European Dermatology Forum/World Allergy

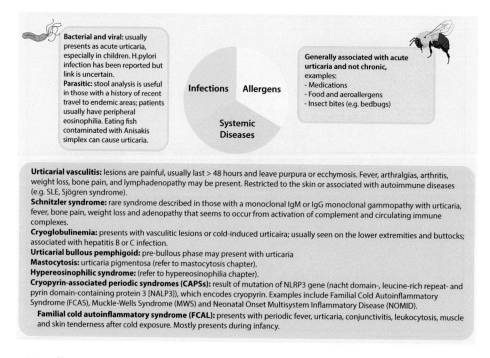

Urticarial vasculitis: lesions are painful, usually last > 48 hours and leave purpura or ecchymosis. Fever, arthralgias, arthritis, weight loss, bone pain, and lymphadenopathy may be present. Restricted to the skin or associated with autoimmune diseases (e.g. SLE, Sjögren syndrome).
Schnitzler syndrome: rare syndrome described in those with a monoclonal IgM or IgG monoclonal gammopathy with urticaria, fever, bone pain, weight loss and adenopathy that seems to occur from activation of complement and circulating immune complexes.
Cryoglobulinemia: presents with vasculitic lesions or cold-induced urticaira; usually seen on the lower extremities and buttocks; associated with hepatitis B or C infection.
Urticarial bullous pemphigoid: pre-bullous phase may present with urticaria
Mastocytosis: urticaria pigmentosa (refer to mastocytosis chapter).
Hypereosinophilic syndrome: (refer to hypereosinophilia chapter).
Cryopyrin-associated periodic syndromes (CAPSs): result of mutation of NLRP3 gene (nacht domain-, leucine-rich repeat- and pyrin domain-containing protein 3 [NALP3]), which encodes cryopyrin. Examples include Familial Cold Autoinflammatory Syndrome (FCAS), Muckle-Wells Syndrome (MWS) and Neonatal Onset Multisystem Inflammatory Disease (NOMID).
   Familial cold autoinflammatory syndrome (FCAL): presents with periodic fever, urticaria, conjunctivitis, leukocytosis, muscle and skin tenderness after cold exposure. Mostly presents during infancy.

Figure 9.3 Differential diagnoses of urticaria. (Figure created with BioRender.com.) [Adapted from (6).]

Organization (EAACI/GA²LEN/EDF/WAO) 2018 adapted from (4), one can do the following:
a. **CSU**
   – Complete blood count (CBC; for eosinophilia)
   – C-reactive protein (CRP) and/or erythrocyte sedimentation rate (ESR; to assess for autoinflammatory conditions)
b. **CIndU** (see table 9.1)
3. **Additional diagnostic tests**: Done based on the patient's history and physical examination and mainly for patients who have *long-standing and/or uncontrolled disease*:
   – Infections: Parasitic workup if eosinophilia and/or history of travel.
   – Functional autoantibodies (e.g., autologous serum skin test or basophil activation test e.g. CD63 levels) typically performed in research settings only.
   – Thyroid autoantibodies and thyroid function test.
   – Allergy (e.g. skin testing): Has little benefit except in rare cases.
      • Although some studies have observed an association between atopic conditions and/or aeroallergen sensitization on skin prick testing in patients

with CSU (7, 8), further mechanistic studies may be needed to elucidate the link.
      • Currently, routine skin prick testing is not a cost-effective diagnostic strategy for screening in CSU patients with normal histories and examinations, even if costs are reduced by identifying a secondary cause (9).
      • Skin testing also presents a practical challenge in CSU due to either dermatographism (causing false positives) or concurrent antihistamine therapy (suppressing skin tests and causing false negatives).
   – Concurrent CIndU: (see Table 9.1 for testing).
   – *Basal serum tryptase level* for systemic symptoms or disease to rule out monoclonal mast cell disease.
   – Consider *skin biopsy* when:
      • Diagnosis is in question and symptoms persist.
      • If the patient fails to respond to usual treatments.
      • If therapies with toxic effects are being considered.

Table 9.1 Diagnostic Testing for Chronic Inducible Urticarias (ClndU)

ClndU types	Definition	Investigations*
Symptomatic Dermographism (urticaria factitia or dermographic urticaria)	Wheal and flare upon firmly stroking the skin	***Provocation test:*** Stroke (moderate) the skin on the volar forearm or upper back with a blunt smooth object (e.g. closed ballpoint pen tip), dermographic tester (36 g/mm^2), or FricTest (longest pin) ***Reading time:*** 10 min after testing ***Positive test:*** Development of a wheal and flare
Cold Urticaria (cold contact urticaria)	Itchy wheals with cold exposure including cold liquids, objects or air; systemic reactions may cause anaphylaxis	***Provocation test:*** Place an ice cube in a thin plastic bag and apply it on the volar forearm for 5 minutes. Remove early if hives develop ***Reading time:*** 10 min post ice-cube removal ***Positive test:*** Development of a wheal and flare response ($)
Heat Urticaria (heat contact urticaria)	Heat-exposed skin provokes hives	***Provocation test:*** Applying a heat source, or using Temp Test (up to 44°C) for 5 min ***Reading time:*** 10 min after testing ***Positive test:*** development of a wheal and flare
Delayed Pressure Urticaria (pressure urticaria)	Hives or angioedema provoked by constant pressure application to the skin (delayed)	***Provocation test:*** Pressure test with suspension of weights on the shoulder (e.g: 7 kg, shoulder strap width 3 cm) for 15 min ***Reading time:*** About 6 hours after testing ***Positive test:*** Development of angioedema and erythema at the site of pressure
Solar Urticaria	Urticaria induced by light exposure (ultraviolet (UV) and/or visible light)	***Provocation test:*** Using ultraviolet (UV) and visible light of different wavelengths. The test is done by exposing the skin (buttock) to UVA 6 J/cm^2, UVB (e.g., Saalmann Multitester SBC LT 400), and visible light (projector) ***Reading time:*** 10 min after the test ***Positive test:*** Development of a wheal and flare (%)
Vibratory Angioedema	Skin swellings immediately after exposure to vibration. Common triggers include mowing the lawn or jackhammer use	***Provocation test:*** Using a vortex vibrator on the volar forearm for 5 min, 1000 rpm ***Reading time:*** 10 min after testing ***Positive test:*** Development of angioedema or wheals
Cholinergic Urticaria	Small hives provoked by change and increase in core body temperature during exercise, with strong emotions, or hot water bath	***Provocation test 1:*** With exercise (e.g. treadmill). Patient exercises for 30 min, with pulse rate rise by 3 beats /min every min. If the exercise test is positive with wheals, a warming test [Test 2] is performed after 24-hours. ***Provocation test 2:*** With bath provocation (warming test) via a wann bath at 42°C and monitoring body temperature rise by ≥ 1°C above baseline ***Reading time:*** Done throughout the test and up to 10 min after the end of the test ***Positive test:*** Described as having urticarial lesions in both test 1 and test 2 provocations

(Continued)

Table 9.1 Diagnostic Testing for Chronic Inducible Urticarias (ClndU) (Continued)

ClndU types	Definition	Investigations*
Aquagenic Urticaria	Itchy wheals or angioedema after skin contact with water; differentiate from cold urticaria	**Provocation test:** Applying a towel/compress soaked with water at 35°C–37°C. The towel is applied to patient skin (upper body) for 40 minutes. Towel/compress are removed earlier if/when the patient develops itchy wheals **Reading time:** During 40-minute observation period up to 10 min post-removal **Positive test:** Development of a wheal and flare

$ CBC and ESR or CRP can be done if indicated to rule out other diseases; ice cube test generally negative in cases of CAPS (Cryopyrin-associated periodic syndromes).

% Rule out other light-induced dermatoses if indicated (e.g. polymorphous light eruption).

* Testing methods adapted from Magerl M et al. The definition, diagnostic testing, and management of chronic inducible urticarias – The EAACI/GA(2) LEN/EDF/UNEV Consensus Recommendations 2016 Update and Revision (57).

Management (4)

Non-Pharmacologic

- Education on disease etiology, prognosis (see below), and treatment strategies is especially important.
- Identify and treat/eliminate underlying cause if present (e.g. thyroid disease, medications).
- Avoid triggering factors such as alcohol, NSAIDs, and patient-specific triggers.
  - Decrease emotional/physical stress. Evidence shows that disease activity and severity are linked with stress levels (10).
  - Foods/pseudoallergens: Controversial; pseudoallergen-free diets have been proposed and may be effective in about 1 in 3 patients. However, they are extremely difficult to follow and are rarely recommended. We do not advise pseudoallergen-free diets unless requested by patients and in this case suggest using the diet published by Magerl et al. (11).
- Avoid physical provocations in CIndU (e.g. pressure, heat, cold).
- Tolerance induction (e.g. cold urticaria, solar urticaria) such as ultraviolet A (UVA) rush therapy are effective within 3 days (12). However, continuous daily exposure may be required given the short duration of tolerance induction (several days).
- For patients with cold urticaria:
  - Avoidance of cold exposure is recommended.
  - Educate patients on activities that are high risk (surgeries, swimming, consumption of cold beverages/food).
  - Epinephrine auto-injector is provided for patients with the following features: Frequent and/or unavoidable cold exposure, systemic symptoms, and/or history of anaphylaxis.

Pharmacologic

Chronic spontaneous urticaria is a heterogeneous disease; therefore patients with similar clinical manifestations will respond differently to treatment options. In general, we follow the international guidelines from the *EAACI/GA²LEN/EDF/WAO Guideline for the definition, classification, diagnosis, and management of urticaria (4).*

Some Important Points on Pharmacologic Treatments

Updosing to Fourfold Second-Generation H1 Antihistamines

- CSU patients can be categorized as (A) responders to standard doses of H1 antihistamines, (B) non-responders to standard doses of H1 antihistamines but responders to higher doses of H1 antihistamines, or (C) non-responders to H1 antihistamines regardless of dose.
- A 2016 systematic review reported that only 38.6% of CSU patients showed controlled disease when treated with *standard licensed doses* of H1 antihistamines (13).
  - However, there was a *63.2% rate of response to updosing* in patients with CSU who were non-responders to standard-dose H1 antihistamines (13).
- There is no evidence for superiority in CU of one second-generation H1 antihistamine over another.

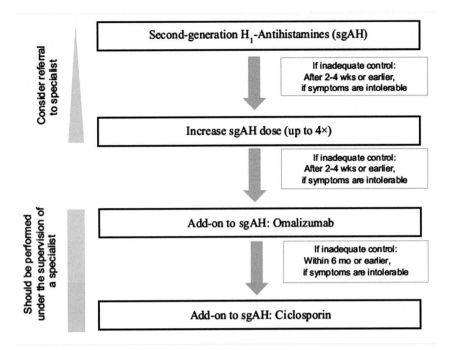

Figure 9.4 Treatment algorithm for chronic urticaria. Omalizumab should be tried before ciclosporin A since the latter is not licensed for urticaria and has an inferior profile of adverse effects. A short course of glucocorticosteroids may be considered in case of severe exacerbation. Other treatment options are available (see below). [Reprinted with permission from Zuberbier et al. The EAACI/GA²LEN/EDF/WAO guideline for the definition, classification, diagnosis and management of urticaria. *Allergy*, 2018; 73:1393–1414. John Wiley & Sons (4).]

- Sedation is a common limiting side effect of updosing (14), and patients should be cautioned.
  - Bilastine causes the least amount of sedation in this drug class.

Leukotriene Receptor Antagonists (LTRAs) (Montelukast) and H2 Antihistamines (Famotidine, Ranitidine) (15)

- Previously third-line treatments, these medications have been removed from the most recent international treatment algorithm (4); however, they may be beneficial in some patients and have a good side effect profile for add-on therapy.
  - A 2012 Cochrane review on the topic of H2 antihistamines for urticaria examined four low-quality, older studies, with 144 participants in which no firm conclusions could be drawn, but the combination of ranitidine with diphenhydramine appeared to be slightly more effective in reducing symptoms of urticaria than diphenhydramine alone (16).
  - A 2018 case series described montelukast reducing symptom severity and frequency in 22 (92%) of 24 patients with angioedema-predominant CSU (17).
- In general, these agents may be considered as a safe temporizing "add-on pharmacotherapy bridge" before omalizumab is initiated, if second-generation non-sedating H1 antihistamines are maximized at quadruple the standard dose.

Anti-IgE (Omalizumab)

- Anti-IgE monoclonal antibody is shown to be safe and effective for CSU treatment (18–23).
- Reported to be effective in CIndU (24, 25) involving cholinergic urticaria (26), cold urticaria (27, 28), solar urticaria (29), heat urticaria (30), symptomatic dermographism (31, 32), and delayed pressure urticaria (33).
- Prevents angioedema development in CSU (34).
- Effective as a long-term treatment option (35).
- Approved for adults and children 12 years and older.

- Dosing in CU: 150 mg or 300 mg subcutaneously (SC) per month.
  - Dosing is independent of serum total IgE level (18), although lower total IgE level is associated with slower or less responsiveness.
  - Recommended dose in CSU is 300 mg SC every 4 weeks.
  - Suboptimal responders may benefit from higher doses (450 mg or 600 mg every 4 weeks) or from more frequent dosing (such as 150 mg every 2 weeks) (18, 36).

Cyclosporine A

- Cyclosporine A may have disease-modifying effects and it is used as adjuvant in the management of difficult to control CSU (4, 38).
- Rapid onset of action and patient symptoms resolve within the first 8 weeks (37).
- Side effects: Hypertension and nephrotoxicity; thus, regular blood pressure and renal function monitoring is advised and use is contraindicated with uncontrolled hypertension or renal disease (37).

Oral Steroids

- A short course may be used during an acute exacerbation of CU that is not controlled with maximum antihistamine dosing (4), but oral steroids should not be routinely recommended as a long-term option due to side effects.
  - The optimal dosing and duration of oral corticosteroids has not been established and patient response differs. Rebound worsening of urticaria with cessation of glucocorticoids may occur and a short taper may be considered.
  - Even short-term use of oral corticosteroids increases the incidence of acute adverse events that result in major morbidity and mortality (i.e. sepsis, venous thromboembolism, fracture) by 2- to 5-fold above background rates in a large retrospective cohort study (38).

Other Immunomodulators/Immunosuppressants

- Rare cases will not respond to initial or approved treatments and may require off-label/experimental treatments previously published in case reports/series such as intravenous immunoglobulin (IVIg), hydroxychloroquine, dapsone, sulfasalazine, colchicine, mycophenolate, azathioprine, and others (4, 39).

Disease Activity Impact and Control (4)

- Assess disease activity and impact on quality of life at each visit.
- The *Urticaria Activity Score for Seven Days (UAS-7)* is the main activity score utilized in clinical practice for CU and helps guide management decisions.
  - Scoring of *daily pruritus and number of wheals* expressed as a weekly score from 0–42.
  - Score <6 per week is considered well-controlled CU.
  - Limitation: Does not account for disease activity of angioedema.
- Other assessment tools:
  - Chronic Urticaria Quality of Life Questionnaire (CU-Q2oL).
  - Angioedema Quality of Life Questionnaire (AE-QoL).
  - Urticaria control test (40).

Prognosis

- CU is a **self-limited condition** in most individuals.
  - 80%–90% of adults and children with CU have **no allergic etiology identified (4)**.
- The average duration of CSU is 2–5 years (41–43).
- Symptoms lasting >5 years occur in ~20% of individuals (41–43).
- Presence of angioedema and positive autoimmune testing is associated with increased disease duration (46).
- The spontaneous remission rate at 1 year for CU patients with unidentified triggers is about 30%–50% (41, 44, 47).
  - In children, the resolution rate for CSU is reported to be ~10% per year (48).

SPECIAL POPULATIONS: PREGNANCY AND LACTATION

General Considerations (49)

- Lack of guidelines on how to manage CSU during pregnancy.
- Many practitioners are uncomfortable managing CSU during pregnancy/lactation and this can lead to disease exacerbation.
- Adequate management during pregnancy/lactation improves patient quality of life.
- While CSU may appear during pregnancy, it is most often a preexisting condition.

- CSU may improve, worsen, or remain the same during pregnancy.
- CSU is unlikely to cause infertility or adverse pregnancy outcomes (expert opinion).

Differential Diagnosis (49, 50)

Other dermatoses specific to pregnancy respond to topical and oral glucocorticoids and must be considered if symptoms occur during gestation (18, 50). These include:

- **Polymorphic eruption of pregnancy (known more commonly as pruritic urticarial papules and plaques of pregnancy [PUPPP]):** Mimics urticarial lesions, occurs in the third trimester, and disappears with delivery. Usually recurs in subsequent pregnancies.
- **Atopic eruption of pregnancy:** Papular or eczematous eruption occurring any time during gestation, likely associated with exacerbation of underlying atopy.
- **Gestational pemphigoid:** Sudden onset of urticaria-like lesions, later generalizing with more herpetic appearing lesions; occurs at any stage of pregnancy; not associated with herpes infection.
- **Intrahepatic cholestasis of pregnancy:** Pruritus associated with liver disease of pregnancy, symptoms resolve with delivery.
- **Prurigo of pregnancy:** Pruritic papules on extensor surfaces, usually occurring after 20 weeks' gestation.
- **Pustular psoriasis of pregnancy:** Impetigo herpetiformis occurring in the second half of pregnancy and resolving after delivery.
- **Progesterone hypersensitivity:** Usually occurs pre-conception, most often is cyclical urticaria. Can rarely present in the first trimester when endogenous progesterone levels are high, improves in the second trimester.

Management During Pregnancy

- Patients benefit from a *pre-conceptual assessment* to review medications and disease control (expert opinion).
- Follow-up with an allergist-immunologist should be done *once a trimester* or more frequently if disease exacerbation (expert opinion).
- Second-generation H1 antihistamines are preferred as first-line management during pregnancy and lactation (49, 51); **use the lowest effective dose**, up to four times recommended dose (49).

- *Preferred during pregnancy and lactation:* Cetirizine and derivatives, loratadine and derivatives, and fexofenadine (49, 51).
- Although not recommended during pregnancy or lactation, emerging data indicate that rupatadine and bilastine are not associated with adverse pregnancy outcomes.
  - If a patient with CSU responds only to rupatadine or bilastine, these should be continued during pregnancy (expert opinion).
- Short course of oral steroids can be prescribed for exacerbations during pregnancy or breastfeeding, but chronic usage should be avoided (49).
- Anti-leukotrienes may be continued during pregnancy.
- Although omalizumab has not been approved for pregnancy, results from the Xolair® Pregnancy Registry and small case series do not show any adverse pregnancy outcomes (52–54).
- Omalizumab should be continued throughout pregnancy if previously effective pre-conception (expert opinion).
- Omalizumab carries a risk of anaphylaxis with the first three doses.
  - It should not be initiated during pregnancy unless absolutely necessary (expert opinion).
- Dapsone, cyclosporine, and mycophenolate mofetil should be avoided during pregnancy and lactation.
  - Discontinue use at least 1 month prior to conception (expert opinion) (55).
- Azathioprine may be continued during pregnancy if no other alternatives are available and disease control is achieved with this agent. Risk/benefits must be assessed on an individualized basis (expert opinion) (55).

REFERENCES

1. Antia C et al., J Am Acad Dermatol. (2018), PMID: 30241623/DOI: 10.1016/j.jaad.2018.01.020.
2. Maurer M et al., Allergy. (2011), PMID: 21083565/ DOI: 10.1111/j.1398-9995.2010.02496.x.
3. Fricke J et al., Allergy. (2020), PMID: 31494963/DOI: 10.1111/all.14037.
4. Zuberbier T et al., Allergy. (2018), PMID: 29336054/ DOI: 10.1111/all.13397.
5. Yu L et al., J Eur Acad Dermatol Venereol. (2019), PMID: 31025425/DOI: 10.1111/jdv.15640.
6. Saini SS. Urticaria and Angioedema. In: Burks AW, Holgate ST, O'Hehir RE, Bacharier LB, Broide DH, Hershey GK, Peebles Jr RS. Middleton's Allergy: Principles and Practice E-Book, Ninth Edition.

Amsterdam: Elsevier. Available at: https://www.clinicalkey.com/dura/browse/bookChapter/3-s2.0-C20161002419 (Accessed: August 24, 2020).

7. Wong MM et al., Allergy Asthma Clin Immunol. (2020), PMID: 32944029/DOI: 10.1186/s13223-020-00461-x.

8. Shalom G et al., Br J Dermatol. (2017), PMID: 28129676/DOI: 10.1111/bjd.15347.

9. Shaker M et al., J Allergy Clin Immunol Pract. (2020), PMID: 31751758/DOI: 10.1016/j.jaip.2019.11.004.

10. Varghese R et al., Ann Allergy Asthma Immunol. (2016), PMID: 26905640/DOI: 10.1016/j.anai.2016.01.016.

11. Magerl M et al., Allergy. (2010), PMID: 19796222/DOI: 10.1111/j.1398-9995.2009.02130.x.

12. Beissert S et al., J Am Acad Dermatol. (2000), PMID: 10827409/DOI: 10.1016/s0190-9622(00)90299-8.

13. Guillén-Aguinaga S et al., Br J Dermatol. (2016), PMID: 27237730/DOI: 10.1111/bjd.14768.

14. van den Elzen MT et al., Clin Transl Allergy. (2017), PMID: 28289538/DOI: 10.1186/s13601-017-0141-3.

15. Dhanya NB et al., Indian J Dermatol Venereol Leprol. (2008), PMID: 19052407/DOI: 10.4103/0378-6323.44303.

16. Fedorowicz Z et al., Cochrane Database Syst Rev. (2012), PMID: 22419335/DOI: 10.1002/14651858.CD008596.pub2.

17. Akenroye AT et al., J Allergy Clin Immunol Pract. (2018), PMID: 29733981/DOI: 10.1016/j.jaip.2018.04.026.

18. Saini S et al., J Allergy Clin Immunol. (2011), PMID: 21762974/DOI: 10.1016/j.jaci.2011.06.010.

19. Maurer M et al., J Allergy Clin Immunol. (2011), PMID: 21636116/DOI: 10.1016/j.jaci.2011.04.038.

20. Saini SS et al., J Invest Dermatol. (2015), PMID: 25501032/DOI: 10.1038/jid.2014.512.

21. Maurer M et al., N Engl J Med. (2013), PMID: 23432142/DOI: 10.1056/NEJMoa1215372.

22. Kaplan A et al., J Allergy Clin Immunol. (2013), PMID: 23810097/DOI: 10.1016/j.jaci.2013.05.013.

23. Zhao ZT et al., J Allergy Clin Immunol. (2016), PMID: 27040372/DOI: 10.1016/j.jaci.2015.12.1342.

24. Maurer M, et al., J Allergy Clin Immunol. (2018), PMID: 28751232/DOI: 10.1016/j.jaci.2017.06.032.

25. Metz M et al., Int Arch Allergy Immunol. (2011), PMID: 20733327/DOI: 10.1159/000320233.

26. Metz M et al., Allergy. (2008), PMID: 18186820/DOI: 10.1111/j.1398-9995.2007.01591.x.

27. Boyce JA, J Allergy Clin Immunol. (2006), PMID: 16751006/DOI: 10.1016/j.jaci.2006.04.003.

28. Metz M et al., J Allergy Clin Immunol. (2017), PMID: 28389393/DOI: 10.1016/j.jaci.2017.01.043.

29. Guzelbey O et al., Allergy. (2008), PMID: 18925897/DOI: 10.1111/j.1398-9995.2008.01879.x.

30. Bullerkotte U et al., Allergy. (2010), PMID: 19930230/DOI: 10.1111/j.1398-9995.2009.02268.x.

31. Maurer M et al., J Allergy Clin Immunol. (2017), PMID: 28389391/DOI: 10.1016/j.jaci.2017.01.042.

32. Krause K et al., Allergy. (2010), PMID: 20560911/DOI: 10.1111/j.1398-9995.2010.02409.x.

33. Bindslev-Jensen C et al., Allergy. (2010), PMID: 19804440/DOI: 10.1111/j.1398-9995.2009.02188.x.

34. Staubach P et al., Allergy. (2016), PMID: 27010957/DOI: 10.1111/all.12870.

35. Maurer M et al., J Allergy Clin Immunol. (2018), PMID: 29132956/DOI: 10.1016/j.jaci.2017.10.018.

36. Saini S et al., J Allergy Clin Immunol. (2011), PMID: 21762974/DOI: 10.1016/j.jaci.2011.06.010.

37. Türk M et al., J Allergy Clin Immunol Pract. (2018), PMID: 29410306/DOI: 10.1016/j.jaip.2018.01.027.

38. Hon KL et al., Recent Pat Inflamm Allergy Drug Discov. (2019), PMID: 30924425/DOI: 10.2174/1872213X13666190328164931.

39. Waljee AK et al., BMJ. (2017), PMID: 28404617/DOI: 10.1136/bmj.j1415.

40. Rutkowski K et al., Clin Exp Allergy. (2017), PMID: 28452145/DOI: 10.1111/cea.12944.

41. Weller K et al., J Allergy Clin Immunol. (2014), PMID: 24522090/DOI: 10.1016/j.jaci.2013.12.1076.

42. Kozel MM et al., J Am Acad Dermatol. (2001), PMID: 11511835/DOI: 10.1067/mjd.2001.116217.

43. Nebiolo F et al., Ann Allergy Asthma Immunol. (2009), PMID: 19927539/DOI: 10.1016/S1081-1206(10)60360-2.

44. Chansakulporn S et al., J Am Acad Dermatol. (2014), PMID: 25023899/DOI: 10.1016/j.jaad.2014.05.069.

45. Champion RH et al., Br J Dermatol. (1969), PMID: 5801331/DOI: 10.1111/j.1365-2133.1969.tb16041.x.

46. Toubi E et al., Allergy. (2004), PMID: 15230821/DOI: 10.1111/j.1398-9995.2004.00473.x.

47. Eun SJ et al., Allergol Int. (2019), PMID: 29945815/DOI: 10.1016/j.alit.2018.05.011.

48. Kulthanan K et al., J Dermatol. (2007), PMID: 17408437/DOI: 10.1111/j.1346-8138.2007.00276.x.

49. Netchiporouk E et al., JAMA Dermatol. (2017), PMID: 28973060/DOI: 10.1001/jamadermatol.2017.3182.

50. Saini S et al., J Allergy Clin Immunol Pract. (2020), PMID: 32298850/DOI: 10.1016/j.jaip.2020.03.030.

51. Danesh M et al., Clin Dermatol. (2016), PMID: 27265068/DOI: 10.1016/j.clindermatol.2016.02.002.

52. Etwel F et al., Drug Saf. (2017), PMID: 27878468/DOI: 10.1007/s40264-016-0479-9.

53. Cuervo-Pardo L et al., Eur Ann Allergy Clin Immunol. (2016), PMID: 27425170.

54. Ensina LF et al., J Investig Allergol Clin Immunol. (2017), PMID: 29057743/DOI: 10.18176/jiaci.0179.

55. Pfaller B et al., Allergy. (2021), PMID: 32189356/DOI: 10.1111/all.14282.

56. Götestam Skorpen C et al., Ann Rheum Dis. (2016), PMID: 26888948/DOI: 10.1136/annrheumdis-2015-208840.

57. Magerl M et al., Allergy. (2016), PMID: 26991006/DOI: 10.1111/all.12884.

58. Kolkhir et al. J Allergy Clin Immunol (2017), PMID: 27777182. DOI: 10.1016/j.jaci.2016.08.050.

Angioedema

ABEER FETEIH, FARIDA ALMARZOOQI, MICHAEL FEIN, GENEVIÈVE GENEST, HOANG PHAM, AND MOSHE BEN-SHOSHAN

HEREDITARY ANGIOEDEMA (HAE)

GENERAL BACKGROUND (PATHOPHYSIOLOGY AND EPIDEMIOLOGY)

- Usually develops from C1 esterase inhibitor (C1INH) deficiency/impairment, which is a SERPINs (*ser*ine *p*rotease *in*hibitor) (1).
- **Mutation:** Autosomal dominant in the *SERPING1* (SERPIN peptidase inhibitor, clade G, member 1; MIM: 606860) gene resulting in C1INH deficiency (quantitative or functional) (1, 2).
- Approximately 75% of patients have a positive family history of HAE and 25% presumably have a de novo mutation (1).
- Main mediator of swelling is **bradykinin** (1–4).
  - C1INH normally regulates activation of the contact system.
  - In cases where C1INH is deficient or dysfunctional, the contact system is destabilized, resulting in the activation of factor XIIa and plasma kallikrein.
  - Activation of plasma kallikrein catalyzes the cleavage of high-molecular-weight kininogen which releases bradykinin.
  - Bradykinin binds to the B2 bradykinin receptor, which increases vascular endothelial permeability.
- **Prevalence: 1:30,000–1:80,000** in the general population (1, 2).
- Delay in diagnosis is common and increases morbidity/mortality.
  - Due to rarity of HAE, disease heterogeneity, cases lacking family history, and when limited to abdominal attacks.
  - Symptoms usually begin in childhood and often worsen in puberty (1, 2).

TYPES OF HAE

- **Type I HAE with reduced C1INH antigenic level:** ~85% of cases (1).
- **Type II HAE with reduced C1INH functional activity:** ~15% of cases (1).
- **HAE with normal C1INH (formerly type III HAE)**
  - As of early 2021, there are five subtypes (2):
    - HAE-FXII due to mutations in the gene for FXII coagulation protein, it represents 20% of HAE with normal C1INH in Europe (2).
    - HAE-PLG due to mutations in the gene for plasminogen.
    - HAE-ANGPT1 due to mutations in the gene for angiopoietin-1.
    - HAE-KNG1 due to a mutation in the kininogen 1 gene.
    - HAE-Unknown (HAE-U) for patients in whom the responsible mutation has not yet been found.
  - Attack onset is usually during late teenage years or early adulthood and in females (2).
  - Attacks affecting the skin (mostly face) and tongue are exacerbated by estrogens such as oral contraceptives, hormonal replacement therapy, or pregnancy (2, 5, 6).
  - This subtype of angioedema is associated with less abdominal attacks compared with the other forms of HAE (2).

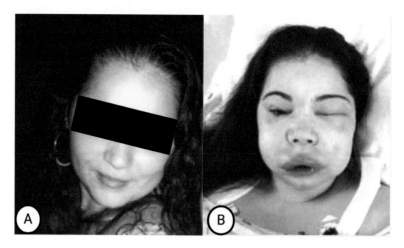

Figure 10.1 Hereditary angioedema (HAE). (A) Patient with HAE before and (B) during an angioedema attack. HAE swelling episodes are unpredictable and lead to significant pain, anxiety, disruption in normal routine, and may be life-threatening. (Figure created with BioRender.com.) (Images reprinted with permission courtesy of U.S. Hereditary Angioedema Association. HAEImages.com.)

Clinical Manifestations

- Recurrent non-pitting swelling of the deep layers of the skin, usually lacking the presence of pruritus or urticaria, and can affect the face, oropharynx, larynx, extremities, abdomen, genitals, and urinary tract (1).
- **Characteristics of swelling**
  - Usually, an acute attack of angioedema will build over 24 hours and then slowly return to baseline after 48–72 hours (1).
  - Attacks usually have a protracted duration of 3–5 days if untreated.
- **Prodromal symptoms:** May manifest hours or even full day before the angioedema attack.
  - For example, **erythema marginatum** (evanescent erythematous non-urticarial skin eruption), localized tingling, tightening sensation in the skin, fatigue, malaise, flu-like symptoms, irritability, mood changes, hyperactivity, thirst, nausea (1, 2).
- Disease severity is **heterogeneous** among individuals: For instance, patients not on prophylactic therapy may experience attacks every 10–20 days lasting for 2–5 days or once a year (1).

Morbidity and Mortality in HAE

- Patients with HAE are at risk of death by asphyxiation from oropharyngeal/laryngeal angioedema (1).
- Mortality rate from laryngeal angioedema is approximately ≥30% in those with HAE (1).

- Abdominal attacks may mimic acute abdomen symptoms that cause the patient to have unnecessary surgical intervention (1).

Precipitating Factors for HAE Attacks (1, 2)

- Emotional stress
- Infections
- Trauma, medical procedures, and surgery
- Angiotensin-converting enzyme (ACE) inhibitors (contraindicated)
- Oral contraceptive pills (with estrogen) and estrogen replacement therapy (contraindicated)

Diagnosis and Investigations

1. **C4 level**
   - Used as a screening test to exclude a diagnosis of HAE (1).
   - Sensitivity is 81%–96% in screening for C1INH-deficient patients (2).
   - C4 level is usually normal in those with HAE who are on treatment (1).
   - C4 levels during an HAE attack should be low.
     - **It is very unlikely** to have HAE if C4 level is normal during an attack but could still be due to HAE with normal C1INH (1).
   - If C4 level is low or suspicion is very high, continue investigations.

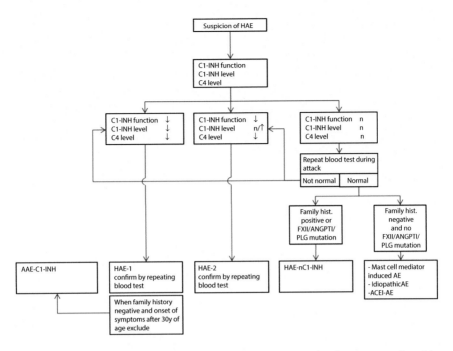

Figure 10.2 Diagnostic algorithm for hereditary angioedema. (Reprinted with permission from Maurer et al. The international WAO/EAACI guideline for the management of hereditary angioedema—The 2017 revision and update. *Allergy.* 2018; 73:1575–1596, Wiley.) (*Abbreviations:* n: normal; ↑: increased; ↓: decreased.)

2. **C1INH antigenic level (and functional level if the antigenic level is normal) (1)**
   - **Functional levels are generally less than 50%–60% of the lower limit in HAE.**
   - Low C4 and C1INH antigenic levels confirm type I HAE.
   - Low C4 level, normal C1INH antigenic level, and low C1INH function confirm type II HAE (1).
   - No **routine** laboratory test targets are available for confirmation of type III HAE causes.
     - Diagnosis based on clinical history of **attacks at later age of onset** and a **positive family history** of autosomal dominant pattern.
     - If history is suggestive, request genetic studies for **FXII/ANGPT1/PLG/KNG1** (1, 6).

Management

- **Goals**
  1. Educate patient to recognize symptoms.
  2. Recognize significant psychosocial impact.
  3. Prevent future episodes (short- and long-term prophylaxis).

  4. Manage acute attacks.
  5. Genetic counseling for family planning.

Non-Pharmacologic Management

- Educate regarding the nature of illness, precipitating factors, and genetic inheritance.
- Assess disease impact on patient quality of life (6).
  - *Recommend* patient support groups (e.g. HAE Canada™).
- Advise the patient on procedures that can exacerbate HAE symptoms (such as dental work and surgical procedures) including the need for prophylaxis.
- Advise to have a MedicAlert™ bracelet or equivalent.

Pharmacologic Management

- Important to distinguish between acute and prophylactic treatment medications, formulations, and dosing. *See product monographs for specific indications, dosing, and side effect profiles.*

A. Acute attacks [Adapted from (1)]
   - Oropharyngeal attacks are a medical emergency and should be treated in a monitored setting.

- Prompt evaluation of patient airway, breathing, vital signs; secure intravenous (IV) lines.
- Acute pharmacologic treatment (*see below.*)
- HAE attacks are not responsive to epinephrine, corticosteroids, and antihistamines.
- HAE attacks should be treated early.

Medication Options Include

1. **Plasma-derived C1INH concentrate**
   - **Dose:** 20 units/kg IV
   - **Side effects:** Anaphylaxis (rare)
2. **Bradykinin (B2) receptor antagonist: Icatibant**
   - **Dose:** 30 mg subcutaneously (SC)
   - **Side effects:** Injection site reactions
3. **Kallikrein inhibitor: Ecallantide**
   - **Dose:** 30 mg SC, three injections of 1 mL each
   - **Side effects:** Anti-drug antibodies and anaphylaxis (uncommon)
4. **Recombinant human C1INH**
   - **Dose:** 50–100 units/kg IV
   - **Side effects:** Anaphylaxis risk in rabbit-sensitized subjects (uncommon)
5. **Fresh frozen plasma (FFP)**
   - **Dose:** 1–2 units IV
   - Effective in acute attacks but can cause an exacerbation of some attacks; may be considered in cases when on-demand first-line treatments are not available (21)

B. *Prophylaxis*

- Decisions to use short- and long-term prophylaxis are individualized based on the patients' history of attack frequency and severity, access to acute medical care, and patient preferences.
- Choice of prophylaxis agents is guided by ease of administration routes, side effect profile, cost/availability, and patient preference.

Short-term prophylaxis (STP)

- Used to protect patients from acute attacks during a certain time frame after the presence of a trigger known to precipitate an HAE attack (e.g. extensive dental work or surgery) (1).
- Ensure that the treating health professional (dentist, surgeon, anesthesiologist, etc.) is aware of patient's condition and that procedure takes place in an appropriate setting with emergency treatments available.

Options Include (2, 7)

1. **C1INH replacement**
   - **Dose:** 1000–2000 units or 20 units/kg in children of plasma-derived C1INH typically given 1 hour prior to intervention
2. **High-dose 17α-alkylated androgens**
   - **Dose:** 6–10 mg/kg/day in divided doses with a maximum dose of 200 mg of danazol, three times/day or equivalent for 5–10 days before the procedure and 2 days after the procedure.
   - Not recommended in children due to hormonal side effects.

Long-term prophylaxis (LTP)

- Used to prevent attacks of angioedema on an ongoing basis.
- Requires regular follow-up to assess level of control, tolerability, and side effects of therapy.
- First-line treatment for LTP is subcutaneous C1NH replacement or lanadelumab (2, 7).

Options Include

1. **Subcutaneous plasma-derived C1INH**
   - **Dose:** 40 or 60 units/kg SC twice weekly and adjust on the basis of patient response
   - **Side effects:** Local injection site reactions, headache, and skin rash
2. **Kallikrein inhibitor monoclonal antibody**
   - **Lanadelumab**
     - **Dose:** 300 mg SC every 2 weeks; and consider decreasing to every 4 weeks in patients who are well controlled
     - **Side effects:** Injection site reaction, upper respiratory infection, headache, myalgias
3. **Intravenous plasma-derived C1INH**
   - **Dose:** C1INH 1000 units IV every 3–4 days to start and adjusted upward as needed
   - **Side effects:** Anaphylaxis (rare), infection transmission (theoretical risk), thrombosis
4. **17α-alkylated androgens**
   - **Danazol**
     - **Adult dose:** 200 mg/day (maximum daily dose: 600 mg/day; once controlled, interval may be reduced to 100 mg every 3 days)
     - **Pediatric dose:** 50 mg/day (maximum daily dose: 200 mg/day; once controlled, interval may be reduced to 50 mg/week)

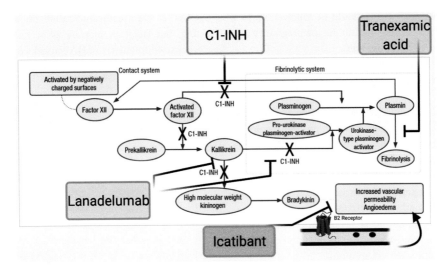

Figure 10.3 Mechanism of action of pharmacologic treatments for HAE. Intravenous C1-INH and icatibant are first-line treatments for acute attacks. Lanadelumab and subcutaneous C1-INH are first-line treatments for long-term prophylaxis. Tranexamic acid is used for long-term prophylaxis but is a less effective option in HAE. (Figure created with BioRender.com.) [Adapted from Longhust, Bork. Hereditary angioedema: An update on causes, manifestations and treatment. *British Journal of Hospital Medicine*, July 2019, 80(22).]

- **Side effects:** Weight gain, masculinization, acne, altered libido, depression, fatigue, nausea, menstrual abnormalities, elevation of liver enzymes, hypertension, and dyslipidemia, and rarely hepatic cancer
  - **Stanozolol**
    - **Adult dose:** 2 mg/day (maximum daily dose: 6 mg/day; once controlled, interval may be reduced to 1 mg every 3 days)
    - **Pediatric dose:** 0.5 mg/day (maximum daily dose: 200 mg/day; once controlled, interval may be reduced to 0.5 mg/week)
5. **Antifibrinolytics**
  - **Tranexamic acid**
    - **Adult dose:** 1 g BID (0.25–1.5 g BID)
    - **Side effects:** Diarrhea, vertigo, postural hypotension, muscle cramps, elevation in muscle enzyme levels, and thrombosis (1)

Management of HAE with Normal C1INH Levels

- Patients may respond to medications used to treat type I and type II HAE based on previous open-label published reports (1).
- There are reports of successful on-demand treatment with C1INH concentrates, ecallantide and icatibant (1).

- Some patients improve with danazol, progesterone, or tranexamic acid as long-term prophylactic treatment (1).
- Corticosteroids and antihistamines are not effective (1).

SPECIAL POPULATIONS: PREGNANCY AND LACTATION

Diagnosis

- If HAE type I/II is suspected during pregnancy, keep in mind that C1INH levels are unreliable during gestation. C1INH levels should be repeated 6–8 weeks postpartum for confirmation (7).
- If a mother has proven HAE type I or II, her offspring has a 50% chance of inheriting the disease and requires screening after the age of 12 months. However, if the mother has a genetic diagnosis, the child may be tested for this variant at any age (7).

Pre-Conception Considerations

- Patients with HAE considering pregnancy should consult their treating physician first for a pre-conceptual consultation and close follow-up during pregnancy (6, 7).

- Patients with HAE should be followed-up in a high-risk obstetrical unit during pregnancy and delivery (expert opinion).
- If the patient is undergoing in vitro fertilization treatments, STP should be considered for egg retrieval.
  - STP is not required for artificial insemination or embryo transfer procedures unless the patient has a history of vaginal swelling from mechanical trauma (expert opinion).
- Attenuated androgens are contraindicated during pregnancy and lactation and should be stopped at least 3 months prior to conception (7, 8).
- The patient considering pregnancy should have well-controlled disease at least 3 months prior to conception (expert opinion).

Pregnancy and Postpartum Considerations

- HAE attacks may improve, worsen, or remain the same during pregnancy. The third trimester may be the most at risk for increased HAE attacks due to mechanical trauma (6–8).
- STP should be considered for chorionic villus sampling or amniocentesis (expert opinion).
- STP is not required in the event of a natural miscarriage but should be considered if surgical evacuation of the pregnancy is required (expert opinion).
- Uncomplicated vaginal delivery does not require STP; however, on-demand treatment should be available in the delivery room and up to 72 hours postpartum. If the delivery is prolonged or requires forceps or vacuum, STP should be administered.
- STP should also be considered in women with additional risk factors (severe HAE attacks, third trimester HAE exacerbation, and history of traumatic vaginal swelling) (6, 7).
- STP is recommended in the case of C-section; supplemental on-demand treatment should also be available in the delivery room (6, 7).
- Labor and uncomplicated delivery rarely induce attacks. However, the patient remains at risk for HAE attacks during labor and 48 hours postpartum. It is recommended to keep the patient under close observation for 72 hours after delivery.
- Complicated vaginal delivery and C-sections can increase the risk of HAE attacks. Care and follow-up of these patients should be individualized (6).

- HAE is not a contraindication for breastfeeding, but lactation may be associated with an increased frequency of HAE attacks (6).

Medical Management during Pregnancy

- If used prior to pregnancy and effective in long-term prevention of HAE attacks, antifibrinolytics may be continued for the duration of pregnancy, delivery, and the postpartum period. Tranexamic acid is safe during breastfeeding (6).
- Plasma-derived C1INH remains the preferred agent for acute treatment, STP and LTP (when indicated) (6–8). Doses for acute treatment, LTP, and STP must be re-evaluated once a trimester and adjusted for weight gain during pregnancy (expert opinion).
- Icatibant is a US Food and Drug Administration (FDA) category C drug during pregnancy. However, emerging data have not demonstrated any adverse effects on the fetus when used during pregnancy (8).
- Icatibant should be used in the case of a life-threatening (laryngeal) or pregnancy-threatening (abdominal) attack refractory to C1INH administration or if C1INH is unavailable (8).
- FFP is safe during pregnancy. FFP and tranexamic acid should only be used to treat acute attacks when other alternatives (C1INH and icatibant) are unavailable as FFP and tranexamic acid are less effective in treating acute attacks (6).

ACQUIRED ANGIOEDEMA (AAE) WITH C1INH DEFICIENCY

Pathogenesis

- AAE-C1INH deficiency hypothesized to be possibly mediated by (1):
  a. enhanced catabolism of C1INH by underlying autoimmunity or neoplastic processes
  b. autoantibodies against C1INH

Clinical Manifestations

- **Age:** Middle age (>40 years) or older (9).
- No family history of angioedema (1).
- **Prevalence:** Very rare. Unknown, but estimated ~1:500,000 (10).
- **Associated underlying diseases:** Autoimmune (e.g. systemic lupus erythematosus) and lymphoproliferative malignancies (e.g. lymphoma, MGUS) (11, 12).

- Angioedema predominantly affects the tongue, uvula, face, and upper airways; may affect gastrointestinal (GI) tract but less so than with HAE (13).

Diagnosis and Investigations

- Decreased C1INH level and function, decreased C4, decreased to normal C3, and decreased C1q levels.
  - C1q levels are low in 80% of AAE-C1INH (2).
- Investigations for underlying illnesses: Complete blood count (CBC) with differential blood count, C-reactive protein, sedimentation rate, serum protein electrophoresis, and urine protein electrophoresis (13).
  - Consider bone marrow biopsy depending on the above workup.
- High titer of anti-C1INH antibodies (test not commercially available).

Management

- Treating the underlying etiology should improve symptoms (1).
- HAE-specific treatments have shown efficacy in some reports (off-label) (13).
- Tranexamic acid is more effective for LTP than androgens in AAE (13).
- Rituximab demonstrated some efficacy in uncontrolled case reports and series (14).

ACE Inhibitor (ACE-I)-Associated Angioedema

Pathogenesis

- The inhibition of ACE prevents the degradation of bradykinin, which then contributes to the development of angioedema (1).

Clinical Manifestations

- In **0.1%–0.7%** of patients who take ACE-Is, the angioedema occurs **without urticaria**, and usually manifests on the **face, tongue, bowel, and extremities** (15).
- Approximately 50% of attacks occur during the first few months of treatment with ACE-I, but it may happen after years of continuous treatment, occasionally with dose adjustments or addition of other medications.

- Higher risk in African Americans than White ethnic groups (16).
  - Other risk factors: Smoking history, older adults, and female sex (16).

Diagnosis and Investigations

- Normal C1INH level, function, C4, C3, and C1q levels (1).
- Screening complement studies (C3, C4) should be obtained for patients with angioedema on an ACE-I because there may be underlying C1INH deficiency.

Management

- **ACE-I discontinuation**: There may be a time lag between stopping the drug and resolution of angioedema (15).
- Patient observation in a monitored setting for acute oral/laryngeal angioedema as they may require intubation.
- Antihistamines, corticosteroids, and epinephrine are not effective (1).
- The efficacy of icatibant and FFP (17, 18) have been described.
  - However, in a published study of a randomized double-blind trial of icatibant for ACE-I-induced upper airway angioedema, it showed a negative result where it had similar efficacy to placebo in those with at least moderately severe upper airway angioedema induced by ACE-I (19).
- Angiotensin receptor blockers (ARBs) can be used safely in most patients without the recurrence of angioedema (20).
- In general, we recommend a wash-out period of several weeks (~6 weeks) before initiation of an ARB given residual attacks are possible after discontinuation of an ACE-I (1).

Idiopathic Angioedema

- Other types of angioedema need to be excluded before making the diagnosis.
- *Management:* Trial of maximum dose antihistamine therapy (4× normal dose) to rule out histamine-mediated angioedema.
- If not responsive to antihistamine therapy, a trial of omalizumab or LTP treatments (e.g. tranexamic acid) for HAE have been used. (*Refer to Chapter 9 for details*).

Table 10.1 Bradykinin-Mediated Angioedema Overview

AE	HAE C1-INH-HAE Type I	HAE C1-INH-HAE Type II	HAE nC1-INH-HAE	C1-INH-AAE	ACE-I-AAE
Triggers/ Factors	Emotional stress; infections; trauma; medical/dental procedures and surgery; ACE-inhibitors (contraindicated); Oral contraceptive pills (with estrogen) and estrogen replacement therapy (contraindicated) [1, 5, 10, 11, 12]			• Associated with systemic autoimmune and malignant diseases: systemic lupus erythematosus (SLE) and lymphoproliferative malignancies • Treating the underlying cause should improve symptoms [1, 11, 12]	*Higher risk factors:* African Americans, smoking history, older adults, and female sex [16]
Clinical Features	• *Prodromal symptoms:* May manifest hours or one day before the angioedema attack; for example: erythema marginatum, localized tingling, or tightening sensation in the skin • *Non-pitting swelling* of the deep layers of the skin, usually lacking the presence of pruritus or urticaria, and can affect the face, oropharynx, larynx, extremities, abdomen, genitals, and urinary tract • Swelling is long-lasting, worsens over the first 24 hours then peaks, and slowly resolves over 48–72 hours. [5, 6, 7, 8]			Similar symptoms as HAE, but occur in middle age or older; with no family history of angioedema [1, 9]	Angioedema occurs without urticaria in 0.1%–0.7% of patients, and usually manifests on the face, tongue, bowel, and extremities [15]
Biological Profile	C4 level **Low**	**Low**	Normal	**Low**	Normal
	C3 level Normal	Normal	Normal	Low-normal	Normal
	C1Inh level **Low**	Normal-high	Normal	**Low**	Normal
	C1Inh function **Low**	**Low**	Normal	**Low**	Normal
	C1q level Normal	Normal	Normal	**Low**	Normal
Genetic Mutation Associated	*SERPING1*	*SERPING1*	*FXII, PLG, ANGPT1, KNG1*	-	-

Abbreviations: AE- Angioedema; ACE-I-AAE Angiotensin-converting enzyme inhibitor-induced AAE; ANGPT1- Angiopoietin 1; C1Inh- C1 inhibitor; C1Inh-HAE- HAE with C1Inhibitor deficiency; C1Inh-AAE- Acquired AE with C1-inhibitor deficiency; FXII- Coagulation factor XII; HAE- Hereditary AE; KNG1-Kininogen 1; nC1Inh-HAE- HAE with normal C1Inh; PLG- Plasminogen;SERPING1- Serpin peptidase inhibitor, clade G, member 1.

Adapted from (1, 5–12, 15, 16).

REFERENCES

1. Zuraw BL et al., J Allergy Clin Immunol. (2013), PMID: 23726531/DOI: 10.1016/j.jaci.2013.03.034.

2. Busse, Paula J et al., J Allergy Clin Immunol Pract. (2021), PMID: 32898710/DOI:10.1016/j.jaip.2020.08.046.

3. Zuraw BL et al., Clin Rev Allergy Immunol. (2016), PMID: 27459852/DOI: 10.1007/s12016-016-8561-8.

4. Kaplan AP et al., Clin Rev Allergy Immunol. (2016), PMID: 27273087/DOI: 10.1007/s12016-016-8555-6.

5. Caballero T et al., J Allergy Clin Immunol. (2012), PMID: 22197274/DOI: 10.1016/j.jaci.2011.11.025.

6. Maurer M et al., Allergy. (2018), PMID: 29318628/DOI: 10.1111/all.13384.

7. Betschel S et al., Allergy Asthma Clin Immunol. (2019), PMID: 31788005/DOI: 10.1186/s13223-019-0376-8.

8. Hakl R et al., J Clin Immunol. (2018), PMID: 30280305/DOI: 10.1007/s10875-018-0553-4.

9. Zingale LC et al., Immunol. Allergy Clin North Am. (2006), PMID: 17085284/DOI: 10.1016/j.iac.2006.08.002.

10. Cicardi M et al., Allergy Asthma Clin Immunol. (2010), PMID: 20667117/DOI: 10.1186/1710-1492-6-14.

11. Caldwell JR et al., Clin Immunol. Immunopathol. (1972), DOI: 10.1016/0090-1229(72)90006-2.

12. Schreiber AD et al., Blood. (1976), PMID: 1085645/DOI: 10.1182/blood.V48.4.567.567.

13. Cicardi M et al., Allergy. (2014), PMID: 24673465/DOI: 10.1111/all.12380.

14. Branellec A et al., J Clin Immunol. (2012), PMID: 22526593/DOI: 10.1007/s10875-012-9691-2.

15. Byrd JB et al., Immunol Allergy Clin North Am. (2006), PMID: 17085287/DOI: 10.1016/j.iac.2006.08.001.

16. Brown NJ et al., Clin Pharmacol Ther. (1996), PMID: 8689816/DOI: 10.1016/S0009-9236(96)90161-7.

17. Bas M et al., Ann Emerg Med. (2010), PMID: 20447725/DOI: 10.1016/j.annemergmed.2010.03.032.

18. Gallitelli M et al., Am J Emerg Med. (2012), PMID: 22100478/DOI: 10.1016/j.ajem.2011.09.014.

19. Sinert R et al., J Allergy Clin Immunol Pract. (2017), PMID: 28552382/DOI: 10.1016/j.jaip.2017.03.003.

20. Rasmussen et al., J Intern Med. (2019), PMID: 30618189/DOI: 10.1111/joim.12867.

21. Prematta M et al., Ann Allergy Asthma Immunol. (2007), PMID: 17458436/DOI: 10.1016/S1081-1206(10)60886-1.

22. Longhurst et al. Br J Hosp Med. (2019), PMID: 31283393. DOI: 10.12968/hmed.2019.80.7.391,

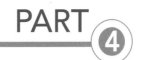
MAST CELL-RELATED DISORDERS/ ANAPHYLAXIS (SYSTEMIC ILLNESSES)

11 Mastocytosis and Mast Cell Activation Syndromes 103
Abeer Feteih, Farida Almarzooqi, Geneviève Genest, Michael Fein, Hoang Pham, and Moshe Ben-Shoshan

12 Anaphylaxis 115
Abeer Feteih, Michael Fein, Natacha Tardio, Geneviève Genest, Lydia Zhang, Hoang Pham, and Moshe Ben-Shoshan

13 Exercise-Induced Anaphylaxis (EIA) and Food-Dependent EIA (FDEIA) 123
Abeer Feteih, Lydia Zhang, Natacha Tardio, and Michael Fein

14 Stinging Insect Hypersensitivity 127
Abeer Feteih, Hoang Pham, Walaa Almasri, and Geneviève Genest

15 Eosinophilia and Hypereosinophilic Syndrome (HES) 135
Abeer Feteih, Hoang Pham, Geneviève Genest, and Natacha Tardio

Mastocytosis and Mast Cell Activation Syndromes

ABEER FETEIH, FARIDA ALMARZOOQI, GENEVIÈVE GENEST,
MICHAEL FEIN, HOANG PHAM, AND MOSHE BEN-SHOSHAN

GENERAL BACKGROUND

- Mast cell (MC) disorders encompass a broad range of disorders, including mastocytosis, MC activation syndromes (MCASs), and hereditary alpha-tryptasemia syndrome (HATS) (1, 2).
- Briefly, MC disorders are related to increased MC infiltration, overactivation, or both (2).
  - Vasoactive mediators including **tryptase and histamine** and cytokines and chemokines are released from activated MCs, resulting in the acute and chronic signs/symptoms seen in MC disorders (see section "Mast Cell Pathobiology") (1, 2).
  - **Serum tryptase**: The most clinically useful biomarker used to diagnose MCASs including mastocytosis.
    - Persistent elevation in serum tryptase is a sign of increased MC number and supports the diagnosis of mastocytosis (1, 2).
    - Transient rise in tryptase (see the section "Investigations") supports the diagnosis of mast cell activation (MCA).
- **Mastocytosis** is the prototypical primary MCAS and involves an abnormal clonal expansion and accumulation of MCs in tissues such as the bone marrow and/or skin (1, 2).
  - There are systemic and cutaneous forms.
  - There are several subtypes of systemic mastocytosis (SM) ranging from benign to malignant and prognosis depends on the subtype.
- *MCAS* is a relatively new diagnostic term and is characterized by clinical and laboratory evidence of MCA secondary to a (1, 2):
  - Monoclonal MC population (primary): Mastocytosis, monoclonal MCAS.
  - Normal MC population responding to triggers (secondary): IgE-mediated allergic/atopic conditions.
  - MC population without clonality or related inflammatory condition (idiopathic).
  - Sometimes "MCAS" is used synonymously with idiopathic MCAS when there is no associated clonal population, inflammatory trigger, or genetic mutations.
- *HATS* is an autosomal dominant MC disorder associated with an increased copy number of the *TPSAB1* gene encoding α-tryptase (1, 2).
  - This disorder with slightly elevated serum tryptase can be, but is not always, associated with MCAS.
- *Prevalence of SM:* ~1 in 10,000 (quite rare), but underdiagnosis is likely (3–5).
  - Most subtypes of SM were middle-age.
  - The male to female ratio ranges from approximately 1:1 to 1:3 depending on the SM subtype.
- Prevalence of monoclonal MCAS and idiopathic MCAS is unknown, but it seems to be low (3).

Mast Cell Pathobiology

- **MCs** are granulocytes and sentinel innate immune cells, which are derived from common myeloid precursors in the bone marrow under the influence of stem cell factor (SCF) (6).
  - SCF is also known as KIT-ligand because it serves as the ligand for CD117, which is a transmembrane receptor tyrosine kinase KIT, encoded by the gene, *KIT* (6).
  - CD117 (KIT) is involved with the regulation of proliferation, migration, survival, and effector function of MCs.

- Gain-of-function *KIT* mutations are observed in 60%–80% of cutaneous mastocytosis (CM) cases and ~80% of indolent SM (ISM) (6).
  - The most common somatic gain-of-function *KIT* point mutation is the substitution of valine for aspartic acid at codon 816 (D816V) which promotes the constitutive activation of *KIT* and subsequent unregulated MC differentiation and survival.
  - There are other *KIT* mutations (e.g. S451C, R634W) as well as other mutations (e.g. *TET2*, *ASXL1*) in patients with SM (6, 7).
- Immature proliferating MC precursors enter the bloodstream and then migrate into various tissues where they are prominent in the skin and mucosal tissues including respiratory and gastrointestinal (GI) tracts, often adjacent to blood vessels and under epithelial surfaces (6, 7).

- MCA can occur through numerous mechanisms due to the diverse receptors they express.
  - *Classic mechanism:* Involves exposure to an antigen (often allergen) that cross-links specific IgE bound to the high-affinity Fc epsilon receptor 1 (FcεRI) on MC surfaces.
  - *Other mechanisms:* Anaphylatoxins (C3a, C5a), aggregated IgG, specific drugs, venoms, physical stimuli, cytokines, and neuropeptides.
- Upon activation, MCs release a variety of mediators that produce a wide range of clinical effects on various organ systems (1, 2, 6, 7) (Figure 11.1).
  - *Preformed molecules:* Histamine, proteases (tryptase, chymase, carboxypeptidase)
  - *Newly synthesized molecules:* Leukotrienes (LTC4), prostaglandins (PGD2), platelet-activating factor (PAF)
  - *Cytokines:* Interleukin (IL)-6, IL-9, IL-13, tumor necrosis factor (TNF)
  - *Chemokines:* CXCL8, CCL2, and CCL5

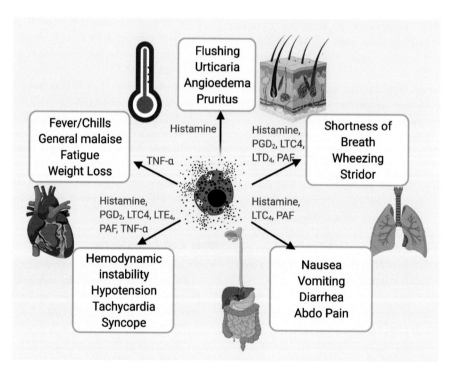

Figure 11.1 Mast cell (MC) mediators and their effects on various organ systems. The diffuse nature of MC mediators is responsible for a wide variety of clinical effects. Blocking specific MC mediators is a key principle of symptomatic management in MC disease. (Figure created with BioRender.com.) [Adapted from (2, 6).]

MAST CELL DISORDERS CLASSIFICATION [ADAPTED FROM (2)]

Primary MCASs

1. **SM**
   a. World Health Organization SM subtypes include (8): (see section "Diagnostic Criteria")
      - ISM
      - Smoldering SM (SSM)
      - SM with an associated hematological neoplasm (SM + AHM)
      - Aggressive SM (ASM)
      - MC leukemia (MCL)
   b. The incidence rate for SM (all subtypes including urticaria pigmentosa [UP]) is 0.89 per 100,000 per year. Cumulative incidence is 12.46 per 100,000 (4).
   c. Disease burden and organopathy typically increase in more advanced forms (ASM/ASM + AHM/MCL), whereas MC mediator symptoms are typically more prominent in ISM/SMM (9).

2. **CM**
   a. The most common form of mastocytosis in children and is defined when abnormal MC accumulation is **limited to the skin**.
   b. Adults with *new-onset* CM usually have systemic forms of the disease (~97%), most often ISM, which tends to persist (10–12).
   c. Subtypes include
      - **UP/maculopapular CM (MPCP):** The most common form presents with red-brown to yellow maculopapular lesions; adult-onset CM is predominantly UP/MPCP (12).
        - **Telangiectasia macularis eruptiva perstans (TMEP):** A variant of MPCP (11).
      - **Diffuse cutaneous mastocytosis (DCM):** Characterized by blistering erosions and crusts.
      - **Mastocytoma of the skin (cutaneous mastocytoma):** Form one or several brown-red plaques or nodular lesions 4–5 cm in diameter (6, 12).
   d. Childhood-onset CM often resolves (~50%–70%) (12, 13).

   e. A 2017 systematic review reaffirmed that (14)
      - UP/MPCM completely resolves at a rate of 1.9% per year.
      - Cutaneous mastocytoma completely resolves at a rate of 10% per year.
      - DCM and SM do not completely resolve.

3. **Monoclonal MCAS (MMCAS) (2)**
   a. Patients have typical symptoms of MCA and evidence of MC clonality (*KIT* D816V mutation and/or CD25+ MCs) **without** meeting full criteria for SM.
   b. Baseline serum tryptase values are normal or mildly increased.

Secondary MCASs

1. MCA secondary to *identifiable triggers*
   a. **Allergic diseases:** IgE-mediated allergies to foods, drugs, and other allergens
   b. **Physical (inducible) forms of urticaria:** See Chapter 9
   c. **Chronic inflammatory/autoimmune diseases:** Lupus and rheumatoid arthritis
   d. **Neoplastic disorders:** Solid tumors and lymphoproliferative diseases
2. MCs are normal in shape (round and fully granulated without spindles), amount, and function.
3. Secondary MCA disorders are significantly more common than other subtypes and may coexist with primary MCASs.

Idiopathic MCASs (IMCASs) (2)

1. Evidence of MCA (clinical and laboratory) without identifiable triggers despite exhaustive history and investigations and without evidence of a monoclonal MC population.
2. Conditions include
   a. Chronic spontaneous urticaria
   b. Idiopathic anaphylaxis (IA)
   c. Idiopathic angioedema (histaminergic)
   d. IMCAS
3. IA and IMCASs are diagnoses of exclusion and require thorough medical history, exam, and investigations to rule out hidden causes of MCA, such as delayed anaphylaxis to red meat allergen galactose-alpha-1,3-galactose or other hidden allergens (see Chapter 12) (15, 16).

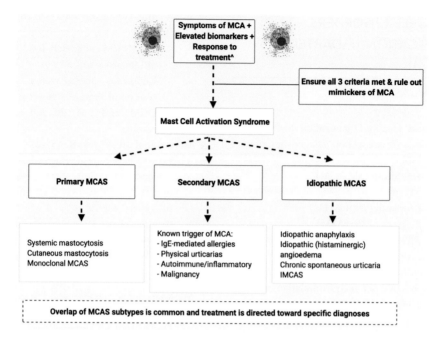

Figure 11.2 Classification of mast cell activation syndromes. (Figure created with BioRender.com.) [Adapted from Valent et al (2).]
^Diagnosis of MCA requires typical symptoms such as flushing, urticaria, angioedema, pruritus, diarrhea, vomiting, and hypotension with evidence of elevated biomarkers such as tryptase (see text) and clinical response to anti-mediator therapy such as anti-histamines.

Other Related Disorders

1. **HAT** is a relatively new disorder first described in 2014 as a genetic trait or syndrome with autosomal dominant inheritance caused by gain of function of the *TPSAB1* gene (tryptase, alpha/beta-1; MIM# 191080) due to duplication or triplication of copy number encoding for alpha-tryptase on a single allele, resulting in overexpression of α-tryptase and increased numbers of MCs in bone marrow biopsy specimens (1, 17, 18).

   – This leads to increased levels of basal serum tryptase (total), as the current widely available commercial tryptase assay measures "total tryptase," which captures both mature and pro-forms of α- and β-tryptase (1).

      • Tryptase is located on chromosome 16 and contains two genes encoding α- or β-tryptase. TPSB2 expresses β-tryptase only, whereas TPSAB1 expresses either α- or β-tryptase. Each is first expressed as a pretryptase before conversion to protryptase forms. Some protryptase portions are constitutively secreted from unstimulated MCs, whereas others are converted to their mature form and spontaneously form homotetramers of mature β-tryptase, which are stored in MC granules (1).

      • The exact mechanism by which increased expression of α-tryptase leads to symptoms is not yet fully understood, but it is hypothesized to be related to increased formation of the α-/β-heterotetramer, which makes MCs more susceptible to activation and might affect risk for anaphylaxis (1).

      • The severity of MCA symptoms correlates to the level of gene copy number and serum tryptase (18).

   – **This is a common trait found in up to 4%–6% of the population (17, 18).**

   – Patients with this trait may report an associated broad range of symptoms and are considered to have HATS (1, 17, 18)

      • *Atopy:* Allergic rhinitis, asthma, anaphylaxis, venom allergy

      • *GI:* Irritable bowel syndrome, gastroesophageal reflux disease, cramping abdominal pain with diarrhea, GI hypomotility

- *Skin:* Flushing and/or pruritus with or without urticaria, vibratory urticaria
- *Skeletal:* Congenital skeletal abnormalities, retained primary teeth
- *Chronic pain:* Arthralgias
- *Connective tissue disorders:* Hyperextensible joints
- *Dysautonomia:* Postural-orthostatic tachycardia syndrome (POTS)
- *Neuropsychiatric:* Anxiety, depression, sleep disturbance

- *Asymptomatic presentation:* Many patients are incidentally discovered when measuring serum tryptase for workup of other symptoms/causes.
- HATS is technically not included in the definition of MCAS, but there is a cluster of HATS patients that overlap with clonal and non-clonal MCAS.

Clinical Manifestations

- **SM/MC disorders should be suspected when the following signs/symptoms occur:**
  1. **Skin, respiratory, and naso-ocular symptoms (2, 9):** Flushing, urticaria, angioedema, pruritus, nasal congestion, dyspnea, and chest tightness.
  2. **GI, cardiovascular, and musculoskeletal symptoms:** Nausea, vomiting, diarrhea, tachycardia, hypotension/hypertension, fatigue, joint pain, bone/muscle pain, and osteoporosis (19).
  3. **Neuropsychiatric symptoms:** Frequently reported as the most debilitating symptoms by patients; includes extreme fatigue, migraines, lack of concentration, "brain fog," loss of memory (20, 21).
  4. **Systemic symptoms:** Anaphylaxis either due to Hymenoptera venom sting or idiopathic (22–24)
     - Insect stings are a trigger for anaphylaxis in about 20% of patients with MC disorders (23).
     - MC disorders have been detected in about 2% of patients with insect sting anaphylaxis (24).
- **CM** (see subtypes described in mast cell disorders classification section).
  1. **Darier's sign:** Urticarial rash develops within a few minutes after direct scratching or stroking around UP/MPCM lesions (11, 25).

  2. **Abdominal cramps or anaphylaxis** may occur even without bone marrow involvement (19).
- **MCA triggers:** Stress, heat (e.g. hot water), alcohol, exercise, insect sting, infection, fatigue, surgical procedures, and medications (e.g. nonsteroidal anti-inflammatory drugs [NSAIDs], antibiotics, opioids, and iodinated contrast agents) (1, 23).

However, cautious long-term use of aspirin is effective in mastocytosis to reduce flushing and hypotension by blocking PGD2 production through the inhibition of cyclooxygenase-1 (COX-1) and COX-2 enzymes (1, 26). Castells et al. outlines a detailed stepwise approach to aspirin initiation (26).

Diagnostic Criteria

- Workup focuses initially on establishing the presence of increased MC mediators (see Investigations) either consistently and/or during acute episodes of MCA.
- Cutaneous and extracutaneous biopsies (e.g. bone marrow) are used to establish the diagnosis of CM, SM, or MMCAS and may require enriched samples specific for MCs.
- If SM confirmed, screening for organ involvement is done with laboratory workup and imaging (see below).

Investigations

- **Labs**
  1. **Serum tryptase level:** If basal tryptase level is elevated >20 ng/mL, there is a high probability of SM (6).
     - If elevated during a symptomatic episode (e.g. anaphylaxis), it should be measured again at least 24 hours after symptom resolution.
     - Abnormally elevated tryptase is defined as serum tryptase level increased by:
       - $(1.2\times$ baseline tryptase) + 2 ng/mL.
         - If elevated compared with baseline within 4 hours after an acute event, this suggests contribution of MCs (7).
  2. **Peripheral blood *KIT* D816V mutation:** A noninvasive way to test for minor, but informative, criteria of SM, especially in those with symptoms that are not clear or with slightly increased serum tryptase levels (6, 27–29).
     - Up to 90% sensitivity for detecting ISM (27).
     - Testing for *KIT* D816V mutation is more efficient in adults than children because children tend to have other *KIT* point mutations (2).

Mast Cell Activation Syndrome (MMCAS/IMCAS)*	1. Clinical symptomatology of mast cell activation such as: dermatographism or hives, diarrhea/abdominal pain, flushing, hypotension, headache, memory and concentration difficulties 2. A transient, measurable increase in either serum tryptase or other mast cell mediators (in urine such as N-methylhistamine [NMH]; prostaglandins [PG] D2 and F2; and leukotrienes [LT] D4, C4, and E4) 3. A response to agents that interferes with mast cell mediators (e.g. second-generation antihistamines or mast cell stabilizers)	
Cutaneous Mastocytosis (CM)^	**Major Criteria:** Typical skin lesions of mastocytosis associated with Darier's sign	**Minor Criteria:** Increased numbers of mast cells in biopsy sections of lesional skin + (Activating) KIT mutation in lesional skin tissue
Systemic Mastocytosis (SM)#	**Major Criteria:** Multifocal dense infiltrates of mast cells (MC) with ≥15 MCs in aggregates in bone marrow (BM) biopsies and/or in sections of other extracutaneous organ(s)	**Minor Criteria:** a. >25% of all MCs are atypical cells (type I or type II) on BM smears or are spindle-shaped in MC infiltrates detected on sections of visceral organs b. KIT point mutation at codon 816 in the BM or another extracutaneous organ c. Mast cells in BM or blood or another extracutaneous organ exhibit CD2 and/or CD25 d. Baseline serum tryptase level >20 ng/ml (in case of and unrelated myeloid neoplasm).

Figure 11.3 Diagnostic criteria of select Mast Cell Disorders.
*All three diagnostic criteria must be met. Significant tryptase elevation is an increase of 2+20% of baseline tryptase value above baseline. (Figure created with BioRender.com.) [Adapted from (6, 10).]
^Refined criteria for cutaneous involvement in patients with mastocytosis according to the "Consensus report of the European Competence Network on Mastocytosis; the American Academy of Allergy, Asthma and Immunology; and the European Academy of Allergology and Clinical Immunology", *Journal of Allergy and Clinical Immunology*, 2016. [Adapted from (27).]
Diagnostic criteria according to the 2016 "updated WHO classification and novel emerging treatment concepts" (13); at least one major plus one minor OR three minor criteria are required to be fulfilled.
(A) Typical red-brown urticaria pigmentosa on the thigh (B) Bone marrow biopsy stained for tryptase showing abnormal spindle-shaped mast cells in aggregates >15 diagnostic of systemic mastocytosis. (Image courtesy (A) of Dr. Michael Fein; Image courtesy (B) of Dr. René P. Michel.)

- However, detection of *KIT* D816V in peripheral blood of children with CM suggests SM (30).

3. **Genetic test** (buccal swab) **for *TPSAB1* gene:** To assess for HATS.
   - Useful as an initial test for patients with mildly elevated serum tryptase.
   - Presence of HATS may reduce need for a bone marrow biopsy; however, some patients with HATS and coexisting MCAS have been described (18, 31).
   - The role of testing for HATS in the diagnostic workup of MCAS in evolving (18):
     - Presently, the 2019 consensus guidelines (2) suggest testing for HATS if symptoms suggest MCA but MCAS criteria are not fulfilled.
     - Other groups have proposed a modified diagnostic algorithm where HATS testing is considered sooner, placing more value on non-invasive testing and only resorting to bone marrow biopsy if peripheral blood *KIT* D816V is negative and if prediction scores indicate a high likelihood of clonality (1, 18).

4. ***FIP1L1-PDGFRA* mutation:** Test in bone marrow or peripheral blood if associated peripheral eosinophilia is present to screen for chronic eosinophilic leukemia, which can present with elevated tryptase, splenomegaly, and MC clusters in bone marrow (2, 9).

5. **Other MC mediators** [Adapted from (26)]
   - 24-hour urine N-methylhistamine
     - Metabolite of serum histamine
     - Normal values vary with age
     - Normal 30–200 µg/g creatinine (age >16 years old)
     - Levels >400 µg/g creatinine correlate with monoclonal MC findings
   - 24-hour urine 11β-PGF2α (metabolite of PGD2)
     - PGD2 causes flushing, rhinitis, bronchoconstriction, vasodilation.
     - Normal reference <1000 ng/24 hours.
     - Level >3500 ng/24 hours correlates with monoclonal MC findings.
     - Aspirin may be effective at reducing flushing in patients with elevated PGD2.

- 24-hour urine leukotriene E4 (LTE4, metabolite of leukotriene C4)
  - Cysteinyl leukotrienes are produced by MCs, basophils, eosinophils, platelets, and endothelial cells and elevated levels are seen in many conditions.
  - Elevated urinary LTE4 >104 pg/mg of creatinine (normal reference 0–104 pg/mg) seen in SM, chronic urticaria, and other conditions.
- **Bone marrow evaluation**
  3. Bone marrow biopsy is currently the standard-of-care exam used to diagnose SM and is required to differentiate among subtypes of SM.
  4. Controversies exist in determining when a bone marrow biopsy is indicated and practice varies by center.
  5. Tryptase level may be used as a guide (see below) as normal levels significantly reduce the likelihood of SM, although do not rule out the diagnosis.
     - *Patients with a diagnosis of MCAS and normal tryptase levels (<8 ng/mL) typically do not require bone marrow biopsies.*

Bone marrow biopsy is recommended in the following cases according to basal serum tryptase levels; adapted from (32):

1. Basal serum tryptase ≥20 ng/mL
   a. Establishing the diagnosis of SM in patients with typical MCA symptoms.
2. Basal serum tryptase ≥15 ng/mL
   a. Identifying if patients with MCA symptoms have ISM or MMCAS.
3. Basal serum tryptase ≥11 ng/mL
   a. Patients with IA or MCAS.
   b. An adult with UP/MPCM.
      - If patients with UP/MPCM and lower tryptase levels develop anaphylaxis, bone marrow biopsy should be considered.
   c. An adult with unexplained hepatosplenomegaly (33) or osteoporosis (34–36).
   d. Patients with anaphylaxis to insect sting (23–24).

- **Imaging**
  1. Bone mineral density scan to evaluate for osteoporosis.
  2. Skeletal X-rays/computed tomography (CT) scans to evaluate for bone fractures.
  3. Abdominal ultrasound to rule out hepatosplenomegaly.

- **Exclusion of other differential diagnosis** (see selected examples below adapted from 1, 2, 14, 18)
  1. **Allergic disease:** Through total IgE and/or serum antigen specific IgE (e.g. Hymenoptera venom), skin-prick testing.
  2. **Endocrine disorders:** Hyperthyroidism, by checking thyroid function test.
  3. **Neuroendocrine disorders**
     - Parathyroid or medullary thyroid cancer (MTC), by testing parathyroid hormone, calcitonin (for MTC).
     - Carcinoid by testing urine 5-hydroxyindoleacetic acid (5-HIAA), chromogranin A.
     - Pheochromocytoma through urine metanephrines and/or catecholamines.
     - VIPoma or other secretory tumors (e.g. gastrinoma, or insulinoma).

Management

- **Avoidance of the potential triggers** causing nonspecific MC degranulation
  - Extremes of temperature, stress, exercise, spicy foods, alcohol.
  - Caution with certain medications: Opiates, vancomycin, radiocontrast media, NSAIDs, certain muscle relaxants.
- Intramuscular epinephrine for anaphylaxis (refer to Chapter 12 for complete management)
  - Patient should always carry their epinephrine auto-injector (two).
  - Anaphylaxis action plan should be provided to the patient.
  - MedicAlert (TM) bracelet and/or wallet cards detailing potential triggers and medications that should be avoided.
- Ask patients about their *quality of life* at each visit and screen for associated depression/anxiety.
  - Consider use of validated tools such as Mastocytosis Quality-of-Life Form (MQLF) or the shorter Mastocytosis Symptom Assessment Form (MSAF) (37).
- Rule out associated conditions and underlying organ damage
  - *Osteoporosis:* Practice varies, consider bone mineral density (BMD) every 2 years in stable patients with SM. Check vitamin D level and supplement as necessary (26).
  - *Venom hypersensitivity:* Testing along with possible immunotherapy in case of systemic/anaphylactic reaction to Hymenoptera venom sting.

- **Special considerations for major surgical/ medical procedures** premedication is typically required with anti-H1 and anti-H2 histamine receptor blockers, leukotriene receptor blocker, and 0.5 mg/kg of prednisone.
  - Anti-H1 combined with anti-H2 antihistamines may suffice for minor procedures (26).

Pharmacotherapy Approach [Adapted from 1, 7, 9, 26]

A. **CM**
  - *Antihistamines:* The most commonly used treatment of UP/MPCM.
    - Clinical results vary from complete resolution of symptoms (mainly pruritus) to no improvement.
  - Topical and oral corticosteroids: Used in DCM and mastocytoma.
    - Rapid regression and remission were observed when oral steroids were used in DCM.
    - Complete resolution and plaque regression was observed with topical steroids in mastocytoma.
  - *Phototherapy:* For UP/MPCM and DCM.

  - Improvement of pruritus but persistent cutaneous lesions in UP/MPCM.
  - Diminished dermographism and disappearance of skin thickening in DCM.

B. **SM**
  - Medical therapy for ISM is aimed at symptom control (see Table 11.1)
  - Cytoreductive therapy is used for aggressive subtypes associated with bone marrow dysfunction, organomegaly, skeletal lytic lesions, and/or malabsorption (9). For severe, refractory symptoms in ISM cytoreductive therapies may be considered.
    - Cytoreductive therapies include (9)
      - Cladribine, midostaurin, imatinib (not effective with *KIT* D816V mutation), interferon-alpha, allogeneic stem cell transplant.

Prognosis and Monitoring (3)

- Mastocytosis in children:
  - *CM:* Majority will regress.
    - Sixty-seven percent complete regression; 20% major regression; 13% partial regression (38).
  - *SM:* Majority will persist (38).

Table 11.1 Common Medications for Symptomatic Treatment in ISM

Drug class	Symptoms targeted and medication examples
H1-Antihistamine	Flushing, pruritus, headache, cognitive impairment. e.g. Cetirizine 10 mg PO daily
H2-Antihistamine	Gastrointestinal symptoms, cognitive impairment. e.g. Famotidine 20 mg PO BID
Leukotriene Antagonist	Pruritus, flushing e.g. Montelukast 10 mg PO daily
Mast Cell Stabilizer	Gastrointestinal symptoms, neuropsychiatric symptoms. e.g. Sodium cromolyn 200 mg PO QID before meals
H1-Antihistamine + Mast Cell Stabilizer	See above e.g. Ketotifen 1–2 mg PO BID
Non steroidal Anti-Inflammatory*	Pruritus, flushing e.g. Aspirin 81–325 mg PO daily
Proton Pump Inhibitor	Gastrointestinal symptoms e.g. Pantoprazole 40 mg PO daily
Bisphosphonate	Osteoporosis e.g. Risedronate 35 m PO weekly
Anti-IgE	Urticaria, anaphylaxis e.g. Omalizumab 300 mg S/C monthly

*Use caution when introducing non-steroidal anti-inflammatories (NSAIDS) if previous tolerance to NSAIDS is unknown.

Adapted from (7, 9, 26).

- Mastocytosis in adults
  - *CM:* Minority of patients will have regression of lesions but this does not correlate with bone marrow MC aggregate regression.
  - ISM in adults (39):
    - Normal to near-normal life expectancy.
    - Small risk of progression to more advanced disease which requires monitoring.
      - Cumulative risk in 10 years according to Escribano et al. (39) is 1.7%.
      - Serum B2-microglobulin and presence of *KIT* mutation in all hematopoietic cell lines independent predictors of progression (39).
  - More aggressive forms of SM have reduced survival depending on subtype and other factors and require more frequent monitoring.
- *Monitoring for progression:* For ISM, yearly monitoring with physical exam (for organomegaly, weight loss, skin changes), serum tryptase level, Complete blood count (CBC) with differential, serum chemistry panel for electrolytes, kidney function, B2-microglobulin, and liver function tests.
  - Consider periodic abdominal ultrasound.

SPECIAL POPULATIONS: PREGNANCY AND LACTATION

General Considerations

- The effect of mastocytosis on pregnancy outcomes and vice versa is unknown (40).
- Limited data from small cohort studies suggest an increased risk of preterm labor and birth (40).
- Patients with mastocytosis benefit from a preconceptual consultation to assess the stability of the disease and review medications prior to pregnancy (expert opinion).

Management during Pregnancy

- Generally, medications should be titrated to the lowest effective dose prior to pregnancy (41).
- First- and second-generation antihistamines have not been associated with an increased risk of birth defects and can be used throughout pregnancy (with preference for class B agents such as loratadine and cetirizine rather than class C agents such as fexofenadine and bilastine) (41).
- However, if adequate control is only achieved with class C agents, they should be continued throughout pregnancy to mitigate risk of mastocytosis exacerbation during pregnancy (expert opinion).
- H2 antihistamines can be continued without interruption during pregnancy (41).
- Glucocorticoids may be continued during pregnancy. Fluorinated glucocorticoids (betamethasone, dexamethasone) should be avoided or used sparingly (41, 42).
- Risks associated with glucocorticoid use during pregnancy include maternal diabetes and hypertension, preterm labor, small-for-gestational-age infants, and possible fetal cleft palate and fetal adrenal suppression at birth (42).
- MC stabilizer cromolyn is a category B drug in pregnancy and can be continued throughout pregnancy. Ketotifen should be used with caution and only when cromolyn is ineffective (41).
- Leukotriene antagonists can be used throughout pregnancy. 5-Lipoxygenase inhibitors should be avoided (41).
- Anti-IgE therapy (omalizumab) has not shown any adverse pregnancy outcomes and can be continued throughout pregnancy if favorable response pre-pregnancy. Omalizumab should not be initiated during pregnancy because of the risk of anaphylaxis (expert opinion).
- The management of anaphylaxis during pregnancy is outlined in Chapter 12.
- Patients requiring cytoreductive treatment (tyrosine kinase inhibitors, cladribine) should not become pregnant (41).
- Pregnant patients with SM benefit from a multidisciplinary team approach. They should be followed closely by allergy-immunology or hematology or maternal fetal medicine and high-risk obstetrics (expert opinion).
- Anesthesia should be consulted prior to delivery for opioid-free labor and delivery/postpartum pain management (41).
- Pre-medication with antihistamines, leukotriene receptor blockers, and corticosteroids should be considered prophylactically prior to delivery (41).

Breastfeeding [Adapted from 40–43]

- Second-generation rather than first-generation antihistamines are generally preferred.
- Famotidine and ranitidine are the preferred H2 antihistamines.

- Cromolyn should be used with precaution and ketotifen should be avoided.
- Glucocorticoids are excreted into breast milk and should be used at the lowest possible dose to control symptoms. Delaying breastfeeding 4 hours after the dose is generally recommended.
- Anti-leukotrienes are probably safe, but should be used with caution. 5-Lipoxygenase inhibitors should be avoided.
- Anti-IgE antibodies are excreted into breast milk. Breastfeeding is not recommended currently; however, data from small cohorts have not shown any harm to the infant.
- Cytoreductive treatments is contraindicated.

ABBREVIATIONS

CM	Cutaneous mastocytosis
COVID-19	Coronavirus disease 2019
DCM	Diffuse cutaneous mastocytosis
HAT	Hereditary alpha tryptasemia
HSCT	Hematopoietic stem cell transplantation
ISM	Indolent systemic mastocytosis
MC	Mast cell
MCA	Mast cell activation
MCL	MC Leukemia
MCAS	Mast cell activation syndrome
MMCAS	Monoclonal MCAS
MPCM	Maculopapular cutaneous mastocytosis
SARS-CoV-2	Severe acute respiratory syndrome coronavirus 2
ASM	Aggressive SM
SM	Systemic mastocytosis
SM-AHN	SM-associated hematologic neoplasm
SSM	Smoldering SM
UP	Urticaria pigmentosa

REFERENCES

1. Weiler CR et al., J Allergy Clin Immunol. (2019), PMID: 31476322/DOI:10.1016/j.jaci.2019.08.023.
2. Valent P et al., J Allergy Clin Immunol Pract. (2019), PMID: 30737190/DOI:10.1016/j.jaip.2019.01.006.
3. Brockow K, Immunol Allergy Clin North Am. (2014), PMID: 24745674/DOI:10.1016/j.iac.2014.01.003.
4. Cohen SS et al., Br J Haematol. (2014), PMID: 24761987/DOI:10.1111/bjh.12916.
5. van Doormaal JJ et al., J Allergy Clin Immunol. (2013), PMID: 23219169/DOI:10.1016/j.jaci.2012.10.015.
6. Theoharides TC et al., N Engl J Med. (2015), PMID: 26154789/DOI: 10.1056/NEJMra1409760.
7. Metcalfe DD. Mastocytosis. In: Burks AW, Holgate ST, O'Hehir RE, Bacharier LB, Broide DH, Hershey GK, Peebles Jr RS. Middleton's Allergy: Principles and Practice E-Book, Ninth Edition. Amsterdam: Elsevier. Available at: https://www.clinicalkey.com/dura/browse/bookChapter/3-s2.0-C20161002419 (Accessed: Jan 29, 2021).
8. Arber DA et al., Blood. (2016), PMID: 27069254/DOI:10.1182/blood-2016-03-643544.
9. Pardanani A, Am J Hematol. (2019), PMID: 30536695/DOI:10.1002/ajh.25371.
10. Berezowska S et al., Mod Pathol. (2014), PMID: 23807778/DOI: 10.1038/modpathol.2013.117.
11. Hartmann K et al., J Allergy Clin Immunol. (2016), PMID: 26476479/DOI: 10.1016/j.jaci.2015.08.034.
12. Caplan RM, Arch Dermatol. (1963), PMID: 14018418/DOI:10.1001/archderm.1963.01590140008002.
13. Ben-Amitai D et al., Isr Med Assoc J. (2005), PMID: 15909466
14. Le M et al., Postgrad Med. (2017), PMID: 28770635/DOI:10.1080/00325481.2017.1364124.
15. Fenny N et al., Immunol Allergy Clin North Am. (2015), PMID: 25841556/DOI:10.1016/j.iac.2015.01.004.
16. Carter MC et al., Ann Allergy Asthma Immunol. (2020), PMID: 31513910/DOI:10.1016/j.anai.2019.08.024.
17. Lyons JJ, Immunol Allergy Clin North Am. (2018), PMID: 30007465/DOI:10.1016/j.iac.2018.04.003.
18. Weiler CR, J Allergy Clin Immunol Pract. (2020), PMID: 31470118/DOI:10.1016/j.jaip.2019.08.022.
19. Sokol H et al., J Allergy Clin Immunol. (2013), PMID: 23890756/DOI:10.1016/j.jaci.2013.05.026.
20. Smith JH et al., Clin Neurol Neurosurg. (2011), PMID: 21664760/DOI:10.1016/j.clineuro.2011.05.002.
21. Moura DS et al., PLOS ONE. (2012), PMID: 22745762/DOI:10.1371/journal.pone.0039468.
22. Akin C et al., Blood. (2007), PMID: 17638853/DOI:10.1182/blood-2006-06-028100.
23. Brockow K et al., Allergy. (2008), PMID: 18186813/DOI:10.1111/j.1398-9995.2007.01569.x.
24. Bonadonna P et al., Allergy. (2009), PMID: 19627274/DOI: 10.1111/j.1398-9995.2009.02108.x.
25. Skrabs CC, Arch Dermatol. (2002), PMID: 12224998/DOI:10.1001/archderm.138.9.1253.
26. Castells M et al., J Allergy Clin Immunol Pract. (2019), PMID: 30961835/DOI:10.1016/j.jaip.2019.02.002.
27. Kristensen T et al., Allergy. (2017), PMID: 28432683/DOI:10.1111/all.13187.

28. Erben P et al., Ann Hematol. (2014), PMID: 24281161/DOI:10.1007/s00277-013-1964-1.

29. Kristensen T et al., J Mol Diagn. (2011), PMID: 21354053/DOI: 10.1016/j.jmoldx.2010.10.004.

30. Carter MC et al., Br J Haematol. (2018), PMID: 30488427/DOI:10.1111/bjh.15624.

31. Sabato V et al., J Allergy Clin Immunol. (2014), PMID: 25086867/DOI:10.1016/j.jaci.2014.06.007.

32. Greenberger PA et al., J Allergy Clin Immunol Pract. (2019), PMID: 30630762/DOI: 10.1016/j.jaip.2018.11.019.

33. Mican JM et al., Hepatology. (1995), PMID: 7557867/DOI:10.1016/0270-9139(95)90625-8.

34. Brumsen C et al., Bone. (2002), PMID: 12477568/DOI:10.1016/s8756-3282(02)00875-x.

35. Guillaume N et al., Am J Med. (2013), PMID: 23200108/DOI: 10.1016/j.amjmed.2012.07.018.

36. Chen CC et al., J Nucl Med. (1994), PMID: 8071694.

37. van Anrooij B et al., Allergy. (2016), PMID: 27089859/DOI:10.1111/all.12920.

38. Uzzaman A et al., Pediatr Blood Cancer. (2009), PMID: 19526526/DOI:10.1002/pbc.22125.

39. Escribano L et al., J Allergy Clin Immunol. (2009), PMID: 19541349/DOI:10.1016/j.jaci.2009.05.003.

40. Matito A et al., Int Arch Allergy Immunol. (2011), PMID: 21447966/DOI:10.1159/000321954.

41. Türk M et al., J Allergy Clin Immunol Pract. (2020), PMID: 31374358/DOI: 10.1016/j.jaip.2019.07.021.

42. Bandoli G et al., Rheum Dis Clin North Am. (2017), PMID: 28711148/DOI: 10.1016/j.rdc.2017.04.013.

43. Lei D et al., J Allergy Clin Immunol Pract. (2017), PMID: 28739366/DOI:10.1016/j.jaip.2017.05.021.

12

Anaphylaxis

ABEER FETEIH, MICHAEL FEIN, NATACHA TARDIO,
GENEVIÈVE GENEST, LYDIA ZHANG, HOANG PHAM,
AND MOSHE BEN-SHOSHAN

GENERAL BACKGROUND

- **Definition:** "Anaphylaxis is a serious allergic reaction that is rapid in onset and may cause death" (1).
- **Lifetime prevalence:** Estimated to be between 1.6% and 5.1% (2).
- **Fatality rate:** Rare outcome with a population prevalence rate of 0.47–0.69 per million persons (0.25%–0.33% of anaphylaxis hospitalization or emergency department [ED] visits) (2).
- Recent studies suggest an increased rate of anaphylaxis visits in Canadian emergency rooms (3, 4).
- The risk of recurrent anaphylaxis in Canada is reported to be almost 20% (5).

Pathogenesis (2, 6)

- The classic mechanism in many cases of anaphylaxis involves mast cell degranulation:
  - In presensitized individuals, subsequent exposure to an allergen results in IgE binding and cross-linking of the high-affinity IgE receptor (FcεRI) on the surface of mast cells (and basophils), stimulating the release of preformed biogenic amines mediators (e.g. histamine, tryptase), the de novo synthesis of lipid mediators (e.g. leukotrienes, prostaglandins, platelet activating factor), and the release of both preformed and newly formed cytokines (e.g. tumor necrosis factor).
  - Histamine (the most important preformed mediator): Causes flushing, airway obstruction, tachycardia, and systemic hypotension.
- May also involve additional cell types such as neutrophils, monocytes, macrophages, and platelets and signaling through additional mediators (e.g. complement-mediated mechanisms involving anaphylatoxins C3a, C4a, C5a).
- As a result of advances in drug hypersensitivity, additional forms of anaphylaxis are now recognized, particularly in the context of hypersensitivity to chemotherapeutics and monoclonal antibodies.
  - Cytokine-storm-like
  - Mixed type with both mast cell involvement and cytokine release

Etiologies (2, 6)

- **Foods**
  - Most common trigger in children, teens, and young adults (e.g. cow's milk, hen's egg, peanut, tree nuts, shellfish, and fish)
- **Medications**
  - Most common trigger in adults (e.g. antimicrobial, antiviral, and antifungal agents; nonsteroidal anti-inflammatories [NSAIDs]; chemotherapeutic agents; biologics)
- **Insect stings**
  - Common trigger in both adults and children (e.g. honey bees, yellow jackets, yellow hornets, white-faced hornets, paper wasps, fire ants)
- **Radiocontrast media**
- **Perioperative agents**
  - Chlorhexidine, latex, neuromuscular blocking agents, local anesthetics, propofol, opioids, sedatives, protamine, colloid plasma expanders, blue dyes
- **Allergy diagnostic tests/interventions**
  - Food or drug provocation challenges, allergy desensitization procedures, allergen or venom immunotherapy, allergy skin tests (particularly intradermal tests)

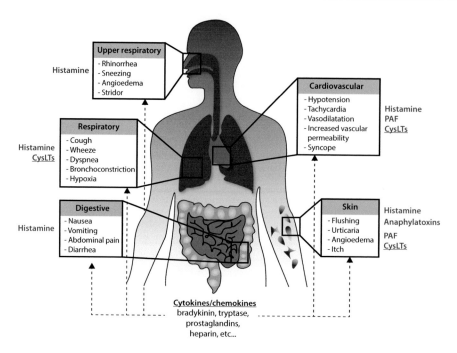

Figure 12.1 Pathophysiology and clinical manifestations of anaphylaxis. [Reprinted with permission from (22) Journal of Allergy and Clinical Immunology, The pathophysiology of anaphylaxis. Laurent L. Reber, Joseph D. Hernandez, Stephen J. Galli, Aug 1, 2017, Volume 140, with permission from Elsevier.]

- **Exercise**
  - Can act as both a cause as well as a cofactor in anaphylaxis
- **Seminal fluid**
  - Rare
- **Aeroallergens**
  - Rare (e.g. systemic reactions to horses have been reported) (7)
- **Idiopathic**
  - Diagnosis of exclusion after a detailed history, allergy skin tests, specific IgE levels, food/drug challenges, screening for previously unrecognized "hidden" triggers (e.g. alpha-1,3 galactose) or clonal mast cell disorders

Clinical Manifestations

- **Onset of symptoms:** Usually occurs within minutes after being exposed to the allergen, but can occur up to a few hours after.
- **Uniphasic course:** Symptoms start resolving within hours of management.
- **Biphasic course**
  - A recurrence of anaphylaxis occurring about 1–72 hours after resolution of initial episode (2).
  - Estimated to occur from less than 1%–20% (2).

Signs and Symptoms of Anaphylaxis [Adapted from 1, 2, 6]

- **Skin:** Urticaria, angioedema, flushing, pruritus
- **Respiratory:**
  - **Upper airway:** Nasal congestion, sneezing, hoarseness, cough, laryngeal edema
  - **Lower airway:** Dyspnea, cough, bronchospasm/wheezing, chest tightness
- **Cardiovascular:** Hypotension, tachycardia, dizziness, syncope
- **Gastrointestinal/genitourinary:** Nausea, vomiting, abdominal pain, diarrhea, uterine cramping
- **Neurologic:** Dizziness, confusion
- **Oropharyngeal:** Pruritus, tingling, angioedema
- **Other:** Anxiety, sense of imminent doom

Important Aspects of the History (6)

- History of symptoms of the anaphylaxis event (see above), including severity of symptoms.
- Time of occurrence of attack.
- Setting of occurrence (home, school, work, and restaurant).
- Treatments administered during the episode (including timing of epinephrine administration).

- Explore possible etiologies (see General Background: Etiologies):
  - Known patient allergies?
  - Ingestants consumed (food, medications) within 6 hours of the event?
  - Sting or bites occurring before the event?
  - Association with sexual activity?
- Explore possible cofactors that may have amplified/augmented the reaction:
  - Exercise, alcohol, NSAIDs, infection, stress, premenstrual status in women
- Review past medical history that may have contributed to the clinical presentation or impact treatment:
  - Prior episodes of anaphylaxis.
  - Atopy (asthma, eczema, allergic rhinitis).
    - Atopy is more common in food-induced, seminal-fluid related, and idiopathic anaphylaxis.
  - Skin disorders (e.g., chronic spontaneous urticaria, hereditary angioedema).
  - Cardiovascular disease (which may reduce physiologic reserve to anaphylaxis).

DIAGNOSIS AND INVESTIGATIONS

Diagnostic Criteria

As stated by the "National Institute of Allergy and Infectious Disease and Food Allergy and Anaphylaxis Network" (Adapted from 1, 2, 6, 21)

- Anaphylaxis is highly likely (sensitivity 95%, specificity 71%) when of one of the following three criteria is met (2):
  - Acute onset of mucocutaneous symptoms PLUS at least one symptom of respiratory compromise OR hypotension in the event of an unwitnessed/unknown exposure.
  - Acute onset of symptoms involving two or more organ systems (mucocutaneous, respiratory, cardiovascular, or gastrointestinal) after exposure to a likely allergen for that patient.
  - Acute onset of hypotension after exposure to known allergy for that patient (1).

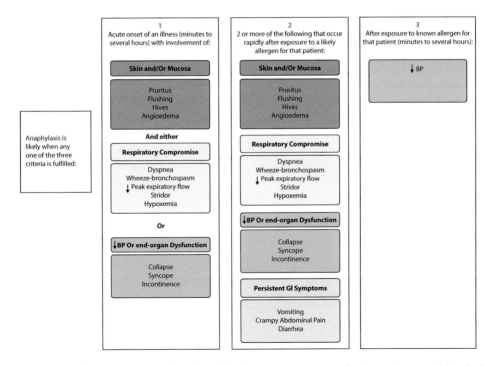

Figure 12.2 Visual representation of the National Institute of Allergy and Infectious Disease and Food Allergy and Anaphylaxis Network criteria for anaphylaxis (21). Diagnosis of anaphylaxis is challenging due to its heterogeneous presentation. Diagnosis is likely when any one of the above three criteria are met. (Image reproduced with permission from Manivannan, V., et al. *Int J Emerg Med* 2, 3–5 (2009). This work is licensed under a Creative Commons Attribution. http://creativecommons.org/licenses/by/4.0/.)

Differential Diagnosis of Anaphylaxis and Its Mimickers [Adapted from the "Anaphylaxis Practice Parameter Update," 2015, Lieberman et al. (6)]

- Vasovagal reaction
- *Flushing syndromes:* Carcinoid, medullary carcinoma of the thyroid, vasointestinal polypeptide (VIP) tumors, mastocytosis and mast cell activation syndrome, rosacea, alcohol-induced flushing
- *Restaurant syndromes:* Scombroid poisoning, monosodium glutamate
- *Nonorganic (selected):* Vocal cord dysfunction syndrome, panic attacks, Munchausen syndrome
- *Other:* hereditary angioedema with rash, paradoxical pheochromocytoma, red man syndrome from vancomycin, capillary leak syndrome

Severity Grading of Anaphylaxis (8)

- It is important to document the severity of anaphylaxis to aid in management, including length of observation period required and creating an anaphylaxis action plan in case of future reactions.

Investigations in Anaphylaxis and Differential Diagnosis [Adapted from (6, 9)]

Tests to Be Done during or Shortly after an Anaphylaxis Attack

- **Serum tryptase level** (most easily attainable): Peaks 60–90 minutes after the symptoms of anaphylaxis start and remains high for at least 5 hours (6).
  - During anaphylaxis, tryptase level should increase by 2 ng/mL + 1.2× (baseline or post 24-hour reaction tryptase level) (9).

- **Plasma histamine:** Remains elevated for only 30–60 minutes.
- **Urine 24-hour histamine metabolites and prostaglandin D2:** May only be available in specialized centers.
- Investigations for alternate causes of symptoms if suspected by the history.

Tests for Determining the Cause of Anaphylaxis

- **Skin prick testing:** In general performed 4–6 weeks after an anaphylactic reaction to a suspected allergen (e.g. food, medication, venom, other). However, some studies suggest that a waiting period as short as 1 week may be sufficient (10).
  - A refractory period lasting up to 6 weeks after an insect sting may occur; therefore, testing should be repeated at this time to avoid a false-negative result (10).
- **Serum-specific IgE:** If indicated (e.g. food, alpha-gal IgE).
- **Other tests:** Depending on the clinical scenario (e.g. basal serum tryptase level/bone marrow biopsy in suspected mastocytosis). (Refer to Chapter 11).

Tests for Alternative Diagnoses (Selected) (6)

- *Carcinoid:* Serum serotonin and urinary 5-hydroxyindoleacetic acid, chromogranin A
- *VIP tumor:* Vasointestinal polypeptide, substance P, urokinase A
- *Pheochromocytoma:* Plasma-free metanephrines, serum catecholamines and 24-hour urinary catecholamines, chromogranin A
- *Imaging for tumors:* Such as computed tomography (CT) scan, positron emission tomography (PET) scan, magnetic resonance imaging (MRI)

Table 12.1 Grading Severity of Anaphylaxis

Mild (skin and subcutaneous tissues only)*
- Generalized erythema, urticaria, periorbital edema, or angioedema

Moderate (features suggesting respiratory, cardiovascular, or gastrointestinal involvement)
- ·Dyspnea, stridor, wheeze, nausea, vomiting, dizziness (presyncope), diaphoresis, chest or throat tightness, or abdominal pain

Severe (hypoxia, hypotension, or neurologic compromise)
- Cyanosis or $SpO_2 < 92\%$ at any stage, hypotension (SBP < 90 mm Hg in adults), confusion, collapse, LOC, or incontinence

Mild reactions can be further subclassified into those with and without angioedema.
Abbreviations: LOC: Loss of consciousness; SBP: Systolic blood pressure
Reprinted with permission from (8) Brown SG. Clinical features and severity grading of anaphylaxis. J Allergy Clin Immunol. 2004 Aug;114(2):371–6, with permission from Elsevier.

Management

Acute Management [Approach Adapted from (1, 2, 6)]

1. Assess the patient's **circulation, airway, breathing (CAB)**, vital signs, and level of consciousness.
2. **Epinephrine**: Should be given immediately to any patient with suspected anaphylaxis. There is no contraindication to the use of epinephrine if medically indicated.
   - Studies support the fact that prompt administration of epinephrine compared with antihistamines/corticosteroids has the highest impact on anaphylaxis management and reduces the risk of uncontrolled reactions and death (11).
   - *Dose:* 0.01 mg/kg (maximum 0.5 mg) given intramuscularly (IM) every 5–15 minutes as needed (1, 2, 6, 12, 13).
   - *Site of injection:* Anterolateral thigh (allows more rapid absorption and higher plasma epinephrine levels compared with subcutaneous or IM administration in the upper arm) (2).
3. **Glucagon**: Consider administering to patients who are taking beta-blockers. Dose range is 1–5 mg IV bolus followed by 5–15 mcg/min infusion.
4. Transfer any patient who receives epinephrine to a hospital ED for evaluation and observation.
5. **Positioning**: Supine position unless there is respiratory compromise; pregnant women should be positioned on their left side (6).
6. **Supportive therapy**
   - **Inhaled beta 2 agonists (e.g. salbutamol)**: For bronchospasm.
   - **Antihistamines**: For hives/skin symptoms.
   - **Supplemental oxygen**: Consider in any patient with anaphylaxis.
   - **Intravenous (IV) crystalloid fluids**: For hypotension if not responding to epinephrine.
   - **Vasopressors**: Such as dopamine, if the patient is still hypotensive despite epinephrine and IV fluids.
   - **Corticosteroids**: Sometimes given empirically but has not been shown to be effective for *acute* treatment; may prevent biphasic/prolonged reactions but there is no definite evidence that they prevent a biphasic response (11).
   - **Further observation**: After acute management, patients need to be observed until symptoms resolve and for a period of time due to the risk of a biphasic response.
     - Recent guidelines suggest 1-hour observation for resolved mild-moderate anaphylaxis and a longer period for severe anaphylaxis (2).
   - **If anaphylaxis fails to respond to the above treatments:**
     - IV epinephrine drip ± intubation with mechanical ventilation depending on the respiratory status.
     - Methylene blue (inhibitor of guanylyl cyclase): can be used in cases of refractory anaphylaxis with observed clinical responses within 20 minutes. Dose range 1.5–2.0 mg/kg bolus and/or infusion (14).

Long-Term Management

- **Educate** on how to recognize and treat an allergic reaction.
- Prescription of an **epinephrine auto-injector** with education on its use and demonstration of technique (6).
- **Evaluation by an allergist** to try to identify the cause of the anaphylaxis (e.g. skin testing with suspected food, drugs, venom), further testing, assessing the need for immunotherapy depending on the cause of the anaphylaxis, and follow-up (6, 10).
- **Avoidance measures** if the cause of anaphylaxis is identified (6).
- Develop an **anaphylaxis action plan** for the patient (6).
- Advise the patient to obtain and wear a medical identifier (such as a **MedicAlert® bracelet**) indicating relevant allergies.

Dose of Epinephrine Auto-Injector

- Given that the weight-based dosing for IM epinephrine for anaphylaxis is 0.01 mg/kg, it is recommended to select an auto-injector dose that approximates the weight-based dosing: 0.15 mg, 0.30 mg, or 0.5mg (based on fixed preloaded auto-injector devices available in Canada, which are EpiPen, Allerject, and Emerade).
  - Weight ≥30 kg: 0.30 mg.
  - Weight between 15 and 30 kg: 0.15 mg.
    - Some sources recommend using the 0.30 mg dose at 25 kg rather than 30 kg (15).

- Weight <15 kg: A dilemma exists for children/infants weighing below 15 kg given no auto-injector is available for this weight range. Some sources suggest it is reasonable to use the 0.15-mg dose while discussing benefits and risks with family (15).

Patient Education and Counseling on Avoidance Measures

- **Educate on cofactors** (can reduce reaction threshold): Exercise, stress, acetylsalicylic acid (ASA), NSAIDs, alcohol, menstruation, and viral infections, among others (6).
- **Instruct to read food labels** carefully and be mindful of hidden ingredients such as "natural flavor" or "spices" that may imply allergen presence (e.g., peanut, tree nuts, milk, egg, shellfish, fish, sesame, soy and wheat), and "may contain" signs (6).

SPECIAL POPULATIONS: PREGNANCY AND LACTATION

Epidemiology

- Anaphylaxis during pregnancy or at birth is a rare event occurring in 3–5 cases per 100,000 hospitalizations while pregnant, but the incidence seems to be increasing (16–18).
- 60% of cases occur during cesarean section (18).
- In patients undergoing cesarean section, the incidence of anaphylaxis can be as high as 7.7 per 100,000 deliveries (18).
- Anaphylaxis during pregnancy and in the postpartum period has a case fatality rate as high as 0.09 per 100,000 maternities (16).
- Prior to labor and delivery, the causes of anaphylaxis mirror those in the general population (17).
- In cases of anaphylaxis during delivery, several agents have been implicated including beta-lactams, oxytocin, and other perioperative drugs (17).
- In cases of anaphylaxis postpartum, these usually occur 72 hours after delivery and can be associated with NSAIDs commonly prescribed for post-delivery pain (17).

Diagnosis

- Skin prick testing is generally acceptable and low-risk in pregnancy. However, caution should be exercised if skin testing is performed with the suspected culprit of an anaphylactic reaction, and skin testing should be delayed until after delivery (expert opinion).
- Intradermal testing carries a risk of anaphylaxis and should be delayed until the postpartum period (17); an exception to this may be penicillin skin testing in a patient without a history of anaphylaxis to penicillin (19).
- Anaphylaxis during pregnancy may manifest predominantly with hypotension and may present with coexistent atypical symptoms such as low back pain, uterine pain (cramps), vaginal itching, and signs of preterm labor or fetal distress. However, most cases present typically as they do in non-pregnant individuals (17).
- The diagnosis of anaphylaxis during pregnancy is more complicated than the non-gravid state as several conditions specific to pregnancy may mimic anaphylaxis:
  - Hypotension can occur during local anesthesia (spinal shock) or with volume depletion (nausea and vomiting) or hemorrhage.
  - Hypotension can also occur in the context of amniotic fluid embolism, peripartum cardiomyopathy, acute myocardial infarction, and pulmonary embolism.
  - Anaphylaxis can usually be distinguished by accompanying symptoms such as bronchospasm and urticaria/angioedema (17).
  - Tryptase is not a reliable marker in peripartum anaphylaxis (20).
  - Tryptase may be elevated in other conditions mimicking anaphylaxis such as peripartum cardiomyopathy, myocardial infarction, and amniotic fluid embolism and pulmonary embolism (17).
  - Laryngopathia gravidarum can present acutely in patients with preeclampsia (usually accompanied by edema and hypertension) and must be differentiated from laryngeal obstruction caused by anaphylaxis (17).

Management

- Pregnant patients with known food or drug allergies should have an anaphylaxis action plan and appropriate medical identification.
- Fetal oxygenation is compromised by maternal hypotension and hypoxemia. Consequences of this may include anoxic encephalopathy.

- The management of anaphylaxis during pregnancy is similar to the non-pregnant state:
  - IM epinephrine should not be delayed and should be given at usual doses and frequency (17, 18).
  - The patient should be placed in the left lower decubitus position if in the second or third trimester with legs elevated (17).
  - High-flow oxygen should be rapidly administered; two peripheral large-bore IV accesses should be installed for volume resuscitation in case of hypotension (17, 18).
  - Continuous fetal monitoring should also be performed in addition to non-invasive maternal monitoring. A minimum maternal systolic blood pressure of 90 mmHg should be maintained (17).
  - If required, endotracheal intubation should be performed by an anesthetist with obstetric experience (potential difficult airway) (17).
  - If protracted hypotension, IV phenylephrine may be most effective to maintain maternal blood pressure without compromising fetal blood flow. However, careful IV epinephrine titration is adequate as well and is still the standard of care (17).
  - Emergency cesarean section may be indicated in the case of severe, refractory and protracted anaphylactic reaction to reduce the fetal risk of hypoxic brain injury. However, significant risks to the fetus include prematurity and maternal risks include those associated with surgery in a medically unstable patient (17).
  - The decision to perform an emergency Cesarean section in this situation must be individualized and performed with input from obstetrics.

REFERENCES

1. Sampson HA et al., J Allergy Clin Immunol. (2006), PMID: 16461139/DOI:10.1016/j.jaci.2005.12.1303.
2. Shaker MS et al., J Allergy Clin Immunol. (2020), PMID: 32001253/DOI:10.1016/j.jaci.2020.01.017.
3. Hochstadter E et al., J Allergy Clin Immunol. (2016), PMID: 27106202/DOI:10.1016/j.jaci.2016.02.016.
4. Miles BT et al., J Allergy Clin Immunol Pract. (2020), PMID: 32244023/DOI:10.1016/j.jaip.2020.03.014.
5. O'Keefe A et al., J Pediatr. (2017), PMID: 27743592/DOI:10.1016/j.jpeds.2016.09.028.
6. Lieberman P et al., Ann Allergy Asthma Immunol. (2015), PMID: 26505932/DOI:10.1016/j.anai.2015.07.019.
7. Davenport J et al., Clin Rev Allergy Immunol. (2020), PMID: 32876923/DOI:10.1007/s12016-020-08807-4.
8. Brown SG, J Allergy Clin Immunol. (2004), PMID: 15316518/DOI:10.1016/j.jaci.2004.04.029.
9. De Schryver S et al., J Allergy Clin Immunol. (2016), PMID: 26478007/DOI:10.1016/j.jaci.2015.09.001.
10. Bernstein IL et al., Ann Allergy Asthma Immunol. (2008), PMID: 18431959/DOI:10.1016/s1081-1206(10)60305-5.
11. Gabrielli S et al., J Allergy Clin Immunol Pract. (2019), PMID: 31035000/DOI:10.1016/j.jaip.2019.04.018.
12. Simons FE et al., J Allergy Clin Immunol. (1998), PMID: 9449498/DOI:10.1016/S0091-6749(98)70190-3.
13. Simons FE et al., J Allergy Clin Immunol. (2001), PMID: 11692118/DOI:10.1067/mai.2001.119409.
14. Evora PR et al., Ann Allergy Asthma Immunol. (2007), PMID: 17941276/DOI:10.1016/S1081-1206(10)60545-5.
15. Sicherer SH et al., Pediatrics. (2017), PMID: 28193791/DOI: 10.1542/peds.2016-4006.
16. McCall SJ et al., BJOG. (2018), PMID: 29193647/DOI:10.1111/1471-0528.15041.
17. Simons FE et al., J Allergy Clin Immunol. (2012), PMID: 22871389/DOI:10.1016/j.jaci.2012.06.035.
18. McCall SJ et al., J Allergy Clin Immunol Pract. (2019), PMID: 31102701/DOI:10.1016/j.jaip.2019.04.047.
19. Blumenthal KG et al., JAMA. (2020), PMID: 32207800/DOI:10.1001/jama.2019.19809.
20. Sleth JC, Int J Obstet Anesth. (2018), PMID: 29653877/DOI:10.1016/j.ijoa.2018.02.007.
21. Manivannan, V. et al., Int J Emerg Med. (2009), PMID: 19390910/DOI:10.1007/s12245-009-0093-z.
22. Reber, Laurent L. et al., J Allergy Clin Immunology. (2017), PMID: 28780941/DOI:10.1016/j.jaci.2017.06.003.

13

Exercise-Induced Anaphylaxis (EIA) and Food-Dependent EIA (FDEIA)

ABEER FETEIH, LYDIA ZHANG, NATACHA TARDIO, AND MICHAEL FEIN

GENERAL BACKGROUND

- Exercise-induced anaphylaxis (EIA) and food-dependent EIA (FDEIA) are rare, potentially life-threatening conditions, characterized by their association with exercise (1).
- Little epidemiologic data exist regarding the prevalence of EIA and FDEIA.
- The prevalence of EIA was estimated at 0.03% in Japanese junior-high students (2). The same group reported the prevalence of FDEIA to be 0.005% in elementary school children and 0.02% in junior high-aged children (3, 4).
- In EIA, the same exercise may not always result in anaphylaxis in the same patient (5).
- In FDEIA, the culprit food is usually consumed **within 4–6 hours prior to exercise** to produce symptoms (5).
- The pathophysiology of EIA and FDEIA is not entirely understood.
  - Different hypotheses exist that relate to the probable influence of exercise on the development of anaphylactic symptoms, which include increased gastrointestinal permeability (6, 7), blood flow redistribution (8), increased osmolality (9, 10), acid-base disturbances, and release of gastrin and endogenous opioids during exercise (26).

Clinical Manifestations

- **Initial symptoms in EIA:** Diffuse warmth, pruritus, fatigue, erythema, hives/urticaria, angioedema, gastrointestinal symptoms, laryngeal edema, and/or cardiovascular collapse if exercise is continued (11, 12).
- **Triggers:** Moderate intensity exercise; however, there is no completely safe level or intensity of exercise for those with EIA (11). In a subgroup of patients with EIA, the association of high humidity and cold and warm environments have been reported (13).
- **Co-triggers that have been reported with EIA:** Any food (15), nonsteroidal anti-inflammatory drugs (NSAIDs) (16, 17), alcohol, menstruation (13), seasonal pollen exposure in those who are sensitized (11), infection, increased body temperature (heat and humidity), and psychological stress (26).
- **FDEIA:** Individuals with a food co-trigger can consume the food without symptoms or exercise without symptoms, but if they eat the food and then exercise, they will develop anaphylaxis (5).

Diagnosis and Investigations

- **EIA and FDEIA are clinical diagnoses (26, 27)**
  - **EIA:** Signs and symptoms compatible with anaphylaxis during or within an hour of exercise and no alternative diagnosis.
  - **FDEIA:** Must meet the above criteria and have an associated food trigger; evidence of IgE-mediated sensitivity to the culprit food; no symptoms upon ingestion of the food in the absence of exercise.
- Detailed history is critical: Focus on the type and intensity of the activity, symptom onset, food consumption, medication use, time of year, and presence of cofactors (26).
- Can be confirmed by a **controlled exercise challenge,** which may trigger usual symptoms (although symptoms may be difficult to reproduce) and if negative, it does not rule out EIA (20, 21).
- Skin prick test (SPT), specific IgE (sIgE) to suspect foods for FDEIA.

DOI: 10.1201/9781003174202-17

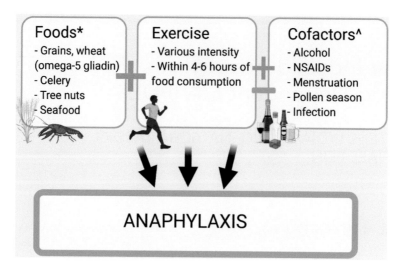

Figure 13.1 Food-dependent exercise-induced anaphylaxis (FDEIA).
* Most common food triggers; many other foods have been reported as well (14, 15, 18). Avoiding culprit foods may allow patients to exercise without developing anaphylaxis (14, 16, 19); patients usually can ingest culprit foods without anaphylaxis if they avoid exercise 4 to 6 hours after consumption (14).
^ Cofactors decrease reaction thresholds in all etiologies of anaphylaxis (FDEIA/EIA). (Figure created with BioRender.com.) [Adapted from (14–16, 18–19).]

Immediate management:

Epinephrine auto-injector (refer to anaphylaxis chapter)

Prior to exercise:

Avoid potential co-factors:
Specific foods (4-6 hours prior)
NSAIDS (avoid 24-48 hours prior)
Extremes of temperature, humid weather, pollen season alcohol

Consider pre-medication:
H1-antihistamines, leukotriene antagonists, mast cell stabilizers may help prevent FDEIA (23-25)

Medic-Alert Bracelet™

During exercise (5):

Carry two epinephrine auto-injectors
Always exercise with someone else educated about EIA/FDEIA or in a supervised location
If any signs or symptoms of anaphylaxis, stop immediately

Figure 13.2 Management of EIA/FDEIA. (Figure created with BioRender.com.) [Adapted from (5, 23–25).]

- sIgE epitope peptides of omega-5 gliadin and high-molecular-weight glutenin for **wheat-dependent EIA** (22).
- Assessment for other diagnoses is recommended, in particular **mastocytosis**, thus evaluation should include a **serum tryptase** and skin examination for cutaneous stigmata of mastocytosis (26, 27).
- Other differential diagnoses of EIA and FDEIA includes idiopathic anaphylaxis, cholinergic urticaria with systemic symptoms, exercise-associated gastroesophageal reflux, postural orthostatic tachycardia syndrome (27).

Management

- Key principles include **education** to prevent reactions, minimizing risk, and preparedness to treat any reactions (Figure 13.2).

REFERENCES

1. Barg W et al., Curr Allergy Asthma Rep. (2011), PMID: 20922508/DOI:10.1007/s11882-010-0150-y.
2. Aihara Y et al., J Allergy Clin Immunol. (2001), PMID: 11742285/DOI:10.1067/mai.2001.119914.
3. Manabe T et al., Allergol Int. (2015), PMID: 26117264/DOI:10.1016/j.alit.2015.01.007.
4. Manabe T et al., Pediatr Int. (2018), PMID: 29341364/DOI:10.1111/ped.13520.
5. Lieberman P et al., Ann Allergy Asthma Immunol. (2015), PMID: 26505932. 2015;115(5):341-84/DOI:10.1016/j.anai.2015.07.019.
6. Hanakawa Y et al., Br J Dermatol. (1998), PMID: 9666843/DOI:10.1046/j.1365-2133.1998.02254.x.
7. Matsuo H et al., Clin Exp Allergy. (2005), PMID: 15836754/DOI:10.1111/j.1365-2222.2005.02213.x.
8. Robson-Ansley P et al., Curr Opin Allergy Clin Immunol. (2010), PMID: 20543674/DOI:10.1097/ACI.0b013e32833b9bb0.
9. Barg W et al., J Investig Allergol Clin Immunol. (2008), PMID: 18714542.
10. Wolanczyk-Medrala A et al., Ann Agric Environ Med. (2009), PMID: 20047266.
11. Shadick NA et al., J Allergy Clin Immunol. (1999), PMID: 10400849/DOI:10.1016/s0091-6749(99)70123-5.
12. Sheffer AL et al., J Allergy Clin Immunol. (1980), PMID: 7400473/DOI:10.1016/0091-6749(80)90056-1.
13. Wade JP et al., Prog Clin Biol Res. (1989), PMID: 2587584
14. Dohi M et al., J Allergy Clin Immunol. (1991), PMID: 1991921/DOI:10.1016/0091-6749(91)90210-f.
15. Kidd JM, 3rd et al., J Allergy Clin Immunol. (1983), PMID: 6833679/DOI:10.1016/0091-6749(83)90070-2.
16. Lewis J et al., J Allergy Clin Immunol. (1981), PMID: 7310010/DOI:10.1016/0091-6749(81)90197-4.
17. Harada S et al., Br J Dermatol. (2001), PMID: 11531805/DOI:10.1046/j.1365-2133.2001.04329.x.
18. Kim CW et al., Nutr Res Pract. (2013), PMID: 24133612/DOI:10.4162/nrp.2013.7.5.347.
19. Novey HS et al., J Allergy Clin Immunol. (1983), PMID: 6841829/DOI:10.1016/0091-6749(83)90468-2.
20. Romano A et al., Int Arch Allergy Immunol. (2001), PMID: 11490160/DOI:10.1159/000053825.
21. Sheffer AL et al., J Allergy Clin Immunol. (1983), PMID:6826991/DOI:10.1016/0091-6749(83)90085-4.
22. Matsuo H et al., J Immunol. (2005), PMID: 16339549/DOI:10.4049/jimmunol.175.12.8116.
23. Peroni DG et al., Ann Allergy Asthma Immunol. (2010), PMID: 20377120/DOI:10.1016/j.anai.2009.12.002.
24. Choi JH et al., Ann Dermatol. (2009), PMID: 20523788/DOI:10.5021/ad.2009.21.2.203.
25. Sugimura T et al., Clin Pediatr (Phila). (2009), PMID: 19483137/DOI:10.1177/0009922809337528.
26. Gianetti MP, Curr Allergy Asthma Rep. (2018), PMID: 30367321/DOI:10.1007/s11882-018-0830-6.
27. Feldweg AM, J Allergy Clin Immunol Pract. (2017), PMID: 28283153/DOI:10.1016/j.jaip.2016.11.022.

14

Stinging Insect Hypersensitivity

ABEER FETEIH, HOANG PHAM, WALAA ALMASRI,
AND GENEVIÈVE GENEST

GENERAL BACKGROUND

- Most reactions to insect stings are local, short-lived, and resolve spontaneously without medical therapy.
- Hypersensitivity reactions include local reactions, large local reactions (LLRs), systemic cutaneous reactions, and systemic reactions (anaphylaxis).
- Venom hypersensitivity is a well-known cause of anaphylaxis, which may be fatal, and subsequently there may be anxiety/uncertainty among the general population regarding need for testing and treatment.
- Patients with *any* hypersensitivity reaction may benefit from consultation with an allergist/immunologist for education on future risk and testing/treatment through a shared decision-making approach.
- Positive serum or skin test results for venom IgE is >20% in healthy adults, especially in the months after a sting (1); therefore, *routine* testing is not indicated.
- Of those individuals who are sensitized (without symptoms), 5%–15% will have a systemic reaction to a later sting, and most will lose the sensitivity over time (2, 3).
- **Mastocytosis** occurs in about 2% of patients with insect sting anaphylaxis, and insect sting anaphylaxis occurs in approximately 25% of patients with mastocytosis (4).
  - May consider screening patients with mastocytosis for venom sensitization without prior history of a sting (5).

STINGING INSECT FAMILIES OF THE ORDER OF HYMENOPTERA (6)

Family Apidae

1. **Honeybee (*Apis mellifera* spp.)**
   - Domestic honeybees: found in commercial hives.
   - Non-domestic honeybees: nest in tree hollows, old logs, buildings.
   - Sting on the feet when walking barefoot in the grass.
   - Usually leave in the skin a barbed stinger with an attached sac of venom.
   - Usually non-aggressive except for **Africanized honeybees**.
2. **Bumblebee (*Bombus* spp.) (7)**
   - An uncommon cause of sting reactions, but anaphylaxis has been reported during occupational exposure in greenhouse workers (8).

Family Vespidae (Vespid Family)

Attracted to sweet food, fruits, and grilled food.

a. **Subfamily Vespinae** [Adapted from (9)]
   A southern yellow jacket (*Vespula squamosa*)

   - **Yellow jacket (*Vespula* spp.)**
     - Stings occur during outdoor activities such as yard work, farming, and gardening.
     - They can build large paper-enclosed nests underground and can also be found in wall tunnels/cracks and in hollow logs.
     - Very aggressive.
     - May sting on the mouth, oropharynx, or esophagus while drinking from a container or cans that contained the insect.

DOI: 10.1201/9781003174202-18

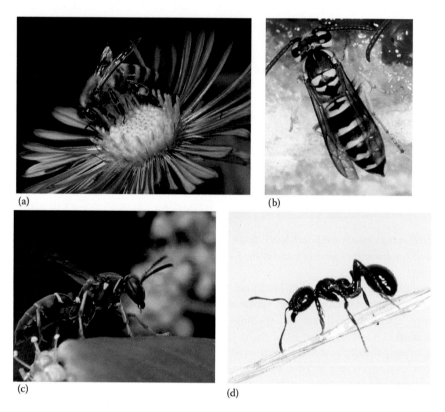

Figure 14.1 Common stinging insects. (a) Honeybee *(Apis mellifera)*, (b) Yellow jacket wasp *(Vespula maculifrons)*, (c) Paper wasp *(Polistes fuscatus)*, (d) Fire ant *(Solenopsis invicta)*. [Reprinted with permission from Taylor & Francis, Lockey et al (39).]

- **Hornets: Yellow hornet *(Dolichovespula arenaria)* and white-faced hornet *(D. maculata)***
  - These build large paper-enclosed nests usually found in bushes and trees.
b. **Subfamily Polistinae: *Polistes* species (paper wasp)**
  - These build open-faced honeycomb nests that are several inches or more in diameter.
  - Nest locations include shrubs, under house eaves, and pipes on playgrounds.

Family Formicidae—Imported Fire Ants Red *(Solenopsis invicta)* or Black *(S. richteri)*

  - Very aggressive.
  - Nest in mounds composed of freshly disturbed soil that can be 6–12 inches high and might extend 1–2 feet in diameter (10).
  - Usually sting individuals many times in a circular pattern leading to *sterile pseudopustules*.
  - *Geography:* Fire ants are only found in select locations (not known to be found in Canada).

Cross-Reactivity and Cross-Sensitization

- *Significant* between venoms of yellow jacket and hornet, and *less* for yellow jacket and hornet with wasp venoms, and *less common* between honeybee and the other venoms (11–15).
- Bumblebee venom contains unique allergens and has variable cross-reactivity with honeybee venom (16).
- There is *limited cross-reactivity* between fire ant venom antigen and those in other venoms of Hymenoptera (17, 18).

Clinical Manifestations (Reaction Types)

- **Local reactions:** Local redness, edema, pruritus, pain
- **LLRs**
  - Painful swelling >10 cm in diameter limited to sting site.
  - Initial increase in swelling over 24–48 hours and resolution around one week (range 3–10 days).

Table 14.1 Stinging Insect Venom Reaction Classifications and Management

Reaction type	Prevalence	Risk of anaphylaxis on subsequent sting	Venom allergy testing	IgE-sensitized	VIT	Epinephrine auto-injector
General Population (no history of a sting)	-	Unknown; 50% of fatal anaphylaxis is on first sting	No	~20%	No	No
Large Local	10% (1)	4–10% (2–5)	No	~80%	No*	No*
Cutaneous Systemic	Adults: 3% Children 0.4–0.8%	Children: <10% Adults: <10%	Consider	Large majority	Consider	Consider
Generalized Systemic (anaphylaxis)	Adults: 3% Children 0.4–0.8%	40–70% (average 50%)** (9–13)	Yes	Large majority	Yes	Yes

*Could consider VIT and/or epinephrine auto-injector if frequent exposures or for quality of life factors, or if patient lives far from medical care.
**If IgE-sensitization demonstrated.
Adapted from (1–5, 9–13, 27).

- **Cutaneous systemic reactions:** Flushing, pruritus, urticaria, and/or angioedema distant from sting site (not involving the tongue, throat, or larynx).
- **Systemic reactions:** Anaphylaxis (refer to Chapter 12).
  - It may be difficult in many cases to differentiate systemic cutaneous versus systemic reactions without documentation of vital signs and a physical exam for wheezing and/or stridor, and testing should be considered if there is any doubt.

History

- An accurate, detailed clinical history is vital in characterizing reaction type and severity as well as relevant clinical factors to determine the need for venom allergen skin testing and possibly desensitization (Figure 14.2).

Diagnosis and Investigations

Testing should typically be considered only if the patient would benefit from venom immunotherapy (VIT).

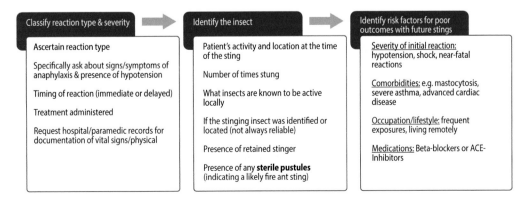

Figure 14.2 Key points to obtain on patient history. [Adapted from (5).]

Skin Testing and/or Specific-IgE (sIgE) Testing

- Test for all five insect species unless a single insect is definitively known/identified (rare).
- Skin testing is the preferred initial test if available, as it is more sensitive than sIgE.
- If skin tests are negative in a patient with a clear history of systemic reaction/anaphylaxis, proceed to check sIgEs.
  - If sIgE is negative, repeat the skin tests in 3–6 months.

1. **Skin prick tests:** Venom extracts with concentrations up to 100 μg/mL.
2. **Intradermal (ID) tests:** Injection of a concentration of 0.001–0.01 μg/mL of about 0.02–0.03 mL.
   - **If the initial ID test is negative:** Increase concentration using 10-fold increments every 20 minutes until the skin test is positive or a maximum concentration of 1.0 μg/mL is reached.
   - Some centers start with ID testing at 1.0 μg/mL without prior skin prick testing, and this approach has been demonstrated to be efficient and safe (19).
   - **Positive ID test:** A wheal of 3–5 mm > the negative control (saline) associated with flare at a concentration of ≤1 μg/mL.

- Venom IgE (by skin test or serum sIgE) is commonly positive for many vespids because of cross-reactivity.
  - **False-positive results:** Can occur at concentrations >1.0 μg/mL from non-specific responses.
  - **Skin testing with fire ant whole body extract (WBE):** A positive test is when the result occurs at ≤1:100 w/v% concentration via skin prick test or ≤1:1000 w/v% by ID skin test.

Basal Serum Tryptase Level

- Increasingly recognized as an important test in venom allergy as there are many implications (Figure 14.3).
- Can be **considered** for any patient who is a candidate for VIT, has a reaction during VIT, or before stopping VIT.
- **Recommended** when high suspicion for underlying mast cell disorder:
  - Severe anaphylaxis to venom sting with:
    - Significant hypotension
    - Lack of urticaria
    - Negative venom-IgE testing

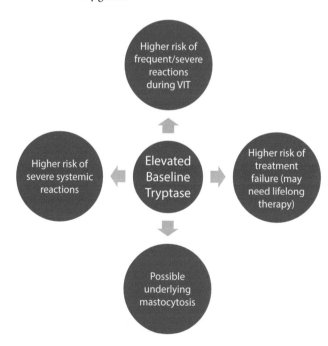

Figure 14.3 Importance of checking baseline serum tryptase level in patients with systemic reaction to venom sting. [Adapted from (5).]

Factors Associated with a Higher Risk of a Reaction [Adapted from (5)]

- History of anaphylaxis to **honeybee sting**.
- History of *near-fatal reactions* to stings.
- Systemic reactions while on VIT (to an injection or a sting).
- **Increased basal serum tryptase level/mastocytosis.**
- *Repeated exposure* to stinging insects that are unavoidable.
- Presence of other medical conditions or concomitant medications.

Management

Key management principles include avoidance strategies, preparedness for/treatment of acute reactions, and venom desensitization in certain situations. Shared decision-making is used between patient and physician to characterize risk of future adverse reactions and consider the risks and benefits of various treatment options such as carrying an epinephrine auto-injector or undergoing VIT.

Acute Management [Adapted from (5)]

a. **Anaphylaxis**
   - Epinephrine (refer to Chapter 12 for complete management)
b. **Local reactions/LLRs**
   - Cold compresses
   - Analgesics
   - Oral antihistamines
   - Oral corticosteroids for LLRs can be used
   - Antibiotics (only if there is evidence of superimposed infection)

Long-Term Management

- Stinging insect avoidance measures: Avoid walking bare-foot outside, wear long sleeves and pants outside, drink beverages from covered containers, use gloves when gardening, be cautious near garbage cans and hollow logs, get a professional to remove nests (5).
- Epinephrine auto-injector: see Figure 14.2
- MedicAlert (TM) bracelet/necklace
- VIT: See Figure 14.2

Patients to Consider for VIT

- For patients with a history of anaphylaxis to insect sting with positive venom-specific IgE testing.
  - Patients with mastocytosis or an increased basal serum tryptase level and anaphylaxis to venom are *highly* recommended to receive VIT.

- Those with LLRs might be considered for VIT for quality-of-life reasons and to reduce the morbidity of frequent or unavoidable sting reactions (20).
- VIT for honeybees, yellow jackets, hornets, and wasps is very effective for those at risk of insect sting anaphylaxis. It lowers the risk systemic reaction later to a sting of about 5% as opposed to up to 60% in those without the VIT (21–23).

Selection of Venoms Used in Immunotherapy

- Two approaches on selecting which venom(s) to use for VIT:
  - *Use only one venom* if the insect that stung was absolutely known, even if there was positive skin or in vitro test results for other stinging insects, relying on venom cross-reactivity and identification of the insect (24, 25, 31).
  - *Use venoms of all insects that were positive* on testing due to the possible reaction to any venoms the patient is sensitized to (25, 26).

VIT Dose and Scheduling

- *Injections:* Given 1–2 times/week with an initial dose of 0.01–1.0 μg then it is increased to a maintenance dose of 100 μg for each insect venom (300 μg with mixed vespid venom).
- *Dosing interval and increments:* It can be modified for better patient convenience.
- *Maintenance dose:* 100 μg is reached in 8–16 weeks by using the US Food and Drug Administration (FDA)-approved dose schedules.
- There are different ways/regimens to reach the maintenance dose:
  - **Conventional** (reached in 4 months) or **modified rush** (in 8 weeks). The risk of systemic reaction is similar using **rush regimens** (2–3 days) but may be slightly greater using **ultrarush regimens** (4–8 hours).
- **Buildup schedules that have more accelerated regimens**
  - **Rush VIT:** Full dose is reached in *days.* This schedule can be used when there is an urgent need for protection, and when there have been repeated systemic reactions impeding progress of VIT; they are optional in all of the cases. Regimens were described by giving a maximum dose between 0.4 and 20 μg on the first day.
  - **Ultrarush VIT:** Done over a period of *hours,* but usually does not achieve the maintenance dose until the second day. Regimens reported include giving a maximum dose of 40–50 μg on the first day.

Interval between Maintenance Dose Injections

- 4-week interval for 12–18 months followed by a 6-week interval for 12–18 months and then 8-week intervals (34–36).
- Intervals can be longer (~12 weeks) between doses in those who stay on VIT for >4 years.

Duration of Treatment with VIT

- 3 to 5 years.
- Even though skin tests remain positive, evidence shows that 80%–90% of patients will not have a systemic reaction to an insect sting if the immunotherapy is stopped after 3–5 years (27–30).

VIT for Imported Fire Ants (IFAs)

- It can be considered in those who have only cutaneous symptoms.
- Duration of treatment is usually 3–5 years.
- Maintenance dose is 0.5 mL of a 1:100 w/v% extract with either *S. invicta* or a mixture of *S. invicta* and *S. richteri* extract, but a higher dose of 0.5 mL of 1:10 w/v% extract has been recommended as well (10, 31–33).

Patients to Consider VIT for an Extended Time, or Indefinitely for Patients with High-Risk Factors

- Very severe reaction before VIT (syncope, hypotension, severe respiratory distress)
- Systemic reaction during VIT
- Honeybee allergy
- Increased basal serum tryptase levels/mastocytosis

Adverse Effects of VIT

- **LLRs**
  - Most common.
  - Size usually is not more than 3–4 inches in diameter.
  - H1 antihistamine pretreatment in the buildup phase of VIT lowers the incidence of local reactions and mild systemic reactions (34).
- **Systemic reactions (anaphylaxis)**
  - *Incidence:*
    - First, modify the dose and schedule.
    - If recurrent reactions, consider a *rush protocol* with H1 antihistamine pretreatment (35).

- If persistent reactions, consider omalizumab (anti-IgE) premedication, which has proven effective (9).

*Note: Benefits of VIT **usually** outweigh the potential risks associated with beta-blockers or angiotensin-converting enzyme inhibitors (ACE) inhibitors in patients who have cardiovascular disease requiring these medications (36).*

Factors with increased risk of relapse after discontinuing VIT (5)

Proven

- Very severe reaction to previous stings
- Elevated basal serum tryptase level
- Systemic reaction during VIT (to injection or sting)
- Less than 5 years of maintenance VIT
- Honeybee anaphylaxis
- Frequent exposure

Possible

- No decrease in venom IgE or skin test size
- Underlying cardiovascular or respiratory disease
- Use of ACEIs or beta-blockers

Risk Factors for Systemic Reactions during VIT (37, 38)

- More frequent in honeybee venom allergic patients
- Those with previous severe reactions to stings
- During rush regimen initial treatment
- With greater time elapsed since the last sting reaction
- Patients with elevated basal serum tryptase levels or mastocytosis

SPECIAL POPULATIONS: PREGNANCY AND LACTATION

- Venom skin testing is relatively contraindicated during pregnancy because of the small risk of anaphylaxis. sIgE testing should be performed as an alternative.
- If the diagnosis of venom allergy is absolutely required during pregnancy and sIgE testing is negative, risk/benefits of venom skin testing must be discussed with the patient. Venom skin testing may be appropriate on an individualized basis and must be performed in a setting equipped to deal with anaphylaxis with patient-informed consent (expert opinion).

- VIT should not be initiated or updosed during pregnancy because of the high risk of adverse reactions during this time (5, 7).
- VIT updosing may be resumed after delivery, but it may be appropriate to wait 6–8 weeks postpartum as hormonal changes may act as cofactors increasing the risk of adverse reaction to VIT (expert opinion).
- However, in pregnant patients with factors associated with a higher risk of a reaction from insect sting the risk of initiating VIT during pregnancy should be weighed with the risk of anaphylaxis from insect sting, and initiation or updosing of VIT may be indicated in certain cases (5).
- In a patient on a maintenance dose of VIT in whom VIT is well tolerated, VIT scheduling should be maintained during pregnancy, the postpartum period, and during lactation (5, 7).

REFERENCES

1. Golden DB et al., JAMA. (1989), PMID: 2739018.
2. Golden DB et al., J Allergy Clin Immunol. (1997), PMID: 9438483/DOI:10.1016/s0091-6749(97)70270-7.
3. Sturm GJ et al., J Allergy Clin Immunol. (2014), PMID: 24365141/DOI:10.1016/j.jaci.2013.10.046.
4. Niedoszytko M et al., Allergy. (2009), PMID: 19627278/DOI:10.1111/j.1398-9995.2009.02118.x.
5. Golden D et al., Ann Allergy Asthma Immunol. (2017), PMID: 28007086/DOI:10.1016/j.anai.2016.10.031.
6. Fitzgerald KT, et al., Clin Tech Small Anim Pract. 2006, PMID: 17265905/DOI:10.1053/j.ctsap.2006.10.002.
7. Sturm GJ et al., Allergy. (2018), PMID: 28748641/DOI: 10.1111/all.13262.
8. de Groot H. Curr Opin Allergy Clin Immunol. (2006), PMID: 16825872/DOI:10.1097/01.all.0000235905.87676.09.
9. Ricciardi L., Int J Immunopathol Pharmacol. (2016), PMID: 27679679/DOI:10.1177/0394632016670920.
10. Steigelman DA et al., Ann Allergy Asthma Immunol. (2013), PMID: 24054357/DOI:10.1016/j.anai.2013.07.006.
11. Hoffman DR., J Allergy Clin Immunol. (1993), PMID: 8227862/DOI:10.1016/0091-6749(93)90014-7.
12. King TP et al., J Allergy Clin Immunol. (1985), PMID: 3989148/DOI:10.1016/0091-6749(85)90040-5.
13. Reisman RE et al., J Allergy Clin Immunol. (1982), PMID: 6801104/DOI:10.1016/s0091-6749(82)80003-1.
14. Reisman RE et al., J Allergy Clin Immunol. (1982), PMID: 6811646/DOI:10.1016/0091-6749(82)90064-1.
15. Reisman RE et al., J Allergy Clin Immunol. (1984), PMID: 6699307/DOI:10.1016/s0091-6749(84)80015-9.
16. Stapel SO et al., Allergy. (1998), PMID: 972222/DOI:10.1111/j.1398-9995.1998.tb03973.x.
17. Hoffman DR et al., J Allergy Clin Immunol. (1988), PMID:3192866/DOI:10.1016/0091-6749(88)90085-1.
18. Rhoades RB et al., Ann Allergy. (1978), PMID: 415642.
19. Quirt JA et al., Ann Allergy Asthma Immunol. (2016), PMID: 26520578/DOI:10.1016/j.anai.2015.10.007.
20. Golden DB et al., J Allergy Clin Immunol. (2009), PMID: 19443022/DOI:10.1016/j.jaci.2009.03.017.
21. Hunt KJ et al., N Engl J Med. (1978), PMID: 78446/DOI:10.1056/NEJM197807272990401.
23. Muller U et al., Allergy. (1979), PMID: 546252/DOI:10.1111/j.1398-9995.1979.tb02006.x.
23. Brown SG et al., Lancet. (2003), PMID: 12660058/DO10.1016/S0140-6736(03)12827-9.
24. Stapel SO et al., Allergy. (1998), PMID: 9722226/DOI: 10.1111/j.1398-9995.1998.tb03973.x.
25. Reisman RE et., J Allergy Clin Immunol. (1992), PMID: 1607552/DOI:10.1016/0091-6749(92)90304-k.
26. Golden DBK. (2014) Insect Allergy. In: Adkinson NF, Yunginger JW, Bochner BS, Busse WW, Holgate ST, Lemanske RF, Simons FER (eds). Middleton's Allergy: Principles and Practice. Eighth Edition, e1260-e1273. Philadelphia, PA: Elsevier.
27. Forester JP et al., Allergy Asthma Proc. (2007), PMID: 17883920/DOI:10.2500/aap.2007.28.3021.
28. Golden DB et al., J Allergy Clin Immunol. (2000), PMID: 10669863/DOI:10.1016/s0091-6749(00)90092-7.
29. Lerch E et al., J Allergy Clin Immunol. (1998), PMID: 9600496/DOI:10.1016/S0091-6749(98)70167-8.
30. Reisman RE., J Allergy Clin Immunol. (1993), PMID: 8258617/DOI:10.1016/0091-6749(93)90060-s.
31. Freeman TM et al., J Allergy Clin Immunol. (1992), PMID: 1500625/DOI:10.1016/0091-6749(92)90073-b.
32. Tankersley MS et al., J Allergy Clin Immunol. (2002), PMID: 11898006/DOI:10.1067/mai.2002.121956.
33. Moffitt JE et al., Ann Allergy Asthma Immunol. (1997), PMID: 9291416/DOI:10.1016/S1081-1206(10)63098-0.
34. Bonifazi F et al., Allergy. (2005), PMID: 16266376/DOI:10.1111/j.1398-9995.2005.00960.x.
35. Goldberg A et al., Ann Allergy Asthma Immunol. (2003), PMID: 14582821.DOI:10.1016/S1081-1206(10)61689-4.
36. Mueller UR. Curr Opin Allergy Clin Immunol. (2007), PMID: 17620826/DOI:10.1097/ACI.0b013e328259c328.
37. Rueff F et al., J Allergy Clin Immunol. (2010), PMID: 20542320/DOI:10.1016/j.jaci.2010.04.025.
38. Korosec P et al., Clin Exp Allergy. (2015), PMID: 26046807/DOI:10.1111/cea.12582.
39. Lockey, R, et al., eds. Allergens and Allergen Immunotherapy. Figure 18.1. Boca Raton, FL: CRC Press.

Eosinophilia and Hypereosinophilic Syndrome (HES)

ABEER FETEIH, HOANG PHAM, GENEVIÈVE GENEST, AND NATACHA TARDIO

GENERAL BACKGROUND

BIOLOGY OF EOSINOPHILS (1–3)

- Bone marrow-derived granulocytes whose proliferation and differentiation are regulated by three main signals: Interleukin (IL-5), IL-3, and granulocyte-macrophage colony-stimulating factor (GM-CSF).
  - IL-5 is a potent signal for eosinophil production and survival.
- Morphologically distinct cells (Figure 15.1): Have unique staining properties (stain bright pink with acidic dye eosin), contain abundant lipid bodies and granules in their cytoplasm, and synthesize and release a wide variety of mediators.
- Mediators produced and released by eosinophils include (select list):
  - *Granule proteins:* Major basic protein (MBP), eosinophilic cationic protein (ECP), eosinophil-derived neurotoxin (EDN), eosinophil peroxidase (EPX), Charcot-Leyden crystal protein.
  - *Cytokines:* IL-5, IL-4, IL-13, transforming growth factor-β (TGF-β), GM-CSF.
  - *Chemokines:* Eotaxin-1, RANTES, CXCL8 (IL-8).

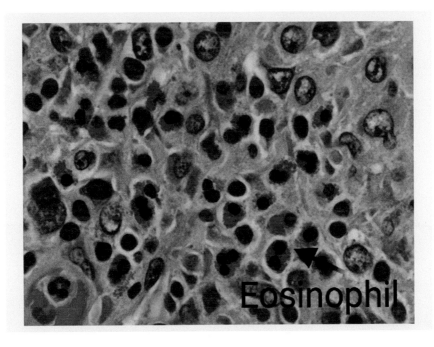

Figure 15.1 Eosinophil. (Image courtesy of Dr. Rene P. Michel.) (Figure created using BioRender.com.)

DOI: 10.1201/9781003174202-19

- *Lipid mediators:* Leukotriene C4 (LTC4), platelet-activating factor (PAF).
- *Oxidative products:* Hydrogen peroxide (H_2O_2), superoxide radical anion.
- *Enzymes:* Metalloproteinase-9 (MMP-9).

• Eosinophils are usually low in the circulation with their migration from the bone marrow to the peripheral blood regulated primarily by IL-5. Mature activated eosinophils (exposed to chemoattractants such as PAF or eotaxin) adhere to endothelial cells, and through the interaction of selectins and integrins, migrate through to tissues (3).

• Play an important role in (1) allergic inflammation and (2) inflammatory response to parasites and viruses.

• Elevated levels can result in tissue damage and inflammation.

DEFINITIONS

• **Eosinophilia:** "Elevation in the absolute eosinophil count (AEC), with severity divided into mild (AEC 500–1500 cells/μL), moderate (AEC 1500–5000 cells/μL), and severe (AEC >5000 cells/μL)" (1).

• **Hypereosinophilia:** "Blood eosinophilia more than or equal to 1500 cells/μL on at least two occasions or evidence of prominent tissue eosinophilia associated with marked blood eosinophilia" (1).

• **Hypereosinophilic syndrome (HES):** "Defined by the association of hypereosinophilia with eosinophil-mediated organ damage and/or dysfunction, provided other potential causes for the damage have been excluded" (1).

Causes of Eosinophilia (Selected) [Adapted from (1, 4)]

• See Figure 15.2 for the causes of eosinophilia.

Classification and Subtypes of HESs [Adapted from (1, 5, 6)]

1. Myeloproliferative
   a. Myeloproliferative hypereosinophilic syndrome (M-HES)
   b. Chronic eosinophilic leukemia (CEL)
2. Lymphocytic hypereosinophilic syndrome (L-HES)
3. Familial HES
4. Overlap disorders
5. Associated HES

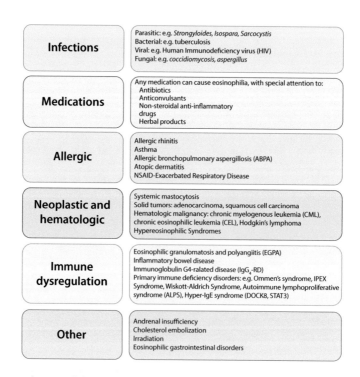

Figure 15.2 Causes of eosinophilia (selected). [Adapted from (1, 3).]

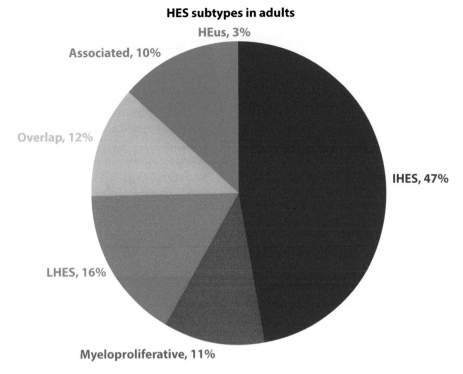

Figure 15.3 Frequency of hypereosinophilic syndrome subtypes in adults. (*Abbreviations:* HE: Hypereosinophilia; HES: Hypereosinophilic syndrome.) [Adapted from Williams et al. (27).]

6. Undefined
   a. Hypereosinophilia of undetermined significance (HEus)
   b. Other

Frequency of HES Subtypes in Adults [Adapted from (27)]

Myeloproliferative

a. **M-HES**
   - Mostly seen in young males (4).
   - Eosinophilia may be associated with a defined myeloid malignancy, whereas others lack a defined myeloid malignancy yet still possess features associated with myeloproliferative disease such as hepatomegaly, splenomegaly, anemia, thrombocytopenia, or tissue damage related to fibrosis (6).
   - Most patients have a gene fusion of Fip1-like 1 (FIP1L1) and platelet-derived growth factor receptor alpha (PDGFRA) (F/P) that can be detected by fluorescence in situ Hybridization (FISH) or reverse transcription polymerase chain reaction (RT-PCR)

tests on bone marrow or peripheral blood (7), and some patients have typical lab and clinical features with a negative PDGFRA screening for the F/P fusion gene or other described fusion partners.

- In those with evidence of M-HES but have a negative F/P screening, they should be evaluated for other mutations such as PDGFRB and FGFR1 (8).
- If testing is negative, patients need to meet four or more of the following criteria to qualify for M-HES diagnosis:
  - Dysplastic eosinophils on peripheral smear.
  - Serum vitamin B_{12} level >1000 pg/mL (due to aberrant B_{12} binding proteins on granulocytes).
  - Serum tryptase level >12 ng/mL.
  - Anemia and/or thrombocytopenia.
  - Hepatosplenomegaly.
  - Bone marrow cellularity >80%.
  - Myelofibrosis.
  - Spindle-shaped mast cells in the bone marrow.

b. **CEL**

M-HES broadly includes CEL, especially if patients are found to be F/P positive or have other cytogenetic abnormalities associated with significant eosinophilia in the presence of >2% blasts in peripheral blood or >5% in the bone marrow; both compartments must be <20% blasts (4).

L-HES

- Occurs in males and females equally (4).
- The most commonly found abnormal T-cell subset in these patients is CD3$^-$CD4$^+$. Other abnormal phenotypes are CD3$^+$CD4$^-$CD8$^-$ and CD3$^+$CD4$^+$CD7$^-$ (9).
- Features that highly support this condition include the identification of T-cell receptor clonality by rearrangement analysis (5, 10).
- Other suggestive features include a high prevalence of dermatologic symptoms (e.g. urticaria, angioedema), obstructive lung disease, gastrointestinal symptoms, elevated total IgE and thymus and activation-regulated chemokine (TARC) (1, 4).
- There are patients who do not have identifiable clonal T-cell populations but may have aberrant T-cell immunophenotyping and evidence of T-cell activation (5, 10).
- Gleich syndrome or episodic angioedema with eosinophilia (EAE): Characterized by episodes of significant eosinophilia with associated angioedema that can occur in a cyclical manner with a CD3$^-$CD4$^+$ T-cell phenotype (1, 11, 12).
- L-HES can progress to overt lymphoma in 5%–25%, such as angioimmunoblastic T-cell lymphoma (1, 4, 13, 14).

Familial HES

- Rare condition that describes eosinophilia of unknown etiology with a strong family history in multiple generations.
- Eosinophilia may be asymptomatic, but some affected families have symptoms similar to F/P-positive HES with cardiac fibrosis and neurologic abnormalities (15).

Overlap Disorders

- Conditions that demonstrate organ-restricted eosinophilia that could be accompanied by peripheral eosinophilia (16).

- **Selected disorders in this category**
  - Eosinophilic gastrointestinal disorders
  - Eosinophilic esophagitis
  - Eosinophilic pneumonia

Associated HES

- Consists of marked peripheral eosinophilia along with conditions that are known to cause eosinophilia.
- Selected conditions: Eosinophilic granulomatosis with polyangiitis (EGPA), systemic mastocytosis, inflammatory bowel disease, sarcoidosis, and human immunodeficiency virus (HIV).

Undefined

a. **HEus (2)**
  - Eosinophilia is considered benign in these cases
  - There could be persistent AEC ≥1500/mm^3 but without developing signs of end-organ damage or dysfunction.

b. **Other:** Patients are usually symptomatic with end-organ dysfunction without the features of L-HES or M-HES.

Clinical Manifestations and Complications Based on Organ/System Involvement in HES
Hematologic (4, 17, 18)

- Anemia, immature eosinophils (e.g. blasts) in the bone marrow and/or peripheral blood, thrombocytopenia, myelofibrosis, hepatosplenomegaly.

Cutaneous

- Skin is very commonly involved, especially in L-HES (4, 19, 20).
- Broad range of skin lesions: Urticaria, angioedema, erythroderma, eczema, pruritus, mucosal ulceration, necrotizing vasculitis, livedo reticularis (20).
- Lesions due to thromboembolic complications: Splinter hemorrhages, nail bed infarcts.

Cardiovascular

- May be present in 40%–60% of patients, and is an important cause of morbidity and mortality (5, 21).
- In HES, cardiac disease is divided into acute necrotic, thrombotic, and late fibrotic stages.
- Valvular dysfunction (3).

- Dilated cardiomyopathy (3).
- Chest pain, dyspnea, embolic events, and arrhythmia (21).

Neurologic

- Transient ischemic attacks (TIA), strokes.
- Primary central nervous system dysfunction (presenting with encephalopathy with behavioral changes, memory loss, and confusion).
- Physical exam findings can include upper motor neuron signs such as increased muscle tone and deep tendon reflexes (22).
- Peripheral neuropathies: Variable in presentation (isolated sensory or motor deficits or both) that can cause numbness, painful paresthesias, weakness, or muscle atrophy (22).
- Less common: Seizures, intracranial hemorrhage, and dementia (19).

Pulmonary

- Pulmonary involvement occurs in about 40% of patients with HES (23).
- Lung complications may happen due to acute or chronic pulmonary embolic disease or accompany cardiac dysfunction (4).
- Shortness of breath, cough, or imaging abnormalities (23), Pleural effusions from cardiac involvement (23) or Fibrotic lung disease (19).

Rheumatologic

- Arthralgias, non-erosive polyarthritis, joint effusions with synovial fluid eosinophilia, Raynaud phenomenon (19).

Gastrointestinal

- Failure to thrive, dysphagia, abdominal pain, vomiting, diarrhea.

Diagnosis and Investigations [Adapted from (4)]

A detailed history and physical exam is recommended to orient investigations. Workup should focus on determining the cause of the eosinophilia as well as the presence of complications/end-organ damage. Below is a list of suggested investigations:

General

- Complete blood count (CBC) with differential; peripheral blood smear; serum total IgE; erythrocyte sedimentation rate (ESR)/C-reactive protein (CRP); vitamin B_{12} serum level; HIV serology; flow cytometry, particularly for T-cell immunophenotyping (CD3, CD4, CD8); serum tryptase level; *Strongyloides* serology; stool ova and parasites, anti-nuclear cytoplasmic antibody (ANCA), anti-nuclear antibodies (ANA)

Screening Tests Recommended for End-Organ Involvement

- **Cardiac:** Serum troponin T, electrocardiogram (ECG), echocardiogram
- **Gastrointestinal:** Liver enzymes
- **Pulmonary:** Chest X-ray, pulmonary function test
- **Renal:** Blood urea nitrogen, creatinine, urinalysis

Further Testing May Be Indicated According to Results of Initial Investigations

- **Cardiac:** Cardiac magnetic resonance imaging (MRI), endomyocardial biopsy
- **Neurologic:** Brain MRI or computed tomography (CT) scan of the head with contrast, electroencephalogram, nerve conduction studies
- **Dermatologic:** Skin biopsy
- **Hematologic:** Bone marrow biopsy, CT scans (chest, abdomen, pelvis), peripheral FISH/RT-PCR for FIP1L1-PDGFRA
- **Pulmonary:** Bronchoalveolar lavage, lung biopsy, chest CT
- **Renal:** Kidney biopsy
- **Gastrointestinal:** Endoscopy with biopsies, abdominal CT scan, amylase/lipase
- **Vascular:** Angiography

MANAGEMENT OPTIONS OF HES

Corticosteroids

- Prednisone 0.5–1 mg/kg daily, lower doses may be tried initially and then titrated (5). Patients with L-HES generally have a good response to steroid treatment.
- Those who have M-HES variants are usually less responsive to steroids (24).

Note: Patients who have a history of possible exposure to Strongyloides *may require treatment with empiric oral ivermectin (200 mg/kg/day) × 2 days to prevent corticosteroid-associated hyperinfection syndrome due to disseminated* Strongyloides *infection (25).*

Hydroxyurea

- Second-line agent.
- Dose: 0.5–2 g oral daily.
- Not usually used as a monotherapy initially and may be most effective with corticosteroids or interferon-α (IFN-α) (5).

IFN-α

- May be considered in a variety of HES subtypes, as it affects many cell lines.
- Clinically, IFN-α initially showed benefit in patients who did not respond to treatment with hydroxyurea and corticosteroids (24).

Tyrosine Kinase Inhibitors (Imatinib)

- First-line therapy in patients with F/P-positive HES.
- Dose: 100–400 mg oral daily (13).
- Many F/P-negative patients will have no response or a partial response to treatment, even at doses higher than those used for treatment of F/P-positive patients (5).

Immunomodulatory Agents

- **Mepolizumab (anti IL-5 monoclonal antibody):** Not approved yet in Canada for HES treatment but clinical trials being conducted to investigate it's efficacy in this setting(5, 25).
- **Reslizumab (humanized anti-IL-5 monoclonal antibody):** Limited published data in HES but has been studied in other eosinophilic conditions.
- **Alemtuzumab** (recombinant humanized monoclonal antibody to CD52): Reserved for patients with severe disease refractory to standard treatments (5).

Cytotoxic Therapies

- Such as cyclophosphamide, cyclosporine, methotrexate, busulfan, and chlorambucil were attempted to be used as maintenance therapy (4).
- There are limited reports of efficacy, and they have major side effects (5).

Allogeneic Stem Cell Transplantation

- May be an option in patients who do not respond to standard treatments.

- Certain subgroups that could be suitable for transplant include F/P-positive patients that are unresponsive to imatinib or patients initially presenting with L-HES that progress to lymphoma.

SPECIAL POPULATIONS: PREGNANCY AND LACTATION

- Information regarding outcomes and management of pregnant women with HES is extremely scarce.
- Patients with HES benefit from pre-conception counseling to determine whether they are medically fit for pregnancy and to review HES medications (26).
- Glucocorticoids may be used throughout pregnancy if absolutely necessary. The lowest effective dose is generally recommended. Significant maternal and fetal side effects are seen with chronic usage (reviewed in Chapter 11).
- Hydroxyurea, tyrosine kinase inhibitors, alemtuzumab, and cytotoxic therapies are contraindicated during pregnancy (1, 26, expert opinion).
- IFN-α and anti-IL-5 therapy may be considered throughout pregnancy if absolutely required to control disease prior to pregnancy (26).

REFERENCES

1. Khoury P, Akuthota P, Weller PF, Klion AD. Eosinophilia and Eosinophil-Related Disorders. In: Burks AW, Holgate ST, O'Hehir RE, Bacharier LB, Broide DH, Hershey GK, Peebles Jr RS. Middleton's Allergy: Principles and Practice E-Book, Ninth Edition. Amsterdam: Elsevier. Available at: https://www.clinicalkey.com/dura/browse/bookChapter/3-s2.0-C20161002419 (Accessed: August 20, 2020).
2. Kita H, Bochner BS. Biology of Eosinophils. In: Burks AW, Holgate ST, O'Hehir RE, Bacharier LB, Broide DH, Hershey GK, Peebles Jr RS. Middleton's Allergy: Principles and Practice E-Book, Ninth Edition. Amsterdam: Elsevier. Available at: https://www.clinicalkey.com/dura/browse/bookChapter/3-s2.0-C20161002419 (Accessed: Jan 24, 2021).

3. Rothenberg ME, N Engl J Med. (1998), PMID: 9603798/DOI:10.1056/NEJM199805283382206.

4. Curtis C et al., Clin Rev Allergy Immunol. (2016), PMID: 26475367/DOI:10.1007/s12016-015-8506-7.

5. Cogan E et al., Expert Rev Hematol. (2012), PMID: 22780208/DOI:10.1586/ehm.12.14.

6. Simon HU et al., J Allergy Clin Immunol. (2010), PMID: 20639008/DOI:10.1016/j.jaci.2010.03.042.

7. Cools J et al., N Engl J Med. (2003), PMID: 12660384/DOI:10.1056/NEJMoa025217.

8. Tefferi A et al., Mayo Clin Proc. (2010), PMID: 20053713/DOI:10.4065/mcp.2009.0503.

9. Roufosse F et al., Immunol Allergy Clin North Am. (2007), PMID: 17868856/DOI:10.1016/j.iac.2007.07.002.

10. Klion A, Annu Rev Med. (2009), PMID: 19630574/DOI:10.1146/annurev.med.60.062107.090340.

11. Gleich GJ et al., N Engl J Med. (1984), PMID: 6727934/DOI:10.1056/NEJM198406213102501.

12. Khoury P et al., Haematologica. (2015), PMID: 25527564/DOI:10.3324/haematol.2013.091264.

13. Klion AD, Blood. (2015), PMID: 25964669/DOI:10.1182/blood-2014-11-551614.

14. Eng V et al., Ann Allergy Asthma Immunol. (2020), PMID: 32044452/DOI:10.1016/j.anai.2020.01.028.

15. Lin AY et al., Am J Med Genet. (1998), PMID: 9508242.

16. Klion AD, Blood. (2009), PMID: 19692700/DOI:DOI:10.1182/blood-2009-07-143552.

17. Chusid MJ et al., Medicine (Baltimore). (1975), PMID: 1090795.

18. Flaum MA et al., Blood. (1981), PMID: 7197565.

19. Weller PF et al., Blood. (1994), PMID: 8180373.

20. Leiferman KM et al., Immunol Allergy Clin North Am. (2007), PMID: 17868857/DOI:10.1016/j.iac.2007.07.009.

21. Ogbogu PU et al., Immunol Allergy Clin North Am. (2007), PMID: 17868859/DOI:10.1016/j.iac.2007.07.001.

22. Moore PM et al., Ann Intern Med. (1985), PMID: 2981493/DOI:10.7326/0003-4819-102-1-109.

23. Akuthota P et al., Immunol Allergy Clin North Am. (2015), PMID: 26209892/DOI:10.1016/j.iac.2015.04.002.

24. Ogbogu PU et al., J Allergy Clin Immunol. (2009), PMID: 19910029/DOI:10.1016/j.jaci.2009.09.022.

25. Mejia R et al., Curr Opin Infect Dis. (2012), PMID: 22691685/DOI:10.1097/QCO.0b013e3283551dbd.

24. Zielinski RM et al., Ann Intern Med. (1990), PMID: 2088325/DOI:10.7326/0003-4819-113-9-716.

25. Mepolizumab: 240563, anti-IL-5 monoclonal antibody - GlaxoSmithKline, anti-interleukin-5 monoclonal antibody-GlaxoSmithKline, SB 240563. Drugs R D. (2008), PMID: 18298130/DOI:10.2165/00126839-200809020-00006.

26. Pfaller B et al., Allergy. (2021), PMID: 32189356/DOI: 10.1111/all.14282.

27. Williams KW et al., J Allergy Clin Immunol Pract. (2016), PMID: 27130711/DOI:10.1016/j.jaip.2016.03.020.

FOOD ALLERGY

16 Food Allergy   145
    Abeer Feteih, Lydia Zhang, Natacha Tardio, Hoang Pham, and Moshe Ben-Shoshan
17 Eosinophilic Esophagitis (EoE)   153
    Abeer Feteih, Hoang Pham, Michael Fein, Serge Mayrand, and Natacha Tardio
18 Celiac Disease and Non-Celiac Gluten Sensitivity   159
    Stephen Tsoukas, Natacha Tardio, and Waqqas Afif

Food Allergy

ABEER FETEIH, LYDIA ZHANG, NATACHA TARDIO,
HOANG PHAM, AND MOSHE BEN-SHOSHAN

GENERAL BACKGROUND

- It is reported that almost 6% of Canadians have IgE-mediated food allergies (6.7% of children and 5.9% of adults) (1).
- Many foods are identified to cause food allergies, but the ones causing the majority of allergic reactions are peanuts, tree nuts, fish, shellfish, milk, egg, wheat, soy, and sesame (2–5).
- Recent studies in Canada suggest that the rate of food-induced anaphylaxis, mainly for tree nuts, is increasing in the last decade (6, 7).
- Patients with food allergies have a higher rate of atopic dermatitis, asthma, and allergic rhinitis (2).

DEFINITIONS

As stated by **the National Institute of Allergy and Infectious Diseases (NIAID) Sponsored Expert Panel.** [Adapted from (2)]:

Food allergy: "is an adverse health effect arising from a specific immune response that occurs reproducibly on exposure to a given food."

Food allergens: "specific components of food or ingredients within food (typically proteins, but sometimes also chemical haptens) that are recognized by allergen specific immune cells and elicit specific immunologic reactions, resulting in characteristic symptoms."

Cross-reactivity: "when an antibody reacts not only with the original allergen, but also with a similar allergen. Cross-reactivity in food allergy ensues when a food allergen shares structural or sequence similarity with a different food allergen or aeroallergen, which may then trigger an adverse reaction similar to that triggered by the original food allergen (e.g. different shellfish or different tree nuts)."

Clinical Manifestations [Adapted from (8)]

1. **Cutaneous**
   - **Acute urticaria**
   - **Angioedema**
   - **Atopic dermatitis**: This is a complex interaction between the skin barrier dysfunction and food exposures, but 30%–40% of infants and young children with eczema may have food allergies as a trigger (9).
     - Mixed IgE- and cell-mediated reaction.
   - **Allergic contact dermatitis**: Pruritus, erythema, papules, vesicles, and edema.
     - Cell-mediated reaction.
   - **Contact urticaria:** At the site of contact with food; typically, not severe.
     - IgE-mediated reaction.

2. **Respiratory (mostly presenting as part of anaphylaxis)**
   - Nasal congestion, rhinorrhea, stridor, tachypnea, cough, wheeze

3. **Gastrointestinal (GI)**
   - **Immediate GI hypersensitivity**
     - Nausea, vomiting, diarrhea, usually with cutaneous and/or respiratory symptoms (as part of anaphylaxis).
   - **Pollen-food allergy syndrome (PFAS) or oral allergy syndrome (OAS)**
     - A special type of localized IgE-mediated food allergy in the oropharynx, usually adult onset, due to ingestion of raw cross-reacting foods in a patient with a primary aeroallergen sensitization who

DOI: 10.1201/9781003174202-21

reports one or several of the following symptoms:

- Oral-pharyngeal pruritus (most common), throat tightness, difficulty swallowing, nausea/vomiting (~5%), dysphonia, nasal and ear pruritus (9).
- PFAS occurs in 47%–70% of those with allergic rhinitis, especially seasonal allergic rhinitis (9).

- Up to 3% of patients with PFAS experience systemic symptoms without oral symptoms, and 1.7% experience anaphylactic shock (9).
- Systemic symptoms are rare in PFAS because cross-reactive food proteins tend to be labile and denature with cooking and food processing, which is why patients often report tolerating processed foods but report symptoms to fresh foods.

- **Food protein-induced enterocolitis syndrome (FPIES)**
  - Presents usually in young infants (10), may be underreported/diagnosed in adults.
  - Symptoms in general include vomiting, diarrhea, and failure to thrive (11).
  - When patients are re-exposed to the offending food after a period of elimination, they can present with repeated projectile vomiting and dehydration usually 2–4 hours after ingestion of that food.
  - Acute FPIES: Repetitive projectile vomiting within 1–3 hours of food ingestion, followed by lethargy, hypothermia (in protracted cases), leukocytosis, high platelet counts, and methemoglobinemia in cases that are severe.
  - Chronic FPIES: Symptoms may include recurrent vomiting, bloody diarrhea, anemia, hypoproteinemia, leukocytosis with eosinophilia, and failure to thrive.

- **Dietary protein-induced proctitis/proctocolitis**
  - Most commonly associated with milk protein, but many food allergens can be involved as well.
  - Symptoms: Blood-streaked stool mixed with mucus in infants who appear healthy.
  - Symptom resolution occurs with dietary avoidance (may include the mother's diet restriction for infants who are breastfeeding).

- The condition usually resolves during infancy.

Note: The most common food allergens in FPIES/procto-colitis/enteropathy are cow's milk and soy proteins in children (2). Adult-onset FPIES is most commonly secondary to crustaceans (shrimp), mollusks, fish, and egg (10).

- **Eosinophilic esophagitis (EoE):** Refer to Chapter 17.
- **Eosinophilic gastroenteritis** (multiple food allergens are usually involved).
  - Abdominal pain, vomiting, diarrhea, failure to thrive/weight loss.

4. Anaphylaxis: Refer to Chapter 12.

Diagnosis and Investigations [Adapted from (8)]

IgE-Mediated Food Allergy

Establishing the diagnosis of an IgE-mediated food allergy requires corroboration of a suggestive history with skin tests, specific IgE (sIgE), or both, and possibly oral food provocations if needed.

- **Details in history:** Food/ingredients ingested, quantity, and its preparation, symptoms associated, timing of onset/resolution of symptoms, medications required for treatment, frequency of symptoms associated with ingestion and if consistently eliciting the manifestations.
- **Presence of cofactors:** Nonsteroidal anti-inflammatory drug (NSAID) use, exercise, stress, alcohol, and fever.
- **Physical examination:** For stigmata of allergic disease (eczema, allergic rhinitis, asthma).
- **Food diary/journal:** With further follow-up can be helpful if there is uncertainty of the culprit food.

1. **Skin tests**
   a. **Skin prick testing (SPT)**
   - Used with commercial extracts for detecting sIgE for the suspected food allergens based on the clinical history.
   - Prick-prick method with fresh food mixed with sterile saline can be used if commercial extracts are not available or in diagnosis of PFAS.
   - This type of food skin testing has a sensitivity of 85% and a specificity of 74% in the presence of supporting history (skin tests done without history of exposure may be falsely positive in 50% of cases and the specificity is accordingly less than 50%) (12).

Table 16.1 Predictive Values of Serum-Specific IgE (sIgE) and Skin Prick Testing (SPT) for Select Food Allergens

Food	>95% Positive		~50% Negative	
	sIgE	SPT	sIgE	SPT wheal (mm)
Egg White	≥7 ≥2 if age <2 y	≥7	≤2	≤3
Cow's Milk	≥15 ≥5 if age <1 y	≥8	≤2	
Peanut	≥14	≥8	≤2 = history of prior reaction ≤5 = no history of prior reaction	≤3
Fish	≥20			

Note: Allergen sensitization often occurs without clinical allergy. Serum-specific IgE levels and skin prick testing for food allergens is used in combination with the clinical history to diagnose food allergy. The above predictive values of a positive food challenge for certain food allergy testing have been established.
Reprinted with permission from Sampson HA et al., J Allergy Clin Immunol. (2014), Elsevier.

- **Positive SPT:** When a wheal and flare develop within 10–20 minutes after applying the allergen with a mean diameter ≥3 mm than the negative control (saline) (13).
- **Negative SPT:** Does not rule out clinical reactivity. If there is still a high degree of clinical suspicion for IgE-mediated food allergy, serum sIgE, and/or oral food challenge (OFC) should be done.

b. **Intradermal skin testing**
  - Not recommended for diagnosing IgE-mediated food allergy due to increased risk of systemic reactions (2, 13).
  - May possibly be used in **alpha-gal hypersensitivity** in those who present with delayed anaphylaxis (alpha-gal is present in mammalian red meats) (14).

2. **Blood tests**
   a. **Serum sIgE to selected food**
     - Not diagnostic of food allergy when used alone and should only be used for selected foods based on clinical history.
     - Performed in those who are highly suspected to have an IgE-mediated food allergy but have a negative SPT.
     - Performed if SPT is avoided (e.g. antihistamine use, generalized urticaria or other skin disease).

- There are predictive thresholds/cutoffs established for peanut, egg, milk, fish, soy, and wheat to decide if an OFC is required.
- If the test is negative then SPTs, OFC, or both to the suspected food may be required.

b. **Component-resolved diagnosis (CRD)**
  - Involves the use of allergenic proteins derived from rDNA technology or purification from natural sources to identify the patient's sIgE reactivity to recombinant allergenic proteins as opposed to the whole allergen (15).
  - May help improve accuracy in the diagnosis and give insight for severity risk in patients, but the clinical utility of component testing has not been fully established yet (8).
  - **Examples (selected)**
    – **Ara h 2 sIgE antibodies:** Most common peanut allergen associated with clinical reactivity (16, 17).
    – **Ara h 1, 2, or 3 sensitizations:** Linked with increased severity of reactions in certain individuals.

3. **OFC**
   - OFCs are resource-intensive procedures and availability may be limited, but they are highly valuable in diagnosis of food allergy.

- There are many types:
  - *Open (unmasked):* Commonly used.
  - *Single-blind with or without placebo:* Commonly used.
  - *Double-blind, placebo-controlled challenges (DBPCFC):* The gold standard and the most difficult type of challenge to conduct (rarely used clinically) (18).
- Graded dosing is recommended regardless of the type of challenge being done (18).
- Informed consent should be obtained from the patient prior to OFC with counseling on the risks and benefits of the procedure.
- It should be done under the supervision of trained medical staff in a health care facility equipped to treat anaphylaxis.
- A positive OFC occurs when there are any **objective symptoms** or signs of an allergic reaction.
- In those who are known allergic who are not consuming baked egg or milk, a food challenge with a muffin (serving portion) or other appropriate food is necessary to ensure safe consumption (19–21).

Patient Factors Associated with an Increased Risk for OFC [Adapted from (23)]

- Uncontrolled asthma
- Respiratory tract infection
- History of a previous severe reaction/reaction after ingesting trace amounts of the causal food
- Uncontrolled urticaria or atopic dermatitis
- Cardiovascular disease, difficult vascular access, or treatment with beta-blockers, angiotensin-converting enzyme inhibitors (ACE-Is)

Food-Dependent Exercise-Induced Anaphylaxis (FDEIA)

- Refer to Chapter 13.

EoE

- Refer to Chapter 17.

PFAS

- Diagnosis is by evidence of allergic sensitization to specific pollen and a history of symptoms consistent with PFAS after consumption of raw

foods (fruits and vegetables) that are indeed cross-reactive with that particular pollen.

- Individuals usually tolerate the cooked form of the food because the proteins that are cross-reactive are heat labile (10).
- SPTs with the suspected fresh fruit (prick-prick method) can be used to help in the diagnosis.
- OFCs if the diagnosis is not certain but the results can be affected by growth conditions/ripening of the fruit that may reduce/destroy the allergenicity of the fruit or vegetable.
- **Clinical entities due to IgE sensitization to cross-reactive aeroallergen and food allergen components are described for many sources of plant, fungal, and invertebrate, mammalian, or avian origin (22):**
  - **Birch-apple syndrome:** Bet v 1 homologue cross-reacting with Mal d 1
  - Cypress-peach syndrome.
  - Celery-mugwort-spice syndrome.
  - Mugwort-peach association.
  - Mugwort-chamomile association.
  - Mugwort-mustard syndrome.
  - Ragweed-melon-banana association.
  - Goosefoot-melon association.
  - Alternaria-spinach syndrome.
  - **Mite-shrimp syndrome: Der p 10** tropomyosin cross-reactivity implicated.
    - Inhaled tropomyosins from house dust mites are hypothesized to be the primary sensitizer for shellfish allergy (23).
  - **Cat-pork syndrome**
  - **Bird-egg syndrome**
  - **Latex-fruit syndrome:** *Hevea brasiliensis* (Hev b 2, Hev b 8, Hev b 10) cross-reacts with banana (Mus xp 5 Mus xp 1), olive pollen (Ole e 2, Ole e 5), pineapple (Ana c 1), and kiwi (Act d 9).

FPIES, Allergic Proctocolitis, Enteropathy

- Detailed history and physical examination.
- **FPIES**
  - Elimination of the suspected food culprit and observe if symptoms resolve.
  - OFC to aid with making an initial diagnosis of FPIES and for future follow-up to determine whether the condition resolved (2). It may not be required for the initial diagnosis when a child presents with recurrent typical symptoms (>2 reactions within 6 months of

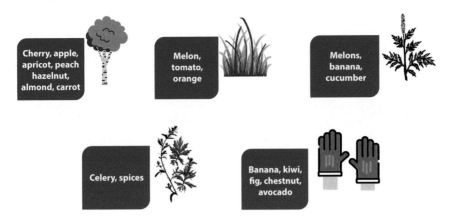

Figure 16.1 Pollen food allergy syndrome. Clockwise from upper left: Birch pollen, grass pollen, ragweed pollen, mugwort pollen, latex.

typical symptoms) and is well when there is elimination of the triggering food.

– Positive OFC in those cases when characteristic symptoms and laboratory results are manifested that can include vomiting and lethargy starting between 1 and 3 hours, diarrhea between 2 and 10 hours, and increased blood neutrophil count (>3500 cells/mL), fecal leukocytes, and/or eosinophil counts, as well as frank or occult blood in stool.

• **Allergic proctocolitis:** Patients have infiltration of eosinophils in the mucosal layers mostly in the lamina propria.

• **Enteropathy:** Endoscopy and biopsy are needed for the definite diagnosis.

• Endoscopy and biopsy may also be required for those with persistent chronic severe FPIES and allergic proctocolitis that do not respond to diet changes.

Differential Diagnosis/Syndromes

Theses can mimic IgE-mediated allergic food reaction: Selected examples adapted from (8)

• Allergic reaction due to medication or insect stings that happen coincidentally at time of food consumption.

• Infectious syndromes: *Staphylococcus aureus* toxin.

• Metabolic disorders: Lactose intolerance.

• Toxic reactions: Scombroid fish toxin, *Salmonella*, *Shigella*, *Escherichia coli* bacteria).

• Chemical effects: Gustatory rhinitis from hot or spicy foods.

• Auriculotemporal syndrome (Frey syndrome) or gustatory flushing syndrome due to foods.

• Pharmacologic reactions: Tryptamine, alcohol, caffeine.

• Others: Sulfites, nitrites, or monosodium glutamate (MSG).

• Mastocytosis: Diagnostic workup can be started with a tryptase level (24).

• Neuroendocrine tumors: Carcinoid syndrome (25).

Management

• **Anaphylaxis:** Refer to Chapter 12. In brief, IgE-mediated food allergy should be treated promptly with epinephrine when anaphylaxis (as defined in the Chapter 12) is suspected, because its clinical course can be unpredictable and rapidly progressive to a severe or fatal extent (26, 27). Non-sedative second-generation antihistamine can complement epinephrine treatment (27).

• **FDEIA:** Refer to Chapter 13.

• **EoE:** Refer to Chapter 17.

• **PFAS:** Avoid consumption of the culprit fruits and vegetables in their raw forms depending on symptom severity, but patients may eat them cooked or baked if well tolerated.

– Strict avoidance may be recommended if symptoms are more severe, progress in severity, or are associated with systemic symptoms (8).

– Strict avoidance AND **epinephrine auto-injector** are recommended in patients with history of laryngeal swelling or respiratory compromise (8).

Non-IgE-Mediated Food Allergy

- Avoidance of the culprit dietary food protein.
- Dietitian/nutritionist referral for nutritional support.
- Acute FPIES treatment:
  - Vigorous intravenous (IV) fluids with normal saline boluses.
  - Ondansetron: A small case series of children with FPIES were successfully treated with it during a supervised OFC (28).
  - Epinephrine can be used if there is severe hypotension (but not helpful as first-line management) (10).
  - IV methylprednisolone: One dose of 1–2 mg/kg can be used in some patients with protracted symptoms (but efficacy not established). Most patients tolerate hypoallergenic casein-based formula but 10%–15% may need to use a formula that is amino acid based (29, 30). Strict maternal diet avoidance of the culprit allergen may be required if symptoms are present during breastfeeding in those with milk/soy FPIES.
- Eczema
  - Elimination diets should not be widely used in cases with eczema with no established history of IgE-mediated food allergy (31–33).
  - Studies report increased risk of food sensitivity in general and in children with eczema particularly. Tree nuts are often eliminated from the diet of multiple-food-allergic patients, despite their low probability for allergy. Sensitization and allergy to most tree nuts exist years later, suggesting that it developed during the period of elimination (31–33).

Long-Term Management of IgE-Mediated Food Reactions

- Avoidance of the culprit food allergen(s).
- Epinephrine auto-injector to carry at all times.
- At each follow-up appointment: Educate on use of epinephrine auto-injector and how to recognize a severe allergic reaction.
- MedicAlert (TM) bracelet.
- Written action plan for the response to anaphylaxis/allergic reactions.
- Individuals who are able to ingest egg and milk in the baked form should regularly continue its consumption and should be followed to reassess symptoms and tolerance.

- Monitoring for evidence of tolerance to the food allergen or development of new food allergies and, if indicated, performing SPTs or allergen sIgE tests.
- Milk and egg allergy (34, 35) can be outgrown quickly but allergy to peanuts, tree nuts, fish, and shellfish are usually more persistent (36–38).
- Testing every 6–12 months is recommended in the first 5 years of life to evaluate for tolerance development (39).
- Interval for testing can be changed to every 2–3 years after that if levels are still high.
- **Oral immunotherapy (OIT):** Has been widely studied and was shown to be effective for several food allergens (e.g. milk, egg, and peanuts) in providing protection through desensitization against life-threatening reactions during therapy, as well as for the possibility of sustained unresponsiveness development when therapy is stopped (40). After considering the benefits and risks associated with this therapy including a potential increase in anaphylactic reactions (41), guidelines have been established for the safe administration of OIT in food-allergic patients (42).

Food Allergy Prevention

From the "Consensus Approach to the Primary Prevention of Food Allergy Through Nutrition: Guidance from the American Academy of Allergy, Asthma and Immunology; American College of Allergy, Asthma, and Immunology; and the Canadian Society for Allergy and Clinical Immunology" (43)

1. Recommendations on relative risk factors of developing food allergy:
   - Consider infants with severe eczema as having the highest risk of developing food allergy.
   - Consider infants with mild-moderate eczema, a family history of atopy in one or both parents, or one known food allergy at an increased risk of developing food allergy (or an additional food allergy).
2. Recommendations for early introduction of peanut, egg, and other potentially allergenic foods (cow's milk, soy, wheat, tree nuts, sesame, fish, shellfish):
   - Introduce these potentially allergenic-containing products to infants, irrespective of their relative risk of developing peanut

allergy, around 6 months of life, but not before 4 months.

- Introduce at home when the infant is developmentally ready for complementary food introduction, in accordance with the family's cultural practice, but not before the infant demonstrates developmental readiness with eating a few other common start foods.
- Use only cooked forms of egg and avoid any raw, pasteurized egg-containing products.

- No requirement to routinely screen with peanut SPT or sIgE and/or perform in-office introduction, but consider these options for families that prefer to not introduce peanuts at home.

- This decision is preference sensitive and should be made taking into account current evidence and family preferences.
- Strongly encourage either home introduction or offer a supervised OFC for any positive SPT or sIgE result.

- Maintain regular ingestion once it is introduced.

3. Recommendation for diverse diets:
- Feed infants a diverse diet as this may help foster prevention of food allergy-based on observational studies.

4. Recommendation against hydrolyzed formulas:
- Do not prescribe or recommend the use of any hydrolyzed formulas for the specific prevention of food allergy.

5. Recommendation against maternal exclusion:
- Do not recommend maternal exclusion of common allergens during pregnancy and lactation as a means to prevent food allergy.

- Although exclusive breastfeeding is universally recommended for all mothers, there is no association between exclusive breastfeeding and the primary prevention of food allergy.

REFERENCES

1. Clarke AE et al., J Allergy Clin Immunol Pract. (2020), PMID: 31706046/DOI:10.1016/j.jaip.2019.10.021.
2. Boyce JA et al., J Allergy Clin Immunol. (2010), PMID: 21134568/DOI:10.1016/j.jaci.2010.10.008.
3. Ben-Shoshan M et al., J Allergy Clin Immunol. (2010), PMID: 20451985/DOI:10.1016/j.jaci.2010.03.015.
4. Sicherer SH et al., J Allergy Clin Immunol. (2010), PMID: 20462634/DOI:10.1016/j.jaci.2010.03.029.
5. Gupta RS et al., Pediatrics. (2011), PMID: 21690110/DOI:10.1542/peds.2011-0204.
6. Miles BT et al., J Allergy Clin Immunol Pract. (2020), PMID: 32244023/DOI:10.1016/j.jaip.2020.03.014.
7. Hochstadter E et al., J Allergy Clin Immunol. (2016), PMID: 27106202/DOI:10.1016/j.jaci.2016.02.016.
8. Sampson HA et al., J Allergy Clin Immunol. (2014), PMID: 25174862/DOI:10.1016/j.jaci.2014.05.013.
9. Carlson G et al., Ann Allergy Asthma Immunol. (2019), PMID: 31376490/DOI:10.1016/j.anai.2019.07.022.
10. Agyemang A et al., Clin Rev Allergy Immunol. (2019), PMID: 30734159/DOI:10.1007/s12016-018-8722-z.
11. Nowak-Wegrzyn A et al., Pediatrics. (2003), PMID: 12671120/DOI:10.1542/peds.111.4.829.
12. Sampson HA et al., J Allergy Clin Immunol. (1984), PMID: 6547461/DOI:10.1016/0091-6749(84)90083-6
13. Bernstein IL et al., Ann Allergy Asthma Immunol. (2008), PMID: 18431959/DOI:10.1016/s1081-1206(10)60305-5.
14. Commins SP et al., J Allergy Clin Immunol. (2009), PMID: 19070355/DOI:10.1016/j.jaci.2008.10.052.
15. Valenta R et al., Clin Exp Allergy. (1999), PMID: 10383589/DOI:10.1046/j.1365-2222.1999.00653.x.
16. Dang TD et al., J Allergy Clin Immunol. (2012), PMID: 22385632/DOI:10.1016/j.jaci.2012.01.056.
17. Nicolaou N et al., J Allergy Clin Immunol. (2010), PMID: 20109746/DOI:10.1016/j.jaci.2009.10.008.
18. Nowak-Wegrzyn A et al., J Allergy Clin Immunol. (2009), PMID: 19500710/DOI:10.1016/j.jaci.2009.03.042.
19. Lemon-Mule H et al., J Allergy Clin Immunol. (2008), PMID: 18851876/DOI:10.1016/j.jaci.2008.09.007.
20. Kim JS et al., J Allergy Clin Immunol. (2011), PMID: 21601913/DOI:10.1016/j.jaci.2011.04.036.
21. Leonard SA et al., J Allergy Clin Immunol. (2012), PMID: 22846751/DOI:10.1016/j.jaci.2012.06.006.
22. Popescu FD, World J Methodol. (2015), PMID: 26140270/DOI:10.5662/wjm.v5.i2.31.
23. Wong L et al., Allergy Asthma Immunol Res. (2016), PMID: 26739402/DOI:10.4168/aair.2016.8.2.101.
24. Schwartz LB, Immunol Allergy Clin North Am. (2006), PMID: 16931288/DOI:10.1016/j.iac.2006.05.010.
25. Pobłocki J et al., Nutrients. (2020), PMID: 32429294/DOI:10.3390/nu12051437.
26. Brown JC et al., J Allergy Clin Immunol Pract. (2020), PMID: 32276687/DOI:10.1016/j.jaip.2019.12.015.

27. Gabrielli S et al., J Allergy Clin Immunol Pract. (2019), PMID: 31035000/DOI:10.1016/j.jaip.2019.04.018.

28. Holbrook T et al., J Allergy Clin Immunol. (2013), PMID: 23890754/DOI:10.1016/j.jaci.2013.06.021.

29. Kelso JM et al., J Allergy Clin Immunol. (1993), PMID: 8258625/DOI:10.1016/0091-6749(93)90069-r.

30. Vanderhoof JA et al., J Pediatr. (1997), PMID: 9403656/DOI:10.1016/s0022-3476(97)70103-3.

31. Du Toit G et al., N Engl J Med. (2015), PMID: 25705822/DOI:10.1056/NEJMoa1414850.

32. Elizur A et al., Pediatr Res. (2017), PMID: 28549059/DOI:10.1038/pr.2017.127.

33. Flinterman AE et al., Allergy. (2006), PMID: 16436148/DOI:10.1111/j.1398-9995.2006.01018.x.

34. Skripak JM et al., J Allergy Clin Immunol. (2007), PMID: 17935766/DOI:10.1016/j.jaci.2007.08.023.

35. Savage JH et al., J Allergy Clin Immunol. (2007), PMID: 18073126/DOI:10.1016/j.jaci.2007.09.040.

36. Fleischer DM et al., J Allergy Clin Immunol. (2005), PMID: 16275381/DOI:10.1016/j.jaci.2005.09.002.

37. Sicherer SH, J Allergy Clin Immunol. (2011), PMID: 21236480/DOI:10.1016/j.jaci.2010.11.044.

38. Fleischer DM et al., J Allergy Clin Immunol. (2003), PMID: 12847497/DOI:10.1067/mai.2003.1517.

39. Ben-Shoshan M, J Allergy Clin Immunol Pract. (2020), PMID: 32389280/DOI:10.1016/j.jaip.2019.12.031.

40. Nurmatov U et al., Allergy. (2017), PMID: 28058751/DOI:10.1111/all.13124.

41. Chu DK et al., Lancet. (2019), PMID: 31030987/DOI:10.1016/S0140-6736(19)30420-9.

42. Bégin P et al., Allergy Asthma Clin Immunol. (2020), PMID: 32206067/DOI:10.1186/s13223-020-0413-7.

43. Fleischer DM et al., J Allergy Clin Immunol Pract. (2021), PMID: 33250376/DOI: 10.1016/j.jaip.2020.11.002.

17

Eosinophilic Esophagitis (EoE)

ABEER FETEIH, HOANG PHAM, MICHAEL FEIN,
SERGE MAYRAND, AND NATACHA TARDIO

GENERAL BACKGROUND

Definition of Eosinophilic Esophagitis (EoE)

- Chronic immune/antigen-mediated esophageal disease characterized by (1) symptoms of esophageal dysfunction, including but not limited to dysphagia and food impaction in adults and feeding intolerance and gastroesophageal reflux disease (GERD) symptoms in children and (2) eosinophil-predominant inflammation in esophageal tissue after exclusion of other disorders associated with similar clinical, histologic, or endoscopic features (1).

Epidemiology

- Increasingly recognized in both children and adults in the past 15–20 years with the first case described in 1968 (2).
- The pooled prevalence is 34.4 cases per 100,000 inhabitants with 34.0 cases per 100,000 in children, and 42.2 cases per 100,000 in adults (3).
- More often observed in males than females by 3:1 in both children and adults (2).

- About 50%–80% of patients with EoE have a personal or family history of atopic disease (e.g. asthma, eczema, allergic rhinitis, and/or food allergies) (4, 5).

Pathogenesis

- In genetically susceptible individuals, EoE arises as a result of food and/or aeroallergen protein antigen interactions with esophageal epithelial cells, which leads to the production of pre-atopic cytokines such as interleukin (IL)-33 and thymic stromal lymphopoietin (TSLP). T-regulatory and CD4+ T-helper type 2 (Th2) cells are then activated to produce transforming growth factor (TGF)-β, IL-4, IL-5, and IL-13. These cytokines signal through downstream transcription factors, which upregulate genes for periostin, calpain 14 (CAPN14), and eotaxin-3 while downregulating genes for desmoglein-1 (DSG1). Collectively, these pathways result in esophageal epithelial barrier dysfunction, tissue remodeling, and eosinophilic inflammation as illustrated in Figure 17.1 (6).

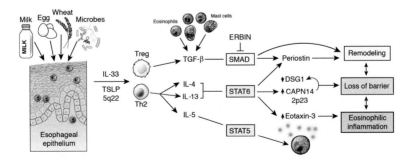

Figure 17.1 Pathophysiology of EoE. Environmental factors, including foods and the microbiome, interact with the esophageal epithelium to elicit production of proatopic cytokines, IL-33 and TSLP. Activated T regulatory and T helper type 2 cells secrete cytokines including TGF-β, IL-4, IL-13, and IL-5, which signal through downstream transcription factors (SMAD, STAT6, STAT5) resulting in epithelial barrier disruption, tissue remodelling, and eosinophilic inflammation. [Reprinted with permission from O'Shea KM et al., Gastroenterology. (2018), Elsevier.

DOI: 10.1201/9781003174202-22

Clinical Manifestations

Signs and Symptoms of EoE Seen Commonly by Age Group (2)

- **Less than 5 years old:** Failure to thrive, feeding difficulties, gagging on solid foods
- **Between 6 and 14 years old:** Vomiting, abdominal pain, and dysphagia
- **More than 15 years old:** Dysphagia, food impaction, and esophageal strictures

Other Signs and Symptoms of EoE

- Heartburn, regurgitation, chest pain, abdominal pain, odynophagia, malnutrition (1)
- Food-induced immediate response of the esophagus (FIRE) (7)
  - Newly reported symptom complex
  - Painful sensation occurring rapidly after esophageal contact with certain foods (mostly fruits, vegetables, nuts, wine), distinct from oral allergy syndrome
  - Pathogenesis and effect on management unknown at this time

Important Questions to Ask on History (2)

- Presence of dysphagia and its characteristics (e.g. solids, liquids, both; intermittent vs. progressive)
- History of food impaction
- Changes in certain eating behaviors (e.g. avoidance of eating meat)
- History of prolonged chewing time
- Increased frequency of drinking fluids with meals to bring down the food
- Required to cut food into small pieces to be able to swallow
- Possible or suspected triggers of symptoms (e.g. specific foods, seasonal variation)
- History of atopic disease (asthma, eczema, allergic rhinitis), history of food allergies
- Undergoing oral immunotherapy (OIT) or sublingual immunotherapy (8)

Diagnosis

All of the following are needed (1):

- Symptoms of esophageal dysfunction (see Clinical Manifestations section above)
- Presence of ≥15 **eosinophils/high-power field (hpf)** in at least 1 esophageal biopsy specimen
- Exclusion of other causes of esophageal eosinophilia

Note: According to the "International Consensus Diagnostic Criteria for Eosinophilic Esophagitis: *Proceedings of the AGREE Conference," a proton pump inhibitor (PPI) trial is no longer required for diagnosis of EoE (1).*

Note on Endoscopy and Esophageal Mucosal Biopsies

- All patients with suspected EoE must undergo esophageal mucosal biopsies to confirm diagnosis (2).
- **Macroscopic esophageal findings:** Rings, furrows, exudates, edema, stricture, narrowing, and crepe paper mucosa (2).
- **Microscopic esophageal findings:** Esophageal eosinophilia, superficial layering could be found on biopsy specimens, eosinophilic microabscess, extracellular eosinophil granules, basal cell hyperplasia, dilated intercellular spaces, and lamina propria fibrosis (2, 9).
- Biopsy specimens need to be obtained from both the proximal or mid and distal esophagus regardless of the gross appearance of the esophageal mucosa, as well as from areas revealing endoscopic abnormalities (2, 10).
- At least 4 biopsies are required to obtain adequate sensitivity for the detection of EoE (5–6 biopsies are generally recommended). One study found that 6 biopsies increases the sensitivity of this investigation to 99% (11).

Differential Diagnosis of Esophageal Eosinophilia (Selected Conditions) (1)

- EoE
- GERD
- Eosinophilic gastritis, gastroenteritis, or colitis with esophageal involvement
- Infections
- Achalasia
- Celiac disease
- Inflammatory bowel disease (e.g. Crohn's disease)
- Hypereosinophilic syndrome
- Hypersensitivity reactions to drugs
- Connective tissue disorders

Additional Investigations to Be Considered According to Clinical History, Differential Diagnosis of Esophageal Eosinophilia, and Nutritional Concerns (1, 12)

- Complete blood count (CBC) with differential
- Tissue transglutaminase (tTG) antibody IgA

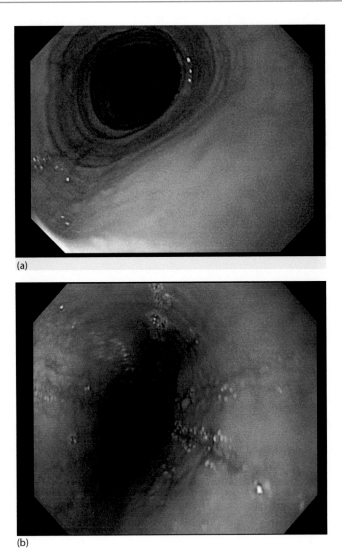

Figure 17.2 Endoscopic images characteristic of EoE. (a) Mid and (b) distal esophagus in two patients with dysphagia showing multiple rings, linear furrows and small whitish papules (eosinophilic abscesses on histology). (Images courtesy of Dr. Serge Mayrand.)

- Ferritin, vitamin B_{12}, 25-hydroxyvitamin D blood levels
- Total IgE
- Erythrocyte sedimentation rate (ESR)
- Stool for ova and parasites (O&P)
- Allergy assessment: Skin prick testing (SPT), serum food-specific IgE (sIgE), atopy patch testing (APT) (12)
  - Allergy testing may help identify causative foods although studies have shown a histological remission of only approximately one-third of adults managed with an allergy-testing directed diet (12). Allergy tests should

be used and interpreted with care in directing management of patients with EoE.

Management

EoE management is complex and requires a multi-faceted, multidisciplinary approach to patient care that includes either one or a combination of the following: Pharmacotherapy with corticosteroid treatment, proton-pump inhibitors (PPIs), restriction in dietary antigens, lifestyle adjustments, and frequent endoscopic diagnostic and therapeutic evaluations (12, 13).

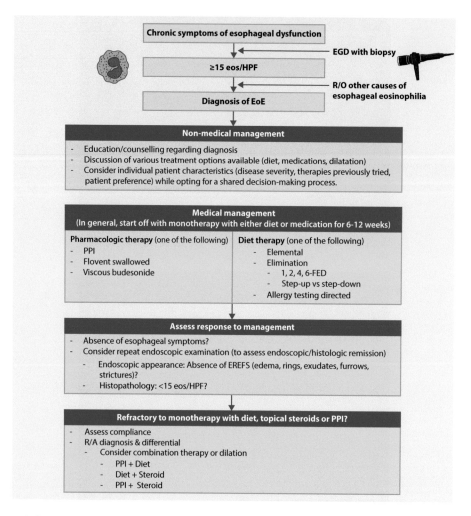

Figure 17.3 Systematic approach to the diagnosis and management of EoE as performed at the McGill University Health Centre (MUHC). (*Abbreviations:* EoE: Eosinophilic esophagitis; EGD: Esophagogastroduodenoscopy; HPF: High power field; PPI: Proton pump inhibiotor; FED: Food elimination diet; R/A: Reassess, R/O: Rule out). (Figure created using BioRender.com.) [Adapted from (1, 12) and (13).]

Diet

- It has been shown that all the types of diets below may be effective with improved clinical symptoms and pathology (6, 12, 13).
- Shared decision-making process is recommended when selecting a regimen (12, 13).
- With all dietary approaches, it remains unclear how long specific foods need to be avoided, which order to reintroduce individual foods, and how often to perform gastroscopy and mucosal biopsies for reassessment (1). Research is ongoing to clarify the most appropriate approach.
- At this time, an upper endoscopy with biopsies is performed to assess response to diet elimination and introduction (13).

- *Elemental diet*
  - Removal of all sources of possibly allergenic protein from the diet by using an amino acid-based formula for nutritional support (12). Generally reserved for severe cases. Compliance to this diet is difficult.
  - If there is favorable clinical and histologic response, one new food is reintroduced in a sequential fashion, starting with the least allergenic foods (fruits and vegetables) to the most highly allergenic (e.g. dairy, soy, egg, wheat, and peanuts) (12).
  - Most effective diet treatment with histological and clinical resolution in greater than 90% of pediatric and adult patients (4, 12).

- May require administration using a nasogastric tube, which may lead to adherence issues and impaired quality of life (12).
- *Targeted elimination diet (allergy-testing directed)*
  - Elimination of food based on SPT, sIgE, or APT to food.
  - Studies suggest a success rate of 45.5% for targeted, test-driven diets overall, and even lower success rates in adults (12).
  - Positive clinically irrelevant results and false-negative results complicate this dietary approach should be used with care in directing management.
- *Empiric food elimination diet*
  - Elimination of the most common food antigens (in the absence of, or regardless of, the results of allergy testing) (12).
  - A step-up versus step-down approach to elimination of dietary antigens has been suggested (12).
    - **Step-down approach**: Involves eliminating all possible food antigen triggers with the re-introduction of one food at a time:
      - Six-food elimination diet (SFED): generally, consists of the avoidance of dairy, egg, soy, wheat, peanut/tree nuts, fish/shellfish (12, 14).
      - Four-food elimination diet: Generally, consists of the avoidance of milk, eggs, wheat, and soy (12, 15).
    - **Step-up approach**: Involves eliminating the most common culprit(s):
      - Dairy is likely the most commonly implicated triggering food (74%), followed by wheat (26%) and egg (17%) (16).
      - In some centers, cow's milk single-food elimination is used as the first trial, based on data suggesting a response rate approaching that of the SFED (~65%) but with greater convenience/feasibility (12, 17).

Pharmacologic Treatment

PPIs

- In general, pharmacological management begins with PPI therapy (13).
- PPI dose: Pantoprazole 40 mg orally QD to BID in adults for 8–12 weeks (1, 2, 10).

Steroids [Adapted from (9)]

Topical Swallowed Steroids

- Remain an important part of EoE management with literature showing efficacy in improving symptoms and reducing disease activity (13).
- Options available include:
  - *Fluticasone propionate* [Adapted from (10)]
    - **Dose:** 880–1760 mcg/day in a divided dose (adults) or 88–440 mcg/day in a divided dose (children).
    - **Preparation/technique:** Given by a pressurized metered-dose inhaler that is activated into the mouth and *swallowed* (without inhaling and without a spacer device). The patient should be instructed not to eat or drink for 30 minutes after taking the medication and can rinse mouth without swallowing.
  - *Budesonide (oral viscous)* [Adapted from (10)]
    - **Dose:** 2 mg/day typically in a divided dose (adults) or 1 mg/day (children).
    - **Preparation/technique:** Given *orally* after mixing the contents of the vial used for nebulization with a thickening agent to increase the viscosity of the solution (e.g. with sucralose, apple sauce, or honey). More convenient and successful treatment option, with high clinical and histologic response rates in pediatric and adult patients with EoE (18, 19).
- **Side effects of topical corticosteroids to be considered**
  - Oral candidiasis: Most common side effect; has been reported in up to 15% of patients treated with topical corticosteroids (13).
  - Growth suppression and adrenal insufficiency: Very limited descriptions in certain populations but prospective long-term studies are ongoing (13).
- **Maintenance therapy** [Adapted from Hirano, 2020]
  - "In patients with EoE in remission after short-term use of topical corticosteroids, the AGA/JTF suggests continuation of topical glucocorticosteroids over discontinuation of treatment. (Conditional recommendation, very low quality evidence)" (13).

– The AGA/JTF does qualify this recommendation by stating that patients who place a high value on avoidance of long-term topical steroid use and possible side effects and/or place a low value on the prevention of potential long-term undesirable outcomes (e.g. recurrent dysphagia, food impaction, and esophageal stricture), could reasonably prefer cessation of treatment after initial remission is achieved, provided clinical follow-up is maintained.

Biologics

- There is currently a knowledge gap in terms of biologic options in EoE and the use of monoclonal antibodies such as anti-IL-5, anti-IL-13, and anti-IL-4 receptor α should be conducted in the setting of a clinical trial (13).
- Dupilumab, a monoclonal antibody against the α-chain of IL-13 and IL-4 receptors, showed major improvements in dysphagia when it was used weekly in adult patients with active moderate to severe EoE in a double blind placebo controlled phase 2 trial (20).
- The American Gastroenterological Association (AGA)/Joint Task Force for Allergy-Immunology Practice Parameters (JTF) suggests against the use of anti-IgE for EoE (13).

Esophageal Dilation Therapy [Adapted from (10, 13)]

- Effective in patients who have symptoms with esophageal strictures that persist despite medical or dietary treatment and in those who present initially with esophageal stenosis with severe symptoms.
- Risks: Post-dilation chest pain (up to 75% of patients), bleeding, and esophageal perforation.

REFERENCES

1. Dellon ES et al., Gastroenterology. (2018), PMID: 30009819/DOI:10.1053/j.gastro.2018.07.009.
2. Cianferoni A et al., Clin Rev Allergy Immunol. (2016), PMID: 26194940/DOI:10.1007/s12016-015-8501-z.
3. Navarro P et al., Aliment Pharmacol Ther. (2019), PMID: 30887555/DOI:10.1111/apt.15231.
4. Liacouras CA et al., Clin Gastroenterol Hepatol. (2005), PMID: 16361045/DOI:10.1016/s1542-3565(05)00885-2.
5. Assa'ad AH et al., J Allergy Clin Immunol. (2007), PMID: 17258309/DOI:10.1016/j.jaci.2006.10.044.
6. O'Shea KM et al., Gastroenterology. (2018), PMID: 28757265/DOI:10.1053/j.gastro.2017.06.065.
7. Biedermann L et al., Allergy. (2021), PMID: 32662110/DOI:10.1111/all.14495.
8. Cafone J et al., Curr Opin Allergy Clin Immunol. (2019), PMID: 31058677/DOI:10.1097/ACI.0000000000000537.
9. Collins MH, Gastrointest Endosc Clin N Am. (2008), PMID: 18061102/DOI:10.1016/j.giec.2007.09.014.
10. Dellon ES et al., Am J Gastroenterol. (2013), PMID: 23567357/DOI: 10.1038/ajg.2013.71.
11. Nielsen JA et al., Am J Gastroenterol. (2014), PMID: 24445569/DOI: 10.1038/ajg.2013.463.
12. Cianferoni A et al., Clin Exp Allergy. (2019), PMID: 30714219/DOI:10.1111/cea.13360.
13. Hirano I et al., Gastroenterology. (2020), PMID: 32359562/DOI:10.1053/j.gastro.2020.02.038.
14. Kagalwalla AF et al., Clin Gastroenterol Hepatol. (2006), PMID: 16860614/DOI:10.1016/j.cgh.2006.05.026.
15. Molina-Infante J et al., J Allergy Clin Immunol. (2014), PMID: 25174868/DOI:10.1016/j.jaci.2014.07.023.
16. Spergel JM et al., J Allergy Clin Immunol. (2012), PMID: 22743304/DOI:10.1016/j.jaci.2012.05.021.
17. Kruszewski PG et al., Dis Esophagus. (2016), PMID: 25721813/DOI:10.1111/dote.12339.
18. Gupta SK et al., Clin Gastroenterol Hepatol. (2015), PMID: 24907502/DOI:10.1016/j.cgh.2014.05.021.
19. Straumann A et al., Gastroenterology. (2010), PMID: 20682320/DOI:10.1053/j.gastro.2010.07.048.
20. Hirano I et al., Gastroenterology. (2020), PMID: 31593702/DOI:10.1053/j.gastro.2019.09.042.

Celiac Disease and Non-Celiac Gluten Sensitivity

STEPHEN TSOUKAS, NATACHA TARDIO, AND WAQQAS AFIF

GENERAL BACKGROUND

- Celiac disease (CD) is an autoimmune gluten-sensitive enteropathy, due to exposure to gliadin protein.
- Traditionally, 1% global prevalence (highest in Scandinavia).
- Recent meta-analysis: pooled global seroprevalence 1.4%, however, biopsy-confirmed CD only 0.7% (1, 2).
  - Female to male ratio is 3:2.
  - Higher prevalence in children.
  - Increasing prevalence 0.6% (1991–2000) to 0.8% (2011–2016) (2).
  - Global distribution correlates with geographic wheat consumption and frequency of HLA-DQ2/DQ8 haplotypes (3).
- More common with concomitant autoimmune disease and genetic syndromes:
  - Autoimmune hepatitis, autoimmune thyroiditis, chromosomal abnormalities (Down syndrome, Turner syndrome), inflammatory bowel disease (IBD), inflammatory myopathies, rheumatoid arthritis (RA), Sjogren syndrome, systemic sclerosis, systemic lupus erythematosus (SLE), type 1 diabetes mellitus (DM) (4–8).
- Risk of CD is unaffected by the timing of gluten introduction in children (9, 10).
- CD has an increased risk of malignancy:
  - Enteropathy-associated T-cell lymphoma (EATL), B-cell non-Hodgkin lymphoma (NHL), small bowel adenocarcinoma, esophageal squamous cell carcinoma (controversial) (11).
- Classically known as the celiac "iceberg" as majority of patients (up to 7/8) remain undiagnosed (12).

DEFINITIONS

- **Classic celiac sprue:** Abnormal serology and histology with gastrointestinal (GI) symptoms
- **"Atypical" celiac sprue:** Abnormal serology and histology with atypical symptoms
- **Silent celiac sprue:** Abnormal serology and histology without symptoms
- **Latent celiac sprue:** Abnormal serology, genetic susceptibility, but normal histology

Pathogenesis and Immunology

- Presentation of gluten peptides to CD4+ Th1 cells leads to downstream activation of intraepithelial lymphocytes (IELs) with intestinal inflammation, crypt hyperplasia, and villous atrophy (13).
- Enzyme tissue transglutaminase (TG2) deamidates gluten peptides including gliadin, increasing affinity for HLA-Class II DQ2 and DQ8 on antigen presenting cells (13).
- HLA Class II DQ2 and DQ8 haplotypes present in 30%–35% of people globally; however, only 2%–5% of these develop CD (13).
  - 95% of CD patients are DQ2+ (14), 5% are DQ8+ (15).
  - Dose-dependent effect of HLA-DQ2 gene: increased binding and immune activation in homozygotes (14).
- Anti-tissue transglutaminase (t-TG) autoantibodies are related to stimulation of gluten-reactive T cells but are not involved in intestinal injury (16).
- Autoantibodies may play a direct role in extraintestinal injury. Dermatitis herpetiformis (DH) involves cutaneous deposition of anti-tTG3 autoantibodies reacting to epidermal transglutaminase (4).

DOI: 10.1201/9781003174202-23

Table 18.1 Associated Features of CD of by Age

Exclusively pediatric	Exclusively adult
Short stature (33%), delayed puberty	Alopecia, infertility, neuropathy, secondary hyperparathyroidism with osteopenia, osteoporosis

Adapted from [4, 17].

Clinical Manifestations

Intestinal Manifestations

Diarrhea, steatorrhea, bloating, abdominal pain, and flatulence.

- Children are more likely to present with malabsorption symptoms compared with adults (2).

Extraintestinal Manifestations (EIMs) (4, 17)

- Present in up to 60%.
- 18% of children and 9% of adults have exclusively EIM at diagnosis.
- Commonly:
  - Weight loss
  - Fatigue (37%)
  - Headache
  - Anemia (48% iron deficient)
  - Abnormal liver enzymes (40%)
  - Arthralgia/arthritis (20–30%), myalgias
  - Alopecia, stomatitis, cutaneous involvement
- **Findings related to vitamin deficiencies (malabsorption)**
  - Koilonychia, glossitis, stomatitis, osteomalacia, poor wound healing, hypogonadism, edema, pellagra, cataracts, easy bleeding

Diagnosis and Investigations

Refer to the 2019 European Society for the Study of Coeliac Disease (ESsCD) and 2013 American Gastroenterological Association (AGA) Guidelines (18, 19).

General Principles

- Recommend testing if:
  - Signs, symptoms, or laboratory evidence suggestive of CD or malabsorption.
  - Asymptomatic with first-degree relative with CD (9).
  - Patient with type 1 DM, or unexplained elevation of serum aminotransferases.
- Diagnostic testing must be done on a gluten-containing diet (GCD):
  - *Gluten challenge:* Traditionally 10 g/day for 6–8 weeks, but 3g/day for 14 days may be sufficient (~2 slices of wheat-based bread) (18, 19).
- Diagnosis relies on a combination of clinical features, serology, genotype, and histology; not solely symptom based.

Serological Testing for CD

See Figure 18.2 for testing algorithm for CD.

- IgA deficiency is more common in CD (2%–3%); may yield false negatives (20).
- If deficient, perform IgG-based testing.
- Anti-gliadin antibodies are **not** recommended (poor sensitivity and specificity).
- Salivary and fecal antibody testing is under investigation (limited sensitivity).

Genotyping

- HLA-DQ2/DQ8 typing is **not** a routine test.
- May be useful to rule out CD (>99% negative predictive value [NPV] if both negative) (5):
  - If already on GFD without prior testing and unable to perform gluten challenge.
  - In asymptomatic patients with first-degree relative with CD.
  - If positive serology but normal histology (on GCD).

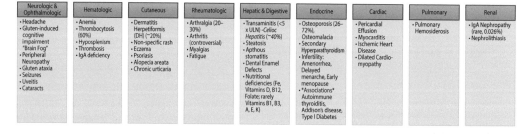

Neurologic & Ophthalmologic	Hematologic	Cutaneous	Rheumatologic	Hepatic & Digestive	Endocrine	Cardiac	Pulmonary	Renal
• Headache • Gluten-induced cognitive impairment "Brain Fog" • Peripheral Neuropathy • Gluten ataxia • Seizures • Uveitis • Cataracts	• Anemia • Thrombocytosis (60%) • Hyposplenism • Thrombosis • IgA deficiency	• Dermatitis Herpetiformis (DH) (~20%) • Non-specific rash • Eczema • Psoriasis • Alopecia areata • Chronic urticaria	• Arthralgia (20–30%) • Arthritis (controversial) • Myalgias • Fatigue	• Transaminitis (<5 x ULN) -Celiac Hepatitis (~40%) • Steatosis • Aphthous stomatitis • Dental Enamel Defects • Nutritional deficiencies (Fe, Vitamins D, B12, Folate; rarely Vitamins B1, B3, A, E, K)	• Osteoporosis (26–72%), Osteomalacia • Secondary Hyperparathyroidism • Infertility: Amenorrhea, Delayed menarche, Early menopause • *Associations* Autoimmune thyroiditis, Addison's disease, Type I Diabetes	• Pericardial Effusion • Myocarditis • Ischemic Heart Disease • Dilated Cardio-myopathy	• Pulmonary Hemosiderosis	• IgA Nephropathy (rare, 0.026%) • Nephrolithiasis

Figure 18.1 Extraintestinal manifestations by system. [Adapted from (4, 17).]

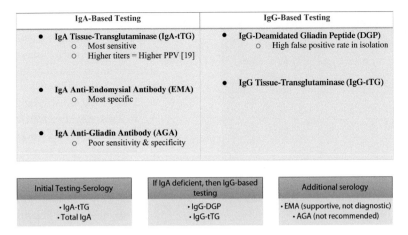

IgA-Based Testing	IgG-Based Testing

• **IgA Tissue-Transglutaminase (IgA-tTG)**
   ○ Most sensitive
   ○ Higher titers = Higher PPV [19]
	• **IgG-Deamidated Gliadin Peptide (DGP)**
	   ○ High false positive rate in isolation

• **IgA Anti-Endomysial Antibody (EMA)** ○ Most specific	• **IgG Tissue-Transglutaminase (IgG-tTG)**
• **IgA Anti-Gliadin Antibody (AGA)** ○ Poor sensitivity & specificity	

Initial Testing-Serology	If IgA deficient, then IgG-based testing	Additional serology
• IgA-tTG • Total IgA	• IgG-DGP • IgG-tTG	• EMA (supportive, not diagnostic) • AGA (not recommended)

Figure 18.2 Serology testing in celiac disease. [Adapted from (18, 19).]

Endoscopy and Biopsy

- Gold standard confirmatory testing: *Upper endoscopy with duodenal biopsies* while on GCD.
  - At least 4 biopsies from the second stage of the duodenum *and* 2 biopsies from the duodenal bulb (13% false-negative rate if only post-bulbar biopsies) (21).

- **Endoscopic appearance (22, 23)**
  - Scalloping or loss of folds, mosaic pattern, micronodules.
  - Normal endoscopy does not exclude CD.
  - Multiple biopsies needed (including duodenal bulb) given patchy distribution.

Table 18.2 Indications for Biopsy

When is endoscopy indicated?	
High clinical suspicion, even with negative serology	**Suggest serology with confirmatory biopsy only if positive**

• Chronic diarrhea (non-bloody, malabsorption)
• High-output ostomy
• Unexplained iron deficiency Anemia
• Biopsy-proven dermatitis herpetiformis
• Villous atrophy on small bowel imaging
• Failure to thrive (Pediatrics)
• Intestinal symptoms *with*:
  • Autoimmune disease
  • IgA deficiency
  • Family history of CD
	• Irritable bowel syndrome
	• Chronic fatigue syndrome
	• Idiopathic acute or chronic pancreatitis
	• Microscopic colitis
	• Thyroid disease (Hashimoto's, Graves)
	• Down or Turner Syndrome
	
	Isolated Extra-Intestinal Features
	• Recurrent aphthous ulcers, enamel defects
	• Unexplained transaminitis
	• Osteoporosis/Osteopenia
	• Hyposplenism, functional asplenia
	• Pulmonary hemosiderosis
	• IgA nephropathy
	• Non-DH skin lesions, psoriasis
	• Infertility, recurrent miscarriage, late menarche, early menopause
	• Unexplained ataxia, peripheral neuropathy, epilepsy, headaches, mood-disorders, ADHD, or cognitive impairment
	• Intestinal symptoms *in absence of*:
	  • Autoimmune disease
	  • Family history of CD

Adapted from (18).

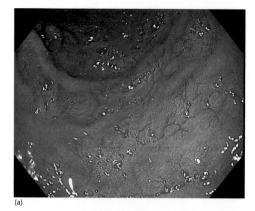

(a)

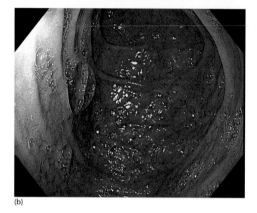

(b)

Figure 18.3 Duodenum: Mosaic pattern, scalloping of folds. (Images courtesy of Dr. Waqqas Afif.)

- **Histologic appearance (21)**
  - *Defining feature*: IELs
  - Crypt hyperplasia
  - Villous atrophy
  - Reactive epithelial changes
  - Intragranulocytic infiltrates
  - Lymphoplasmacytic inflammation
  - Increased crypt apoptotic activity
- **Similar histologic features of IELs and Villous atrophy can be seen in other conditions**
  - Infectious (Whipple's disease, Tropical sprue, Giardiasis), Inflammatory bowel diseases, Enteropathy Associated T-Cell Lymphoma (EATL), Auto-immune enteropathies, Immune-deficiencies (CVID, AIDS enteropathy), Infiltrative diseases, Medications (Mycophenolate Mofetil, Colchicine, Angiotensin-Receptor Blockers, Chemotherapeutics, Checkpoint inhibitors) [24–26]

Diagnostic Considerations: Special Groups

- If elevated anti-tTG but normal histology:
  - Review biopsies, test for other autoantibodies (anti-endomysial antibody [EMA]) ± HLA typing.
    - Likely CD if EMA and anti-tTG positive.
    - If EMA negative, test for HLA DQ2/DQ8. CD excluded if negative; however, if positive, repeat serology needed.
- Diagnosis in children (27):
  - Diagnosis without biopsy:
    - Only if **symptomatic** with **anti-tTG titers >10× upper limit of normal (ULN)** and **positive anti-EMA serology**.
    - **Lower titers still require biopsy**.
- Asymptomatic screening for CD in high-risk groups (family history, type 1 DM, genetic syndromes) (27)
  - Consider HLA testing, if positive → standard serology and specialist referral ± biopsy.
    - May not be cost-effective; alternatively opt for first-line serology.

Management

- **Mainstay of treatment is lifelong gluten avoidance/gluten-free diet (GFD)**
  - Avoid barley, rye, wheat.
    - Oats may be safely tolerated, but caution given risk of cross-contamination with gluten (19, 28).
  - Improved outcomes with dietician involvement and patient education.
- **Test for concurrent nutritional deficiencies (Iron, folate, B_{12}, vitamin D, calcium, micronutrients)**
  - Most levels normalize with GFD alone, but may require temporary supplementation.
  - GFD is typically low in folate and fiber.
- **Management of EIMs**
  - Most EIM resolve with GFD, but may fail in up to 26% of children and 49% of adults (17).
  - DH: May respond to GFD, however, dapsone 50–100 mg PO daily is used as first-line therapy (contraindicated in G6PD deficiency) (29).
  - Osteopenia/osteoporosis: Typically has improvement on GFD alone. Limited evidence suggests bisphosphonates not superior to GFD alone (30, 31).
    - Screening dual energy x-ray absorptiometry (DEXA) recommended after 1 year of GFD (4).
  - Gluten ataxia may be irreversible if GFD not initiated early (4).

- **Adjunctive treatment of uncomplicated CD**
  - Pharmacologic treatment including steroids is reserved for refractory disease.
  - Further research has looked into genetic modification or pre-treatment of wheat, enzyme supplementation, and tight junction modification (32–34).

Long-Term Monitoring: Multidisciplinary Follow-Up (Physician, Dietician)

- **Clinical assessment**
  - Residual or new symptoms.
  - GFD adherence.
  - Screening: Malnutrition, liver disease, associated autoimmune conditions.
- **Confirm normalization of laboratory abnormalities used in diagnosis**
  - Serology is useful in confirming treatment response: 82% seronegative by 6–12 months of strict GFD; 93% negative at 5 years (35, 36).
    - ESsCD proposes to repeat serology every 3 months for 1 year then annually (18).
    - Prior American College of Gastroenterology (ACG) guideline recommends annual serology (19).
- **No absolute routine follow-up biopsy if asymptomatic, although reasonable to repeat endoscopy in 1–2 years (especially if age >40, severe index presentation, or seronegative CD)**
  - Seronegativity ≠ histologic healing.
  - Mucosal healing may take a median of 2 years (children) to 3 years (adults) (37, 38).

Slow-Responders (Previously "Non-Responsive CD")

Persistent symptoms, signs, or laboratory abnormalities *despite ≥ 6–12 months of GFD* (19, 26).

- Incidence 7%–30% of CD.
- Most continue to improve on GFD, or have an alternative cause for symptoms.
- If possible, reassess initial serology and histology to confirm correct diagnosis of CD.
- If confirmed, 36%–51% are associated with ongoing gluten exposure and require careful dietician evaluation.
  - Consider repeating serology for further evidence.
- In absence of dietary causes, repeat endoscopy looking for persistence of villous atrophy (see above).

- Normal histology suggests benign disease: food intolerance, small intestinal bacterial overgrowth (SIBO), pancreatic insufficiency, microscopic colitis, or irritable bowel syndrome (IBS).

Refractory Celiac Disease (RCD)

- Persistent symptoms, signs or laboratory abnormalities *despite ≥ 12 months of GFD* in absence of other disorders including overt lymphoma [18]
  - Incidence 0.04–1.5% of CD; mean age 50; 2–3x more common in women [39]
  - Main symptoms: diarrhea, abdominal pain, weight loss, night sweats
  - Diagnosis: confirm initial diagnosis of CD; repeat serology and biopsies to exclude other causes of villous atrophy
  - RCD Type II involves aberrant monoclonal IELs with a 33–52% chance of EATL and a 44–58% 5 year survival. Referral to specialized center is indicated. (25, 26, 41)

Non-Celiac Gluten Sensitivity (NCGS)

- IBS-like symptoms and EIM with rapid onset following gluten exposure and abrupt improvement with GFD.
  - Exclude wheat allergy (allergy consult, skin test) and CD (serology, genotyping, and histology).
  - NCGS excluded if no symptomatic response to 6 weeks of GFD.
- No increased risk of malignancy, severe malabsorption, or any association with autoimmune disease.
- Mild, non-celiac enteropathy could be a continuum with later development of CD.
- No diagnostic test is proven or available at this time.
- There is evidence of symptomatic/serologic/histologic improvement with GFD in seropositive patients with mild enteropathy but non-diagnostic for CD (43, 44).

REFERENCES

1. Singh P et al., Clin Gastroenterol Hepatol. (2018), PMID: 29551598/DOI:10.1016/j.cgh.2017.06.037.
2. Reilly NR et al., Semin Immunopathol. (2012), PMID: 22526468/DOI:10.1007/s00281-012-0311-2.
3. Lionetti E et al., Best Pract Res Clin Gastroenterol. (2015), PMID: 26060103/DOI:10.1016/j.bpg.2015.05.004.
4. Therrien A et al., J Clin Gastroenterol. (2020), PMID: 31513026/DOI:10.1097/MCG.0000000000001267.

5. Sollid LM et al., Clin Gastroenterol Hepatol. (2005), PMID: 16234020/DOI:10.1016/s1542-3565(05)00532-x.

6. Page SR et al., QJM. (1994), PMID: 7987659.

7. Kylökäs A et al. BMC Gastroenterol. (2016), PMID: 27457377/DOI:10.1186/s12876-016-0488-2.

8. Lauret E et al., Biomed Res Int. (2013), PMID: 23984314/DOI:10.1155/2013/127589.

9. Crespo Escobar P et al., Rev Esp Enferm Dig. (2018), PMID: 29699403/DOI:10.17235/reed.2018.5324/2017.

10. Lionetti E et al., N Engl J Med. (2014), PMID: 25271602/DOI:10.1056/NEJMoa1400697.

11. Freeman HJ, World J Gastroenterol. (2009), PMID: 19340898/DOI:10.3748/wjg.15.1581.

12. Newnham ED, J Gastroenterol Hepatol. (2017), PMID: 28244672/DOI:10.1111/jgh.13704.

13. Schuppan D et al., Gastroenterology. (2009), PMID: 19766641/DOI:10.1053/j.gastro.2009.09.008.

14. Vader W et al., Proc Natl Acad Sci U S A. (2003), PMID: 14530392/DOI:10.1073/pnas.2135229100.

15. Megiorni F et al., J Biomed Sci. (2012), PMID: 23050549/DOI:10.1186/1423-0127-19-88.

16. Stepniak D et al., Hum Immunol. (2006), PMID: 16728270/DOI:10.1016/j.humimm.2006.03.011.

17. Jericho H et al., J Pediatr Gastroenterol Nutr. (2017), PMID: 28644353/DOI:10.1097/MPG.0000000000001420.

18. Al-Toma A et al., United European Gastroenterol J. (2019),PMID:31210940/DOI:10.1177/2050640619844125.

19. Rubio-Tapia et al., Am J Gastroenterol. (2013), PMID: 23609613/DOI:10.1038/ajg.2013.79.

20. Dickey W et al., Eur J Gastroenterol Hepatol. (1997), PMID: 9222726/DOI:10.1097/00042737-199706000-00002.

21. Lagana SM et al., Gastroenterol Clin North Am. (2019), PMID: 30711210/DOI:10.1016/j.gtc.2018.09.003.

22. Bonatto MW et al., Endosc Int Open. (2016), PMID: 27556094/DOI:10.1055/s-0042-108190.

23. Ravelli AM et al., Gastrointest Endosc. (2001), PMID: 11726850/DOI:10.1067/mge.2001.119217.

24. Mahadev S et al., Aliment Pharmacol Ther. (2017), PMID: 28220520/DOI:10.1111/apt.13988.

25. Hujoel IA et al., Curr Gastroenterol Rep. (2020), PMID: 32185560/DOI:10.1007/s11894-020-0756-8.

26. Rubio-Tapia A et al., Gut. (2010), PMID: 20332526/DOI:10.1136/gut.2009.195131.

27. Husby S et al., J Pediatr Gastroenterol Nutr. (2020), PMID:31568151/DOI:10.1097/MPG.0000000000002497.

28. Pinto-Sánchez MI et al., Gastroenterology. (2017), PMID: 28431885/DOI:10.1053/j.gastro.2017.04.009.

29. Antiga E et al., Front Immunol. (2019), PMID: 31244841/DOI:10.3389/fimmu.2019.01290.

30. Mautalen C et al., Am J Gastroenterol. (1997), PMID: 9040213.

31. Kumar M et al., Indian J Med Res. (2013), PMID: 24521630.

32. Cornell HJ et al., Scand J Gastroenterol. (2005), PMID: 16243716/DOI:10.1080/00365520510023855.

33. Leffler DA et al., Gastroenterology. (2015), PMID: 25683116/DOI:10.1053/j.gastro.2015.02.008.

34. Greco L et al., Clin Gastroenterol Hepatol. (2011), PMID: 20951830/DOI:10.1016/j.cgh.2010.09.025.

35. Zanini B et al., Dig Liver Dis. (2010), PMID: 20598661/DOI:10.1016/j.dld.2010.05.009.

36. Sugai E et al., Dig Liver Dis. (2010), PMID: 19679520/DOI:10.1016/j.dld.2009.07.011.

37. Wahab PJ et al., Am J Clin Pathol. (2002), PMID: 12219789/DOI:10.1309/EVXT-851X-WHLC-RLX9.

38. Rubio-Tapia A et al., Am J Gastroenterol. (2010), PMID: 20145607/DOI:10.1038/ajg.2010.10.

39. Malamut G et al., Dig Dis. (2015), PMID: 25925926/DOI:10.1159/000369519.

40. Mukewar SS et al., Am J Gastroenterol. (2017), PMID: 28323276/DOI:10.1038/ajg.2017.71.

41. Bagdi E et al., Blood. (1999), PMID: 10381521.

42. Cellier C et al., Lancet Gastroenterol Hepatol. (2019), PMID:31494097/DOI:10.1016/S2468-1253(19)30265-1.

43. Kurppa K et al., Gastroenterology. (2009), PMID: 19111551/DOI:10.1053/j.gastro.2008.11.040.

44. Kurppa K et al., Gastroenterology. (2014), PMID: 24837306/DOI:10.1053/j.gastro.2014.05.003.

PART 6

DRUG ALLERGY

19 Drug Allergy   167
    Abeer Feteih, Hoang Pham, and Ghislaine Annie Clarisse Isabwe

20 Adverse Reactions to Nonsteroidal Anti-Inflammatory Drugs and Aspirin   177
    Abeer Feteih, Lydia Zhang, Geneviève Genest, and Ghislaine Annie Clarisse Isabwe

21 Adverse Reactions to Vaccines   183
    Abeer Feteih, Lydia Zhang, and Geneviève Genest

Drug Allergy

ABEER FETEIH, HOANG PHAM, AND GHISLAINE
ANNIE CLARISSE ISABWE

GENERAL BACKGROUND

- Many drugs, dyes, and antiseptics can contribute to allergic reactions such as antibiotics, anesthetics (local and general), biologics, chemotherapy, chlorhexidine, nonsteroidal anti-inflammatory drugs (NSAIDs), etc.
- Drug hypersensitivity accounts for about 5%–10% of all adverse drug reactions (ADRs) (1).
- It is important to make a correct diagnosis of drug allergy for the identification of the culprit drug and also for investigating all cross-reactive structures and find an alternative that is a safer option (2).

DEFINITIONS

- **Drug allergies:** "are drug hypersensitivity reactions (DHRs) for which a definite immunological mechanism (either drug-specific antibody or T cell) is demonstrated." As stated by the International Consensus on drug allergy (ICON) (3).
- **Adverse Drug Reactions (ADRs):** "All unintended pharmacologic effects of a drug except therapeutic failures, intentional over- dosage, abuse of the drug, or errors in administration." **Definition as stated from the Joint Task Force on Practice Parameters: American Academy of Allergy, Asthma and Immunology (AAAAI); American College of Allergy, Asthma and Immunology (ACAAI); and Joint Council of Allergy, Asthma and Immunology Drug Allergy: An Updated Practice Parameter (4).**
  - **ADRs classification (4)**
    - **Predictable (type A):** Usually dose dependent, are related to the known pharmacological actions of the drug and occur in otherwise healthy individuals.
    - **Unpredictable (type B):** Defined by the World Health Organization (WHO) as "the dose-independent, unpredictable, noxious, and unintended response to a drug taken at a dose normally used in humans" (5, 6).
      - Drug idiosyncrasy
      - Drug intolerance
      - Drug allergy
      - Pseudoallergic reactions

CLASSIFICATIONS OF DRUG ALLERGY

The Gell and Coombs' Classification is the most well-known classification (see Figure 19.1 and 19.2) (7,8), but a more recent drug allergy classification was proposed by Muraro et al. according to the phenotypes and endotypes (9)

- **Phenotypes**
  - *Immediate*
    - *IgE mediated*
      - Reactions that occur after multiple dose exposures (e.g. penicillin)
      - Reactions that occur on first exposure with unrecognized prior sensitization (e.g. cetuximab and prior sensitization to galactose-alpha-1,3-galactose [alpha-gal])
    - *Direct mast cell/basophil activation:*
      - Complement activation and anaphylatoxins (C3a and C5a)
      - Mas-related G-protein-coupled receptor-X2 (MRGPRX2)

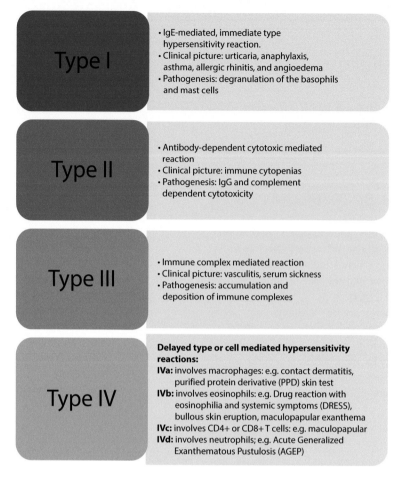

Figure 19.1 Drug Hypersensitivity reaction types according to Gell and Coombs' Classification. [Adapted from (3, 7, 8, 71).]

– e.g. quinolones, neuromuscular blocking agents, icatibant (10)

- *Cyclooxygenase-1 (COX-1) inhibition:* e.g. NSAIDs

– *Delayed:* Single-organ or multi-organ involvement

- *Cutaneous reactions:* Most common
- *Other organs:* Hepatic, pulmonary, renal, hematologic

Hypersensitivity reactions to monoclonal antibodies (biologics) (11)

- **Phenotypes and Endotypes (amenable to desensitization)**
  – *Type I (IgE/non-IgE):* Mast cell, basophils
  – *Cytokine release:* T cell
  – *Mixed reactions:* Type I and cytokine release
  – *Type IV:* Macrophage, T cell

CLINICAL CLASSIFICATION OF DHRs [ADAPTED FROM ICON ON DRUG ALLERGY (3)]

- **Immediate drug hypersensitivity reactions (IDHRs)**
  – **Onset:** Within 1–6 hours after the last drug administration (9, 12), but usually within 1 hour after receiving a new course of a medication
  – **Mechanism of the reaction:** Mostly IgE mediated
  – **Clinical picture**
    - Urticaria, angioedema, conjunctivitis, rhinitis, bronchospasm, nausea/vomiting, diarrhea, abdominal pain, anaphylaxis

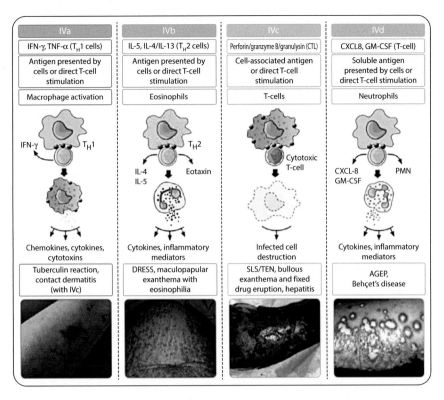

Figure 19.2 Extended Gell & Coombs classification of delayed T cell–mediated ADRs. Reprinted from (71) J *Allergy Clin Immunol*, 143 (1), Controversies in Drug Allergy: Testing for Delayed Reactions(2019), 66–73, with permission from Elsevier. (*Abbreviations:* AGEP: Acute generalized exanthematous pustulosis; CTLs: Cytotoxic T lymphocytes; CXCL8: C-X-C Motif Chemokine Ligand 8; DRESS: Drug reaction with eosinophilia and systemic symptoms; GM-CSF: Granulocyte-macrophage colony-stimulating factor; IFN-γ: Interferon gamma; IL: Interleukin; PMN: Polymorphonuclear leukocytes; SJS: Stevens-Johnson syndrome; TEN: Toxic epidermal necrolysis; Th1: T helper type 1 cells; Th2: T helper type 2 cells; TNF-α: Tumor necrosis factor alpha.)

- **Non-immediate drug hypersensitivity reactions (NIDHRs)**
  - **Onset:** Usually appears several hours to days after starting treatment
  - **Mechanism of the reaction:** Usually T-cell dependent
  - **Clinical picture**
    - Maculopapular rash
    - Delayed urticaria
    - Fixed drug eruption (FDE)
    - Drug rash with eosinophilia and systemic symptoms (DRESS) or drug-induced hypersensitivity syndrome (DiHS)
    - Toxic epidermal necrolysis (TEN)
    - Stevens-Johnson syndrome (SJS)
    - Acute generalized exanthematous pustulosis (AGEP)
    - Hepatitis, anemia, nephritis: Can occur without or with skin symptoms (e.g. DRESS)

Note: Severe cutaneous adverse reactions (SCARs) include DRESS/DiHS, SJS, TEN, and AGEP.

CLINICAL MANIFESTATIONS AND APPROACH

History (Focused)

- Identification, ethnicity
- Past medical history and past surgical history
- Medications (including aspirin, NSAIDs, beta-blockers, angiotensin-converting enzyme inhibitor (ACE-I) and any other medication)
- Allergies
- Drug(s) that potentially cause the reaction(s): Name of the drug(s), date of initiation and termination of the drug or drugs if more than one with a proper timeline, route of administration (e.g. oral versus intravenous versus subcutaneous)

- Identify which symptoms developed: Urticaria, angioedema, delayed rash and its description, respiratory symptoms, gastrointestinal symptoms, decrease level of consciousness, low blood pressure, fever, joint symptoms, ask about photos of the reaction if available from the patient
- Sequence and chronology of symptoms: Onset (acute vs. delayed), duration, resolution, other associated symptoms
- Reason/context of receiving the drug(s) at each event (e.g. perioperative/surgery)
- Determine whether this was the first exposure to the drug or has been previously received
- Any intervention required at the time of the suspected drug reaction (e.g. emergency department visit, hospitalization, intubation/critical care admission, epinephrine, vasopressors, antihistamines) as this might help gage the severity of the reaction
- Determine whether previous testing and investigation was done for suspected allergy to a drug(s) during any previous reaction (if any)
- Determine whether the patient was "re-exposed" to the same drug after the suspected reaction
- Question the patient on other possible causes of the suspected allergic reaction to exclude other causes (e.g. food, latex, insect sting, exercise) that may have been associated with the reaction around the same time

Physical Examination

Especially when the suspected drug reaction occurred in a hospitalized patient or an acute reaction bringing the patient to the emergency department; a complete physical exam is required including:

- General assessment: Patient's appearance, airway, signs of respiratory distress, mental status, vital signs including temperature
- Face/oropharynx: Angioedema, facial swelling, oral ulcers or lesions, laryngeal edema
- Respiratory exam: For wheezing, stridor
- Cardiac examination
- Abdominal exam
- Skin including mucous membranes: Rashes (e.g. erythema, hives, papules, ulcers, vesicles, blisters, pustules, bullae, Nikolsky sign, skin desquamation, purpuric lesions, discoloration)
- Lymph nodes
- Joints for signs of arthritis/synovitis

Selected Specific Delayed-Type DHRs

DRESS Syndrome

- "Drug-induced, multi-organ inflammatory response that may be life-threatening" (4).
- **Clinical manifestations**: Fever, cutaneous eruptions (exanthems, erythema multiforme, purpura), eosinophilia (most but not all cases), hepatic dysfunction, renal dysfunction, lymphadenopathy (13).
- **Diagnostic criteria:** There is the Japanese group criteria and the European Registry of Severe Cutaneous Adverse (drug) Reaction (RegiSCAR) criteria to assist with establishing the diagnosis along with clinical judgment (see Figures 19.1 and 19.3) (14–16).
- **Onset of the reaction:** 2–8 weeks after initiating treatment; the symptoms may get worse after stopping the drug and symptoms may continue for a number of weeks/months after the drug has been discontinued (4).
- **Human herpesvirus 6 (HHV-6) reactivation:** May signify higher severity of the disease and is found in many patients within 2–3 weeks of the eruption (17).
- **Contributing drugs (selected drugs):** Sulfonamides, allopurinol, sulfasalazine anticonvulsants, abacavir, minocycline, and dapsone, among others (4).
- **Management:** Includes stopping the culprit drug, corticosteroids with a slow taper (but efficacy is unknown), and other treatments including intravenous immunoglobulin (IVIg) (4).
- **Monitor for possible delayed autoimmune sequelae:** Two retrospective studies have described onset of new autoimmune conditions after DRESS, such as type 1 diabetes, thyroiditis, and systemic lupus erythematosus (18, 19).

RegiSCAR Scoring System for DRESS (16, 70)

- SJS
  - **Clinical manifestations**
    - High-grade fever, constitutional symptoms, confluent purpuric macules (on face and trunk) with severe mucosal erosions in >1 mucosal surface usually, they can have serious eye involvement, other organs can be involved as well such as the kidney, liver, and the lungs (4).

Table 19.1 European Registry of Severe Cutaneous Adverse [Drug] Reactions (RegiSCAR) Scoring System for DRESS (Drug Reaction with Eosinophilia and Systemic Symptoms). (This scoring system has been validated.)

RegiSCAR Scoring System for DRESS			
Criteria	No	Yes	Unknown/ Unclassifiable
Fever (>38.5°C)	−1	0	−1
Lymphadenopathy (>2 sites; >1 cm)	0	1	0
Circulating Atypical Lymphocytes	0	1	0
Peripheral Hypereosinophilia	0		0
0.7–1.499 × 10⁹/L - or - 10–19.9%*		1	
>1.5 × 10⁹/L - or - >20%*		2	
Skin Involvement			
* Extent of cutaneous eruption > 50% BSA	0	1	0
* Cutaneous eruption suggestive of DRESS**	−1	1	0
* Biopsy suggests DRESS	−1	0	0
Internal Organs Involved†	0		0
One		1	
Two or more		2	
Resolution in >15 days	−1	0	−1
Laboratory results negative for at least three of the following (and none positive): (1) ANA; (2) Blood cultures; (3) HAV/HBV/HCV serology; and (4) Chlamydia and Mycoplasma serology	0	1	0

* If leukocytes <4.0 × 10⁹/L.
** At least two of the following: Edema, infiltration, purpura, scaling.
† Liver, kidney, lung, muscle/heart, pancreas, or other organ and after exclusion of other explanations.
Note: Final score: < 2, no case; 2–3, possible case; 4–5, probable case; >5, definite case.
Abbreviations: ANA: Antinuclear antibody; BSA: Body surface area; HAV: Hepatitis A virus; HBV: Hepatitis B virus; HCV: Hepatitis C virus.
Reprinted with permission. From Laurence Valeyrie-Allanore, Grace. Dermatology: (2). Obeid, JeanRevuz, Elsevier.

- Epidermal detachment <10% (when it is ≥30% the diagnosis is TEN according to Bastuji-Garin et al.) (20).
- **Contributing drugs (selected drugs):** Sulfonamides, carbamazepine, phenytoin, valproic acid, cephalosporins, imidazole agents, vancomycin (4).
- **Management:** Early recognition, discontinuation of the offending drug is the first step and supportive care in intensive care unit (ICU) or burn unit are the mainstays of management with close attention to fluid status, nutritional support, electrolyte balance, and wound care (4).
  - Multidisciplinary care is needed (e.g. dermatology for wound care and ophthalmology consult is recommended to optimal ocular care).
  - Corticosteroid therapy remains controversial (21–23), but if used, it is recommended to give early and in high doses (24).
  - IVIg) has fallen out of favor after a meta-analysis of nine independent studies comparing IVIg versus supportive care did not find a mortality benefit (25).
  - Etanercept may be a promising potential therapy in the future (25).
- **TEN**
  - **Clinical manifestations:** Patients manifest with confluent erythema in widespread areas then develop epidermal necrosis and detachment (≥30%) with severe mucosal involvement with major loss of skin leading to an equivalent of a third-degree burn (4).
  - Glucocorticosteroids are contraindicated and patients are managed in the burn unit (21).

- Patients have a high risk of developing infection, with mortality rates up to 50% (26).
- **Contributing drugs:** Same drugs as with SJS.
- **Management:** Same as with SJS.
- **FDE**
  - **Clinical manifestations**
    - Eruptions usually involve the lips, acral regions (hands, feet), and genitalia. They may also present as vesicles, and mucosal lesions are usually bullous (4).
    - Typical eruptions present with sharply demarcated, round or oval, red, slightly elevated plaques, ranging from a few millimeters to several centimeters in diameter (4).
    - They recur at the same site (skin or mucosal) on reintroduction of the causative drug (4).
  - **Contributing drugs (selected drugs):** NSAIDs, carbamazepine, tetracycline, cotrimoxazole (27).
  - **Management:** Discontinuation of the drug and avoidance.
- **AGEP**
  - **Clinical manifestations**
    - Starts with erythema or edema in the intertriginous areas or the face and then fine non-follicular sterile pustules develop (4).
    - Fever, neutrophilia, and, in one-third of cases, eosinophilia may also be present (28).
  - **Contributing drugs:** Calcium channel blockers, antibiotics (4).
  - **Management:** Discontinuation of the drug and avoidance.

Diagnosis and Investigations [Adapted from (3, 4, 29)]

After an evaluation by history and physical exam (in an acute case), the following are tests used for drug allergy investigation (in general) depending on the type of the reaction.

1. **Skin testing**
   - Usually done for IgE-mediated immediate drug reactions.
   - Methods:
     - **Skin prick test (SPT) to the suspected drug (if available):** Skin test to penicillin is the only validated skin test in drug allergy (known sensitivity, specificity, negative predictive value [NPV], and positive predictive value [PPV]). For other drugs, non-irritating concentrations for skin testing is available in the literature but have not been validated. SPT is read 15–20 minutes after applying the drug allergen on the volar aspect of the arm. There must be a proper negative control (saline) and a positive control (histamine). Positive test is when the result is 3 mm greater than the negative control.
     - **Intradermal (ID) skin testing:** Done if the SPT is negative. ID testing is done by using 10- to 1000-fold more dilute than the concentration of allergen used in SPT, with 0.02–0.05 mL injected intradermally. Test is read after 10–15 minutes (29).
   - There are many different protocols/regimens proposed in the literature for skin test concentrations that can be used for many drugs, some examples suggested for reading are available in the following references:
   - **For penicillin:** Macy E et al. (30).
   - **For other drugs:** Empedrad et al. (31) and Brockow et al. (32).
   - If the skin tests are positive, it generally suggests drug allergy. If the skin tests are negative, proceed to the next step.

Note: Skin testing should be done 4–6 weeks after the reaction (3).

2. **Drug provocation testing (DPT)/graded dose drug challenge**
   - Gold standard test.
   - Usually done to rule out immediate drug reactions (IgE and non-IgE mediated).
   - This is done to the suspected drug that caused the reaction after weighing patient risk versus benefit.
   - Testing is usually done in a clinical setting where there is immediate access to lifesaving treatment (e.g. epinephrine, crash cart) should there be any life-threatening reaction such as anaphylaxis.
   - It usually involves giving the patient between 1 and 2 doses of the medication (e.g. divided into two doses), first 10% of

the total dose then 90% of the total dose (30-minute interval between doses) followed by 1 hour to observe for any immediate reaction (and longer with some medications e.g. NSAIDs).

- If the DPT is negative, then the patient is unlikely to have an IgE-/non-IgE-mediated immediate hypersensitivity reaction to the drug and can receive it safely should the patient ever require it.
- If the DPT is positive or is deemed to be unsafe due to risks outweighing the benefit, then an alternative should be chosen, or drug desensitization should be done if the patient absolutely needs that specific drug.
- A follow-up assessment should be arranged to rule out any delayed reaction following the DPT.
- Selected examples on DPT suggested for reading include (4, 33, 34).

3. **Patch testing or delayed ID testing**
- May be considered for delayed drug reactions, although yield appears modest (35).
- Should be done at least 4–6 weeks after the acute reaction to avoid false-positive reactions, false-negative reactions, and flaring up of systemic reactions.
- Patch testing for drug hypersensitivity is only available in certain centers and test positivity varies depending on the skin eruption and culprit drugs (35).

4. **Additional tests: Remain an area of ongoing study and currently available in research settings (2)**
- Basophil activation tests (BATs)
- HLA makers
- Cytokines
- Lymphocyte transformation test

5. **Skin biopsy (4)**
- In complex cases, a skin biopsy may be helpful in generating a differential diagnosis when multiple drugs are involved or if other non-drug hypersensitivity skin disorders are suspected (e.g. cutaneous lupus).
  - Sometimes cutaneous drug reactions can resemble one another in early stages (e.g. FDE and early SJS may be hard to discern).

HLA Markers and Disease Associations (Some Examples) [Adapted from (2)]

Screening for the following can be recommended in patients who are at risk:
- In abacavir-induced DHR 45.5%–80% for HLAB*57:01 (36–38)
- In carbamazepine-induced DHR 75%–100% for HLA-B*15:02 (39, 40)

Contraindications to Drug Challenge (As per McGill University Health Centre Pre-Risk Assessment Protocol)

- SCARs (SJS, TEN, AGEP, DRESS/DiHS)
- Exfoliative dermatitis
- Serum sickness
- Severe blood cytopenias
- Agranulocytosis
- Medication-induced vasculitis or autoimmunity to tested medication
- Medication-induced internal organ involvement
- Severe anaphylaxis (high-probability suspicion)
- Pregnancy

Management (General)

1. **Avoidance:** Of the culprit drug once diagnosis of the drug allergy is confirmed.
2. **Clear labeling/de-labeling:** The patient's drug allergy status must be clearly documented after confirmation. This includes changing the allergy status on the medical chart/record, pharmacy chart, and a note to the patient to keep as a reminder as well as a note to the referring physician/family physician (if applicable).
3. **Drug desensitization: (Usually for IgE-mediated immediate hypersensitivity reactions)**
- Usually performed in a monitored setting (e.g. critical care unit or emergency department) if the specific drug is absolutely needed without an available alternative (e.g. neurosyphilis in a pregnant woman with allergy to penicillin).
- There are several regimens proposed in the literature for drug desensitization; in general, starting dose concentration should be decided depending on the severity of the reaction (41–45).
4. **Alternative drug choice:** If there is no absolute indication for the specific culprit drug, an alternative drug should carefully be selected after assessing risk/benefit and cross-reactivity of the

drug(s) or choosing a different class of drug that has no cross-reactivity with the culprit drug.

5. **For type II, III, and IV hypersensitivity reactions:** Additional management other than drug avoidance depends on which reaction the patient had, usually treatment may involve symptomatic supportive treatment or topical or oral steroids (e.g. DRESS).

A Brief Note on Beta-Lactam (BL) Allergy

- The most common BLs associated with DHRs are penicillins (46, 47).
- BL allergy prevalence is 0.7%–10% of the general population (46, 47).
- The true incidence of penicillin allergy in those who report that they are allergic is <10% (48–53).
- DHRs to BLs are categorized into immediate reactions (IRs) and non-immediate (NIRs) based on symptom-onset timing after the first dose of the last therapeutic course (46, 54, 55).
- At least one exposure to the drug should be present before having a reaction, but a previous sensitization can be unsuspected or due to cross-reactivity (56).
- Diagnosis for IgE-mediated IRs (46): SPT followed by ID testing, if negative, the next step is a DPT if there are no contraindications.
- When an allergy to penicillin or another beta lactam antibiotic is suspected, it is important to confirm and verify whether an actual true allergy exists. Improper labelling of patients with penicillin or other beta lactam allergy may lead to unnecessary use of alternative antibiotics that are broader spectrum in coverage, increases the risk of resistant infectious organisms, unfavorable clinical outcomes, increased treatment cost and healthcare utilization, increased patient morbidity, and longer hospital stay for the patient (46).

Penicillin and Cephalosporins

- Cross-reactivity between penicillins and cephalosporins can in part be predicted upon the presence of shared R1, and to lesser degree R2 side chains (59).
- The pattern of cross-reactivity between penicillin and cephalosporin may also be based on the Thiazolidine ring in context of delayed severe cutaneous reactions; this ring maybe an important component in generation of the primary antigen (59).

Penicillins-Cephalosporins and Carbapenems

- Based on prospective studies of carbapenems, cross-reactivity is very unlikely or absent between carbapenems and penicillins-cephalosporins and it is as low as < 1% (57–59).

Penicillin-Cephalosporins and Monobactams

- There is no cross-reactivity between monobactams and the majority of penicillin–cephalosporins (4); however, aztreonam has a cross-reaction with ceftazidime as both drugs have similar side chains (60).

Risk of Anaphylaxis

- Anaphylaxis incidence to penicillins is 0.015%–0.004% and fatality rate of 0.002%–0.0015% according to an international survey adapted from (49).
- More limited data suggest the rate of anaphylaxis from cephalosporins is 0.1%–0.0001% (61).

Radiocontrast Media (RCM) Reactions

Immediate Severe Reaction

- Mostly secondary to non-IgE-mediated release of mediators from mast cells and basophils.
- It occurs in about 1%–3% of patients who receive ionic RCM and <0.5% of those who receive non-ionic agents (62, 63).
- Risk factors for this reaction: Previous history of reactions to RCM, females, using beta-blockers, asthma, and atopy (4).
- Skin testing has been recommended by certain authors (64); however, its validity remains controversial.
- To decrease the risk of a future severe reaction, nonionic, iso-osmolar agents should be used and the patient should be premedicated with systemic steroids and antihistamines (H1 blockers) (4, 65).

Delayed Reactions

Usually present with cutaneous eruptions that are mild and do not need management (66).

- *Perioperative drugs/allergens that can cause allergic reactions* (67)
  - Neuromuscular blocking agents: Atracurium, rocuronium, suxamethonium
  - Powdered natural rubber latex gloves

- – Antibiotics: BLs
- – Propofol
- – Chlorhexidine
- – Opioids
- – NSAIDs
- – Dyes
- *Chemotherapy drugs that can cause allergic reactions* (68)
  - – Taxanes: Such as paclitaxel and docetaxel
  - – Platinum compounds: Cisplatin, carboplatin, oxaliplatin
  - – Asparaginases: *Erwinia carotovora* asparaginase and polyethylene glycol-modified *Escherichia coli* asparaginase (PEG-asparaginase)
  - – Epipodophyllotoxins: Etoposide and teniposide
- *Hypersensitivity reactions to NSAIDs and aspirin*
  - – Refer to Chapter 20.
- *Hypersensitivity to other specific drugs*
  - – We refer to "Practical Guidance for the Evaluation and Management of Drug Hypersensitivity: Specific Drugs" (69).

REFERENCES

1. Riedl MA et al., Am Fam Physician. (2003), PMID:14620598.
2. Mayorga C et al., J Allergy Clin Immunol. (2019), PMID: 30573343/DOI:10.1016/j.jaci.2018.09.022.
3. Demoly P et al., Allergy. (2014), PMID: 24697291/DOI:10.1111/all.12350.
4. Joint Task Force on Practice Parameters et al., Ann Allergy Asthma Immunol. (2010), PMID: 20934625/DOI:10.1016/j.anai.2010.08.002.
5. International Drug Monitoring: The Role of National Centres. Report of a WHO meeting., World Health Organ Tech Rep Ser. (1972), PMID: 4625548.
6. Davies DM et al., Br Med J. (1977), PMID: 832025/DOI:10.1136/bmj.1.6053.89.
7. Coombs PR, Gell PG. (1968) Classification of Allergic Reactions Responsible for Clinical Hypersensitivity and Disease. In: Gell RR, ed. Clinical Aspects of Immunology, 575–96. Oxford, UK: Oxford University Press.
8. Pichler WJ et al., Ann Intern Med. (2003), PMID: 14568857/DOI:10.7326/0003-4819-139-8-200310210-00012.
9. Muraro A et al., Allergy. (2017), PMID: 28122115/DOI:10.1111/all.13132.
10. McNeil BD et al., Nature. (2015), PMID: 25517090/DOI:10.1038/nature14022.
11. Isabwe GAC et al., J Allergy Clin Immunol. (2018), PMID: 29518427/DOI:10.1016/j.jaci.2018.02.018.
12. Bircher AJ et al., J Allergy Clin Immunol. (2012), PMID: 21982115/DOI:10.1016/j.jaci.2011.08.042.
13. Peyrière H et al., Br J Dermatol. (2006), PMID: 16882184/DOI:10.1111/j.1365-2133.2006.07284.x.
14. Eshki M et al., Arch Dermatol. (2009), PMID: 19153346/DOI:10.1001/archderm.145.1.67.
15. Choudhary S et al., J Clin Aesthet Dermatol. (2013), PMID: 23882307.
16. Kardaun SH et al., Br J Dermatol. (2007), PMID: 17300272/DOI:10.1111/j.1365-2133.2006.07704.x.
17. Shiohara T et al., Br J Dermatol. (2007), PMID: 17381452/DOI:10.1111/j.1365-2133.2007.07807.x.
18. Chen YC et al., J Am Acad Dermatol. (2013), PMID: 22959230/DOI:10.1016/j.jaad.2012.08.009.
19. Ushigome Y et al., J Am Acad Dermatol. (2013), PMID: 23182063/DOI:10.1016/j.jaad.2012.10.017.
20. Bastuji-Garin S et al., Arch Dermatol. (1993), PMID: 8420497.
21. Roujeau JC et al., N Engl J Med. (1994), PMID: 7794310/DOI:10.1056/NEJM199411103311906.
22. Fine JD et al., N Engl J Med. (1995), PMID: 7477149/DOI:10.1056/NEJM199511303332207.
23. Cheriyan S et al., Allergy Proc. (1995), PMID: 8566720/DOI:10.2500/108854195778666793.
24. Tripathi A et al., Allergy Asthma Proc. (2000), PMID: 10791111/DOI:10.2500/108854100778250914.
25. Noe MH et al., Clin Dermatol. (2020), PMID: 33341195/DOI:10.1016/j.clindermatol.2020.06.016.
26. Bastuji-Garin S et al., Age Ageing. (1993), PMID: 8310891/DOI:10.1093/ageing/22.6.450.
27. Stubb S et al., Br J Dermatol. (1989), PMID: 2525047/DOI:10.1111/j.1365-2133.1989.tb01337.x.
28. Sidoroff A et al., J Cutan Pathol. (2001), PMID: 11168761/DOI:10.1034/j.1600-0560.2001.028003113.x.
29. Bernstein IL et al., Ann Allergy Asthma Immunol. (2008), PMID: 18431959/DOI:10.1016/s1081-1206(10)60305-5.
30 Macy E, Ngor EW et al., J Allergy Clin Immunol Pract. (2013), PMID: 24565482/DOI:10.1016/j.jaip.2013.02.002.
31. Empedrad R et al., J Allergy Clin Immunol. (2003),PMID:13679828/DOI:10.1016/s0091-6749(03)01783-4.
32. Brockow K et al., Allergy. (2013), PMID: 23617635/DOI:10.1111/all.12142.
33. Kao L et al., Ann Allergy Asthma Immunol. (2013), PMID: 23352526/DOI:10.1016/j.anai.2012.11.007.
34. Iammatteo M et al., J Allergy Clin Immunol Pract. (2014), PMID: 25439369/DOI:10.1016/j.jaip.2014.08.001.
35. Barbaud A et al., Br J Dermatol. (2013), PMID: 23136927/DOI:10.1111/bjd.12125.
36. Phillips EJ et al., J Allergy Clin Immunol. (2011), PMID: 21354501/DOI:10.1016/j.jaci.2010.11.046.

37. Mallal S et al., N Engl J Med. (2008), PMID: 18256392/DOI:10.1056/NEJMoa0706135.
38. Colombo S et al., J Infect Dis. (2008), PMID: 18684101/DOI:10.1086/591184.
39. Mehta TY et al., Indian J Dermatol Venereol Leprol. (2009), PMID: 19915237/DOI:10.4103/0378-6323.57718.
40. Locharernkul C et al., Epilepsia. (2008), PMID: 18637831/DOI:10.1111/j.1528-1167.2008.01719.x.
41. Castells MC et al., J Allergy Clin Immunol. (2008), PMID: 18502492/DOI:10.1016/j.jaci.2008.02.044.
42. Limsuwan T et al., Expert Opin Drug Saf. (2010), PMID: 20001753/DOI:10.1517/14740330903446936.
43. Sancho-Serra Mdel C et al., Eur J Immunol. (2011), PMID: 21360700/DOI:10.1002/eji.201040810.
44. Wendel GD Jr et al., N Engl J Med. (1985), PMID: 3921835/DOI:10.1056/NEJM198505093121905.
45. Brown SG et al., J Allergy Clin Immunol. (2004), PMID: 15316518/DOI:10.1016/j.jaci.2004.04.029.
46. Torres MJ et al., J Allergy Clin Immunol Pract. (2019), PMID: 30245291/DOI:10.1016/j.jaip.2018.07.051.
47. Doña I et al., J Investig Allergol Clin Immunol. (2014), PMID: 25011351.
48. Smith JW et al., N Engl J Med. (1966), PMID: 5909744/DOI:10.1056/NEJM196605052741804.
49. Idsoe O et al., Bull World Health Organ. (1968), PMID: 5302296.
50. Sogn DD et al., Arch Intern Med. (1992), PMID: 1580706.
51. Solley GO et al., J Allergy Clin Immunol. (1982), PMID:7056954/DOI:10.1016/0091-6749(82)90105-1.
52. Warrington RJ et al., Can Med Assoc J. (1978), PMID: 638909.
53. Sullivan TJ et al., J Allergy Clin Immunol. (1981), PMID: 6267115/DOI:10.1016/0091-6749(81)90180-9.
54. Blanca M et al., Allergy. (2009), PMID: 19133923/DOI:10.1111/j.1398-9995.2008.01916.x.
55. Torres MJ et al., Curr Opin Allergy Clin Immunol. (2016), PMID: 27285487/DOI:10.1097/ACI.0000000000000285.
56. Ariza A et al., J Investig Allergol Clin Immunol. (2015), PMID: 25898690.
57. Atanasković-Marković M et al., J Allergy Clin Immunol. (2009), PMID: 19368966/DOI:10.1016/j.jaci.2009.02.031.
58. Atanasković-Marković M et al., Allergy. (2008), PMID: 18186815/DOI:10.1111/j.1398-9995.2007.01532.x.
59. Pichichero ME et al., Ann Allergy Asthma Immunol. (2014), PMID: 24767695/DOI:10.1016/j.anai.2014.02.005.
60. Frumin et al., Ann Pharmacother. (2009), PMID: 19193579/DOI:10.1345/aph.1L486.
61. Kelkar PS et al., N Engl J Med. (2001), PMID: 11556301/DOI:10.1056/NEJMra993637.
62. Coleman WP et al., South Med J. (1964), PMID: 14226898/DOI:10.1097/00007611-196412000-00004.
63. Wolf GL et al., Invest Radiol. (1991), PMID: 2055736/DOI:10.1097/00004424-199105000-00003.
64. Greenberger PA et al., J Allergy Clin Immunol. (1991), PMID: 2013681/DOI:10.1016/0091-6749(91)90135-b.
65. Sánchez-Borges M et al., J Allergy Clin Immunol Pract. (2019), PMID: 30573421/DOI:10.1016/j.jaip.2018.06.030.
66. Webb JA et al., Eur Radiol. (2003), PMID: 12541128/DOI:10.1007/s00330-002-1650-5.
67. Pfützner W et al., Allergo J Int. (2018), PMID: 29974032/DOI:10.1007/s40629-018-0071-1.
68. Zanotti KM et al., Drug Saf. (2001), PMID: 11676304/DOI:10.2165/00002018-200124100-00005.
69. Broyles AD et al., J Allergy Clin Immunol Pract. (2020), DOI:10.1016/j.jaip.2020.08.006.
70. Valeyrie-Allanoire L, Obeid, Revuz J. (2017) Drug Reactions. In: Bolognia J, Schaffer JV, Cerroni L. Dermatology E-book, Fourth Edition. Philadelphia, PA: Elsevier. Available at: https://www-clinicalkey-com.proxy3.library.mcgill.ca/#!/browse/book/3-s2.0-C20131144449 (Accessed Feb 7, 2020)
71. Phillips EJ et al., J Allergy Clin Immunol. (2019), PMID: 30573342/DOI:10.1016/j.jaci.2018.10.030.

20

Adverse Reactions to Nonsteroidal Anti-Inflammatory Drugs and Aspirin

ABEER FETEIH, LYDIA ZHANG, GENEVIÈVE GENEST, AND GHISLAINE ANNIE CLARISSE ISABWE

GENERAL BACKGROUND

- Up to 1.9% of the general adult population reports nonsteroidal anti-inflammatory drug (NSAID) allergy (1).
- Aspirin and NSAIDs can cause many reactions, including exacerbation of underlying respiratory disease, urticaria, angioedema, anaphylaxis, and rarely pneumonitis and meningitis (2).
- Prevalence of aspirin-exacerbated respiratory disease (AERD) is 7.2% in adults with asthma overall, and about 14.9% in patients with severe asthma (3).

CLASSIFICATION OF NSAID ALLERGIES

1. **AERD**
   Other names: Samter's triad, Widal syndrome, aspirin-sensitive asthma, and aspirin-induced asthma.

- **Characteristics (4)**
  - Triad of asthma, recurrent eosinophilic nasal polyps that may lead to hyposmia, and respiratory reactions triggered by aspirin and all cyclooxygenase-1 (COX-1) inhibitor drugs.
  - Reactions are considered to be non-immune mediated (pseudoallergic).
- **Clinical manifestations**
  - Reactions start within 30–120 minutes of drug consumption (4).
  - *Respiratory signs/symptoms (upper and lower):* Rhinorrhea, nasal congestion, eye redness, chest tightness, and bronchospasm.
  - *Other signs/symptoms:* Flushing, nausea, abdominal pain, diarrhea, and macular eruption (pruritic) on the distal extremities (5–7).
- **Diagnosis and investigations**
  - Based on history and clinical manifestations.
  - Gold standard for definite diagnosis: Aspirin oral challenge (4).
  - Elevated levels of urinary leukotriene E4 (LTE4) and prostaglandin (PG) D2 at baseline and higher during acute episodes (4).
- **Aspirin challenge and desensitization in AERD (see Table 20.2)**
  - In the literature, the majority of protocols involve an overlap between aspirin challenge and desensitization, as patients with AERD typically have a reaction during desensitization.
  - The patient should be able to perform the procedure, and should be informed about risks, benefits, alternatives, and the steps of the challenge/desensitization.
- **Management options**
  - Avoidance of all COX-1 inhibitors and use of an alternative if needed.
  - Acetaminophen could be used if needed but cautiously because about one-third of these patients will develop some reaction to ≥1000 mg (4).
  - Patients can almost always tolerate celecoxib (COX-2 inhibitor) (9); however, an oral challenge should be performed to confirm tolerance.
  - *Aspirin desensitization if indicated:* After desensitization, continue aspirin 650 mg

DOI: 10.1201/9781003174202-26

Table 20.1 Classification of NSAID Allergies

Reaction type	Timing	Proposed mechanism	Cross-reactivity	Underlying disease	Desensitization effective
NSAIDs/Aspirin-exacerbated respiratory disease (NERD/AERD)	Acute	*Pseudoallergic:* COX-1 Inhibition	Yes	Asthma and rhinosinusitis	Yes
NSAID-exacerbated cutaneous disease (NECD)	Acute	*Pseudoallergic:* COX-1 Inhibition	Yes	Chronic urticaria	Controversial
NSAID-induced urticaria/angioedema (NIUA)	Acute	*Pseudoallergic:* COX-1 Inhibition	Yes	None	Yes
Single NSAID-induced urticaria/angioedema or anaphylaxis (SNIUAA)	Acute	*Allergic:* IgE-mediated	No	None	Not reported
Single NSAID-induced delayed reactions (SNIDR)	Delayed	*Allergic:* T-Cell mediated	No	None	Not reported

Adapted from Kowalski et al. (16).

twice a day for the first month then decrease the dose to 325 mg twice a day if the patient is doing well (nasal congestion resolved and return of sense of smell) (8).
- Giving montelukast before aspirin desensitization has been shown to reduce the extent of aspirin-induced bronchoconstriction and allows for a safer procedure (10).
- Aspirin desensitization in AERD meaningfully improves upper respiratory symptoms and disease-related quality of life. However, there are increased adverse events leading to treatment discontinuation (major bleeding, gastritis, asthma exacerbation, and rash). **Discontinuation rate is up to 38%** (20).

2. **Multiple NSAID-exacerbated urticaria/angioedema in patients with underlying chronic urticaria**
   - Defined as "an increase in the frequency or severity of chronic urticaria and/or angioedema with the use of any COX-1 inhibitor" (4).
   - There is cross-reactivity by which exposure to any COX-1 inhibitor worsens the patient's chronic cutaneous disease.

   Clinical manifestations
   - Symptoms are limited to the dermis and subcutaneous structures and manifest within minutes to hours of exposure to the drug.

- 12%–30% of adults and children with chronic idiopathic urticaria develop exacerbations of their underlying disease with the use of COX-1 inhibitors (12–14).

Diagnosis and investigations (4)
- History of chronic urticaria (>6 weeks) and history of symptom exacerbation after COX-1 inhibitor consumption.
- Oral drug challenge to a COX-1 inhibitor (e.g. aspirin) when the patient is asymptomatic for at least 2 weeks to confirm the diagnosis.

Management (4)
- Treatment of the underlying chronic urticaria.
- Avoid all COX-1 inhibitors.
- Use selective COX-2 inhibitors for pain if needed.

3. **Multiple NSAID-induced urticaria/angioedema in otherwise asymptomatic patients**
   Clinical manifestations
   - Urticaria and/or angioedema within **1–6 hours** after the consumption of an NSAID.

   Diagnosis and investigations
   - History of ≥2 different NSAIDs triggering a cutaneous reaction (4).
   - Aspirin challenge: When there is a history of a reaction to a single NSAID not caused by aspirin, because single NSAID-induced

Table 20.2 Aspirin Challenge and Desensitization in AERD: 1- or 2-Day Outpatient Options

Inform the patient about risks, benefits, alternatives, and steps of the challenge or desensitization.

Scripps protocol for aspirin challenge and desensitization in an outpatient setting (8):

- Ensure safety and document airway stability *1–7 days before the challenge*:
  - FEV^1 >60% of predicted value (>1.5 L absolute)
  - FEV^1 every hour for 3 hours—<10% variability
  - Start or continue montelukast, 10 mg every day
  - Start or continue inhaled corticosteroids (ICSs)/long acting bronchodilators (LABAs)
  - Start systemic corticosteroid (SCS) burst for low FEV^1 or any bronchial instability
  - Discontinue antihistamines 48 hours before challenge
- *Procedure done over two days to reach 650 mg of aspirin* [see (8) for full protocol].
  - Start with 20.25–40.5 mg of aspirin PO and increase *every 3 hours* over two days.
  - E.g.: *Day 1:* 20–40 mg, 40–60 mg, 60–100 mg; *Day 2:* 100 mg, 160 mg, 325 mg
- Reactions typically occur between 20–100 mg and once treated and patient stabilized, desensitization is continued by repeating provoking dose.

Protocol used at the Brigham and Women's Hospital AERD Center (4, 21):

- Can be safely accomplished in *1 day*; average time to protocol completion: ~9.5 hours
- *Inclusion criteria:* Baseline $FEV^1 \geq 70\%$, no hospital visit for asthma in the previous 6 months, stable asthma treatment for 4 weeks and montelukast 10 mg daily for a minimum of 2 weeks before aspirin challenge
- Administer oral aspirin in escalating doses (40.5, 81, 162.5, and 325 mg) with *90-minute intervals* between doses
- Measure FEV^1 every 90 minutes before proceeding with dose escalation, and with any symptoms
- A challenge is "positive" if there is a 15% decrease in FEV^1 from baseline, and/or an acute and physician-observable increase in at least 2 of the following:
  - Nasal congestion, rhinorrhea, sneezing, nasal or eye itching, or eye redness or tearing
- To achieve desensitization, the dose that provoked a reaction is repeated after patient stabilization and the protocol continues until the patient has tolerated 325 mg of aspirin (cumulative) without evidence of worsening respiratory symptoms

Points to consider:

- 1-day desensitization procedures may take ~9 hours or longer and may require an additional day depending on clinic hours
- 1-day desensitization only performed/studied in patients with baseline FEV^1 > 70%

Adapted from (4, 8, 21).

hypersensitivity reactions limited to the skin have been reported (15).
- Oral aspirin challenge: Standard for confirming this diagnosis.

Management
- NSAID (COX-1 inhibitors) avoidance.
- Use a selective COX-2 inhibitor if needed.
- Successful aspirin desensitization has been reported.

4. **Single NSAID-induced anaphylactic reactions**
   - Anaphylaxis, urticaria, or angioedema induced by a single NSAID.

   Clinical manifestations (4)
   - Symptoms occur **within minutes to an hour** following exposure to the drug.
   - Other associated symptoms: Pruritus, bronchospasm, and hypotension.

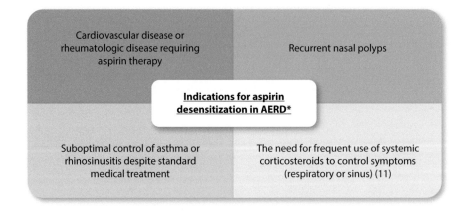

Figure 20.1 Indications for aspirin desensitization in AERD. [Adapted from (4).]
*Important to discuss risks/benefits and alternatives with patient as well as requirement for long-term high-dose aspirin therapy. Asthma should be well controlled before attempting desensitization.

Diagnosis and investigations
- Clinical history alone can usually detect the culprit agent and a negative challenge to aspirin or alternative NSAID is helpful to confirm that the reactions are non-cross-reactive (15).

Management
- Avoidance of the culprit drug and any NSAID with similar structure (4).
- No successful desensitizations to the anaphylaxis-inducing culprit NSAID have been documented. As there are many alternatives, desensitization is not recommended (4).

5. **Delayed reactions to NSAIDs:** Any cutaneous or systemic reaction manifesting after ≥24 hours of drug exposure.

   Clinical Manifestations (4)
   - **Maculopapular rash**: Usually mild and occurs about 1 week after exposure to the drug and resolve after discontinuation.
   - **Fixed drug eruptions:** *Refer to Chapter 19 for rash description.*
   - **Drug rash with eosinophilia and systemic symptoms (DRESS):** *Refer to Chapter 19 for details.*
   - **Stevens-Johnson syndrome (SJS) and toxic epidermal necrolysis (TEN):** *Refer to Chapter 19 for rash description.*
   - **Acute generalized exanthematous pustulosis (AGEP):** *Refer to Chapter 19 for rash description.*
   - **Contact dermatitis.**

Diagnosis
- History/clinical manifestations.
- Patch testing has been used in some cases of fixed drug eruptions, DRESS, and AGEP, although testing is not standardized and the positive and negative predictive values remain unclear.
- All other testing and drug challenges are contraindicated in SJS/TEN, AGEP, and DRESS (16).

Management
- Avoidance of the culprit drug.
- An alternative NSAID will need to be determined depending on each clinical case.

SPECIAL POPULATIONS: PREGNANCY AND ASPIRIN DESENSITIZATION

- Aspirin desensitization during pregnancy is contraindicated unless absolutely necessary for the wellbeing of the patient.
- Aspirin doses up to 160 mg daily are safe and well tolerated during pregnancy (17, 18).
- Desensitization maintenance can be continued at doses of up to 160 mg daily for the entire pregnancy, delivery, and the postpartum period unless indicated otherwise by the treating obstetrician (expert opinion).
- The treating obstetrician must be made aware of the reason for aspirin desensitization.

- If the patient needs to stop aspirin during pregnancy, re-desensitization may be attempted 6–8 weeks post-delivery, with clearance from the obstetrician (expert opinion).
- Doses exceeding 160 mg per day have been associated with congenital anomalies and should be avoided during pregnancy (19).

REFERENCES

1. Gomes E et al., Clin Exp Allergy. (2004), PMID: 15479276/DOI:10.1111/j.1365-2222.2004.02070.x.
2. Joint Task Force on Practice Parameters et al., Ann Allergy Asthma Immunol. (2010), PMID: 20934625/DOI:10.1016/j.anai.2010.08.002.
3. Rajan JP et al., J Allergy Clin Immunol. (2015), PMID: 25282015/DOI:10.1016/j.jaci.2014.08.020.
4. Laidlaw TM et al., J Allergy Clin Immunol Pract. (2017), PMID: 28483309/DOI:10.1016/j.jaip.2016.10.021.
5. Szczeklik A et al., Eur Respir J. (2000), PMID: 11028656/DOI:10.1034/j.1399-3003.2000.016003432.x.
6. Samter M et al., Ann Intern Med. (1968), PMID: 5646829/DOI:10.7326/0003-4819-68-5-975.
7. Cahill KN et al., J Allergy Clin Immunol. (2015), PMID: 25218285/DOI:10.1016/j.jaci.2014.07.031.
8. Stevenson DD et al., J Allergy Clin Immunol. (2006), PMID: 17030229/DOI:10.1016/j.jaci.2006.06.019.
9. Dahlen B et al., N Engl J Med. (2001), PMID: 11188419/DOI:10.1056/NEJM200101113440215.
10. Berges-Gimeno MP et al., Clin Exp Allergy. (2002), PMID: 12372130/DOI:10.1046/j.1365-2745.2002.01501.x.
11. Macy E et al., Ann Allergy Asthma Immunol. (2007), PMID: 17304886/DOI:10.1016/S1081-1206(10)60692-8.
12. Cavkaytar O et al., Allergy. (2015), PMID: 25353369/DOI:10.1111/all.12539.
13. Szczeklik A et al., J Allergy Clin Immunol. (1977), PMID: 410857/DOI:10.1016/0091-6749(77)90106-3.
14. Sanchez-Borges M et al., J Eur Acad Dermatol Venereol. (2015), PMID: 25263736/DOI:10.1111/jdv.12658.
15. Zisa G et al., Allergy Asthma Proc. (2012), PMID: 23026184/DOI:10.2500/aap.2012.33.3590.
16. Kowalski ML et al., Allergy. (2013), PMID: 24117484/DOI:10.1111/all.12260.
17. Duley L et al., Cochrane Database Syst Rev. (2019), PMID: 31684684/DOI:10.1002/14651858.
18. Rolnik DL et al., N Engl J Med. (2017), PMID: 28657417/DOI:10.1056/NEJMoa1704559.
19. Aspirin product monograph (2014).
20. Chu DK et al., Int Forum Allergy Rhinol. (2019), PMID: 31518069/DOI:10.1002/alr.22428.
21. DeGregorio GA et al., J Allergy Clin Immunol Pract. (2019), PMID: 30391549/DOI:10.1016/j.jaip.2018.10.032.

Adverse Reactions to Vaccines

ABEER FETEIH, LYDIA ZHANG, AND GENEVIÈVE GENEST

GENERAL BACKGROUND

- Vaccines are one of the most successful interventions in public health (1, 2, 16, 17).
- Most adverse reactions to vaccines consist of mild local reactions and/or constitutional symptoms (2), which do not contraindicate future doses (4).
- Severe anaphylactic or systemic cutaneous adverse reactions to vaccines occur infrequently (3).

TYPES OF ADVERSE REACTIONS TO VACCINES (4)

LOCAL INJECTION SITE REACTIONS AND OTHER MILD TRANSIENT VACCINE-ASSOCIATED REACTIONS

- Swelling, redness, soreness.
- Transient skin rash in 5% of individuals who receive the measles vaccine, possibly due to the modified vaccine itself (5).

- Fever (late onset) starting 5–12 days after vaccination, occurs in 5%–15% of those who receive the measles, mumps, rubella (MMR) vaccine (6).
- Thrombocytopenia can occur post-MMR vaccine. Rare cases of hemorrhage have been reported (6, 7).
- Arthritis/arthralgia: in about 15% of adult women receiving rubella vaccine (8).

All the above reactions are not contraindications to future immunization with the culprit vaccine (9).

IgE-MEDIATED REACTIONS TO VACCINES (4)

- Usually caused by additives or residual vaccine components, such as gelatin, rather than the microbial immunizing agent itself.
- Occur within 4 hours of exposure to culprit vaccine, most commonly within 15 minutes.
- Anaphylaxis to vaccines occurs at an estimated rate of around **1.3 per million** doses (10).
- Mortality from anaphylaxis caused by vaccines is extremely rare (7).

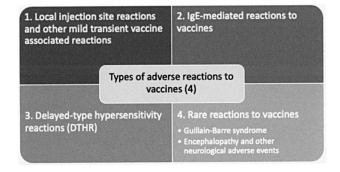

Figure 21.1 Classification of adverse reactions to vaccines. Mild local reactions and mild constitutional symptoms are the most common adverse reactions to vaccines. Thorough history is important to characterize reaction in order to guide management. (This figure is created using BioRender.com.) [Adapted from (4).]

DOI: 10.1201/9781003174202-27

ADDITIVES OR RESIDUAL COMPONENTS OF VACCINES

Gelatin

- Stabilizer in some vaccines and origins from beef or pork.
- Can cause anaphylactic reactions to varicella vaccine, MMR, and Japanese encephalitis vaccine (11, 12).
- There are some countries that have removed gelatin from MMR and varicella vaccines or changed it to a less allergenic gelatin; these include Japan and Germany (13, 14).
- Patients who are allergic to pork/beef or patients with galactose-α-1,3-galactose (alpha-gal) allergy are at risk of developing reactions to vaccines containing gelatin (15).

Egg/Chicken Protein

- Certain vaccines (influenza, yellow fever, rabies) are made using an egg-based manufacturing process and can contain small amounts of residual egg protein (ovalbumin) (3).
- *Influenza vaccines* should be administered to individuals with egg allergy of any severity, just as they would be to individuals without egg allergy (40).
- Consultation with an allergist is recommended prior to administering the yellow fever vaccine (YFV) in egg-allergic patients (4); desensitization protocols to the YFV have been developed for egg-allergic patients and are recommended in case of yellow fever outbreaks (41).
- Urgent consultation with an allergist should be considered for post-exposure prophylaxis (PEP) with rabies vaccine in egg allergic patients; however, the risk of not administering PEP largely outweighs the rare risk of anaphylaxis and PEP should not be delayed (42).
- Chicken protein can be present in the YFV and could cause IgE-mediated reaction in patients allergic to chicken (22).
- Measles or MMR vaccines can be given to children with egg allergy without adverse reactions (18, 19). Examples of vaccine that grow in chick embryo fibroblast cultures and contain almost no egg protein are Measles, Mumps and type of rabies vaccine (16, 17).

Yeast Protein

- Hepatitis B vaccines are grown in *Saccharomyces cerevisiae* (baker's yeast or brewer's yeast) (20).
- Adverse reactions are rare (21).
- Yeast protein may be present in quadrivalent human papillomavirus vaccine (HPV4) (20).

Milk Protein (Casein)

- Used as a stabilizer in certain vaccines [DTaP (Diphtheria, Tetanus, Pertussis Vaccine) and Tdap (Tetanus, Diphtheria, Pertussis Vaccine)].
- However, most cases of anaphylaxis to DTaP and Tdap are caused by the toxoid component.
- In highly milk-sensitized children, there is a theoretical possibility of allergic reaction to DTaP or Tdap, and these vaccines should be administered under enhanced surveillance (3).

Dry Natural Rubber (DNR) Latex

- DNR is found in the rubber of vaccine vial stoppers or syringe plungers and could in theory cause a reaction when administered to latex-allergic patients.
- Other vaccine vial stoppers and syringe plungers made of synthetic rubber pose no risk to latex-allergic persons.

DELAYED-TYPE HYPERSENSITIVITY REACTIONS (DTHRS): CONTACT DERMATITIS

Some DTHRs are related to vaccine additives.

Neomycin

- It is a constituent of many vaccines.
- It may cause a transient local small papule at the injection site in some patients (23, 24).
- Immunization may proceed normally in patients reporting a delayed-type contact dermatitis to neomycin (23).

Thimerosal

- Preservative used in trace amounts in certain vaccines (3).
- Even in patients with intradermal (ID)-proven or patch test-proven hypersensitivity to thimerosal, thimerosal-containing vaccines rarely cause hypersensitivity (3).
- Patch-test proven hypersensitivity to thimerosal could lead to large local reactions from thimerosal-containing vaccines (25, 26), but it is not a contraindication for receiving them (9).

Aluminum

- Is used as an adjuvant to enhance the immune response of the vaccinated subject (boost T-cell immunity) (3).
- Persistent nodules may develop at the injection site from nonspecific inflammation or irritant reactions (3).

RARE REACTIONS TO VACCINES: FUTURE DOSES MAY BE CONTRAINDICATED (9)

Guillain-Barré Syndrome (GBS)

- If GBS develops *within 6 weeks* of receiving the influenza vaccine, patients need to avoid further vaccination with influenza (27).
- GBS history in an individual that was unrelated to influenza infection or other vaccines can receive further vaccination (27).
- Tetanus toxoid has potential association with GBS and brachial neuritis, but neither are contraindications to receiving additional doses of tetanus-containing vaccines (4).

Encephalopathy and Other Neurological Adverse Events

- A very serious reaction to pertussis vaccine is encephalopathy (7).
- Usual onset is within 7 days of immunization.
- Presentation: altered mental status, unresponsiveness, seizures that can last several hours without recovery within 24 hours (7); this can have permanent neurological sequelae.
- This is an absolute contraindication for further vaccination with pertussis.
- Other selected reactions to pertussis vaccine: febrile seizures (28) and hypotonic-hyporesponsive episodes (29); these do not result in permanent adverse outcomes, and they are not contraindications for further doses of the pertussis vaccine (6, 9, 30).

SPECIAL PATIENT POPULATIONS

Pregnant Women

- *Live virus vaccines are contraindicated* because of the risk of live agent vertical transmission of the live vaccine agent (31).

- According to Centers for Disease Control and Prevention (CDC), women should avoid becoming pregnant 1 month after receiving the varicella, MMR, or YFVs (32, 33).
- Women who are pregnant or are trying to conceive should receive the inactivated influenza vaccine (34).
- Pregnant individuals can take the hepatitis B, diphtheria, and tetanus vaccines as required (31).
- Vaccine challenge/desensitization should only be performed under extreme circumstances during pregnancy; when the benefit of the vaccine administration clearly surpasses the risk of anaphylaxis. This should be done under expert council (consultation with pharmacy is recommended) in appropriate settings (intensive care unit) with assistance from appropriate consultants as needed (anesthesia for airway management and obstetrics for continuous fetal monitoring). Neonatology consultation should be considered if the patient is >24 weeks pregnant (expert opinion).

Immunocompromised Patients

- Live vaccines are contraindicated in patients with severe humoral or cellular immune deficiency, whether primary or secondary, due to the risk of fulminant vaccine strain-induced disease (9, 35, 36).
- **Includes**
  - Severe combined immune deficiency (SCID)
  - Common variable immune deficiency (CVID)
  - Severe HIV infection
  - X-linked agammaglobulinemia (XLA)
  - Leukemia, lymphoma

Diagnosis and Management of Suspected Anaphylaxis to Vaccine or Vaccine Components (4)

1. **Skin testing to the vaccine**
   - **Skin prick test (SPT):** With full-strength vaccine. Diluted vaccine concentration can be used in patients with a previous life-threatening reaction. If the full-strength SPT is negative (with appropriate negative/positive controls), then
   - **ID test:** With vaccine 0.02 mL diluted 1:100.

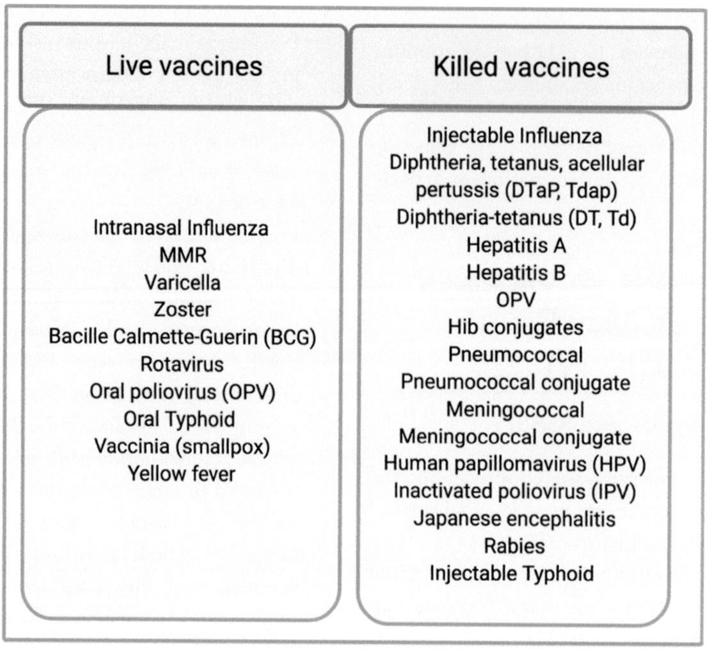

Live vaccines	Killed vaccines
Intranasal Influenza MMR Varicella Zoster Bacille Calmette-Guerin (BCG) Rotavirus Oral poliovirus (OPV) Oral Typhoid Vaccinia (smallpox) Yellow fever	Injectable Influenza Diphtheria, tetanus, acellular pertussis (DTaP, Tdap) Diphtheria-tetanus (DT, Td) Hepatitis A Hepatitis B OPV Hib conjugates Pneumococcal Pneumococcal conjugate Meningococcal Meningococcal conjugate Human papillomavirus (HPV) Inactivated poliovirus (IPV) Japanese encephalitis Rabies Injectable Typhoid

Figure 21.2 Examples of live and killed vaccines. (Figure created with BioRender.com.) [Adapted with permission from (4).]

2. **Skin testing to vaccine components**
   - SPT with commercial extracts of egg and *S. cerevisiae* yeast
   - SPT with commercial gelatin or serum-specific IgE to gelatin
   - Specific IgE testing to latex
   - Patch testing to aluminum/thimerosal for delayed reactions

3. **Skin testing results**

   - **If negative results:** The patient can receive the vaccine but requires observation for 30 minutes post-vaccination (37, 38).
   - **If positive results:** To the vaccine or component(s) of the vaccine, and if the patient requires more doses, the vaccine needs to be given by graded doses/desensitization (35).
   - If IgG antibodies are available for the culprit immunizing agent, protective antibody responses can be measured to determine whether further vaccination is essential.

Method of Graded Intramuscular Vaccine Dosing with 15-Minute Intervals

- 0.05 mL of a 1:10 dilution
- 0.05 mL full strength
- 0.1 mL full strength
- 0.15 mL full strength
- 0.2 mL full strength, then observe the patient for 30 minutes after
- This should all be done under the care of a physician who is trained and equipped to treat anaphylaxis (39)

Note:

- *DTHR can occur after ID skin testing with tetanus toxoid (39).*
- *Skin testing with vaccines can lead to irritant or false-positive results; skin test interpretation should always be done with a previous understanding of the pre-test probability of allergic reaction to the culprit vaccine (4).*

REFERENCES

1. National Vaccine Advisory Committee. Public Health Rep. (2013), PMID: 23450872/DOI:10.1177/003335491312800203.
2. Caubet JC et al., Immunol Allergy Clin North Am. (2014), PMID: 25017679/DOI:10.1016/j.iac.2014.04.004.
3. McNeil MM et al., J Allergy Clin Immunol. (2018), PMID: 29413255/DOI:10.1016/j.jaci.2017.12.971.

4. Kelso JM et al., J Allergy Clin Immunol. (2012), PMID: 22608573/DOI:10.1016/j.jaci.2012.04.003.

5. Strebel MJP, Dayan GH, Halsey NA. (2008) Measles Vaccine. In: Plotkin SA, Orenstein W, Offit P, eds. Vaccines, 353–398. Philadelphia, PA: WB Saunders Elsevier.

6. Centers for Disease Control and Prevention, MMWR Recomm Rep. (1996) PMID: 8801442.

7. Stratton KR et al., JAMA. (1994), PMID: 8182813.

8. Howson CP et al., JAMA. (1992), PMID: 1727962.

9. National Center for Immunization and Respiratory Diseases. MMWR Recomm Rep. (2011), PMID: 21293327.

10. Nilsson L et al., Pediatr Allergy Immunol. (2017), PMID: 28779496/DOI:10.1111/pai.12762.

11. Kelso JM et al., J Allergy Clin Immunol. (1993), PMID: 8473675/DOI:10.1016/0091-6749(93)90344-f.

12. Sakaguchi M et al., Allergy. (2001), PMID: 11421899/DOI:10.1034/j.1398-9995.2001.056006536.x.

13. Nakayama T et al., J Allergy Clin Immunol. (2000), PMID: 10984383/DOI:10.1067/mai.2000.108433.

14. Zent O et al., Vaccine. (2004), PMID: 15542177/DOI:10.1016/j.vaccine.2004.07.016.

15. Bogdanovic J et al., J Allergy Clin Immunol. (2009), PMID: 19665767/DOI:10.1016/j.jaci.2009.06.021.

16. Fasano MB et al., J Pediatr. (1992), PMID: 1593346/DOI:10.1016/s0022-3476(05)81953-5.

17. O'Brien TC et al., Appl Microbiol. (1971), PMID: 4995854.

18. Baxter DN, Vaccine. (1996), PMID: 8852409/DOI:10.1016/0264-410x(95)00154-s.

19. James JM et al., N Engl J Med. (1995), PMID: 7708070/DOI:10.1056/NEJM199505113321904.

20. Vaccine Excipient and Media Summary, by Excipient. (2011) In: Atkinson W, Wolfe S, Hamborsky J, eds. Centers for Disease Control and Prevention. Epidemiology and Prevention of Vaccine-Preventable Diseases, 12th Edition. Washington, DC: Public Health Foundation.

21. DiMiceli L et al., Vaccine. (2006), PMID: 16154669/DOI:10.1016/j.vaccine.2005.07.069.

22. Kelso JM et al., J Allergy Clin Immunol. (1999), PMID: 10400862/DOI:10.1016/s0091-6749(99)70136-3.

23. Rietschel RL et al., JAMA. (1981), PMID: 7452881/DOI:10.1001/jama.245.6.571b.

24. Elliman D et al., Lancet. (1991), PMID: 1671258/DOI:10.1016/0140-6736(91)90995-2.

25. Noel I et al., Lancet. (1991), PMID: 1679511/DOI:10.1016/0140-6736(91)91289-7.

26. Rietschel RL et al., Dermatol Clin. (1990), PMID: 2137393.

27. Fiore AE et al., MMWR Recomm Rep. (2010), PMID: 20689501.

28. Barlow WE et al., N Engl J Med. (2001), PMID: 11547719/DOI:10.1056/NEJMoa003077.

29. Cody CL et al., Pediatrics. (1981), PMID: 7031583.

30. DuVernoy TS et al., Pediatrics. (2000), PMID: 11015547/DOI:10.1542/peds.106.4.e52.

31. Bhole MV et al., Immunol Allergy Clin North Am. (2008), PMID: 18940576/DOI:10.1016/j.iac.2008.06.005.

32. McLean HQ et al., MMWR Recomm Rep. (2013), PMID: 23760231.

33. Marin M et al., MMWR Recomm Rep. (2007), PMID: 17585291.

34. Centers for Disease Control and Prevention (CDC), MMWR Recomm Rep. (2013), PMID: 24048214.

35. American Academy of Pediatrics. (2009) Red Book: Report of the Committee on Infectious Diseases, 28th Edition. Elk Grove Village (IL): American Academy of Pediatrics.

36. Moss WJ et al., Bull World Health Organ. (2003), PMID: 12640478.

37. Buckley RH et al., N Engl J Med. (1991), PMID: 2052044/DOI:10.1056/NEJM199107113250207.

38. Wood RA et al., Pediatrics. (2008), PMID: 18762513/DOI:10.1542/peds.2008-1002.

39. Bernstein IL et al., Ann Allergy Asthma Immunol. (2008), PMID: 18431959/DOI:10.1016/s1081-1206(10)60305-5.

40. Greenhawt M et al., Ann Allergy Asthma Immunol. (2018), PMID: 29273128/DOI:10.1016/j.anai.2017.10.020.

41. Cancado B et al., Lancet Infect Dis. (2019), PMID: 31345456/DOI:10.1016/S1473-3099(19)30355-X.

42. Moro PL et al., Travel Med Infect Dis. (2019), PMID: 31203930/DOI:10.1016/j.tmaid.2018.10.016.

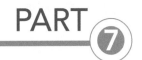
CLINICAL IMMUNOLOGY

22 General Approach to Primary Immunodeficiency (PID) in Adults   191
    Abeer Feteih, Lydia Zhang, Reza Alizadehfar, and Christos Tsoukas
23 Immunoglobulin Replacement Therapy   199
    Abeer Feteih, Farida Almarzooqi, Reza Alizadehfar, and Christos Tsoukas

General Approach to Primary Immunodeficiency (PID) in Adults

ABEER FETEIH, LYDIA ZHANG, REZA ALIZADEHFAR,
AND CHRISTOS TSOUKAS

DEFINITION AND BACKGROUND

- Primary immunodeficiencies (PIDs) are a group of inherited disorders of the immune system that predispose affected individuals to an increased frequency and severity of infection, abnormal inflammatory responses, autoimmune disease, and malignancy (1).
- Initially, PID in children was thought to be rare, and even more rare in adults, however it is now increasingly recognized.

- Prevalence estimation: ~1:2000 live births (1).
- There are >350 discovered PIDs.
- Lack of general awareness of these disorders often results in a delay in diagnosis.
- Secondary causes of immunodeficiency must be ruled out before a diagnosis of a PID is made.
- To increase general awareness among the medical community, ten warning signs of PID have been proposed by the "Jeffrey Modell Foundation" (see Table 22.1) (2).

Table 22.1 Jeffrey Modell Foundation: 10 Warning Signs of Primary Immunodeficiency (PID)

In adults	In children
≥ 2 new ear infections within 1 year	≥ 4 new ears infections within 1 year
≥ 2 new sinus infections within 1 year, in the absence of allergy	≥ 2 serious sinus infections within 1 year
1 pneumonia per year for more than 1 year	≥ 2 pneumonias within 1 year
Chronic diarrhoea with weight loss	≥ 2 months of antibiotics with little effect
Recurrent viral infections (colds, herpes, warts, condyloma)	Failure of an infant to gain weight or grow normally
Recurrent need for IV antibiotics to clear infections	Need for IV antibiotics to clear infections
Recurrent deep abscesses of the skin or internal organs	Recurrent, deep skin or organ abscesses
Persistent thrush or fungal infection on skin or elsewhere	Persistent thrush in mouth or fungal infection on skin
Infection with normally harmless tuberculosis-like bacteria	≥ 2 deep-seated infections including septicemia
A family history of primary immunodeficiency	A family history of primary immunodeficiency

Note: Delay in diagnosis is common in PID. Morbidity and mortality may be greatly reduced with early diagnosis through heightened awareness of PID and the use of warning signs.
Reprinted with permission from the Jeffrey Modell Foundation (2).

Classification

Based on the "International Union of Immunological Societies: 2017 Primary Immunodeficiency Diseases Committee Report on Inborn Errors of Immunity" (3)

Note: For the purpose of this chapter, only selected sub-classifications and examples are mentioned, therefore, for more details, please refer to the main cited reference.

1. **"Immunodeficiencies affecting cellular and humoral immunity" (selected diseases and examples):**
   - **Severe combined immunodeficiency (SCID):**
     - T-B+ SCID (e.g. gamma chain deficiency with a mutation in the IL2RG gene, JAK3 deficiency, IL7Rα deficiency)
     - T-B– SCID (e.g. RAG1/RAG2 deficiency, Artemis deficiency, adenosine deaminase [ADA] deficiency)
   - **Combined immunodeficiencies (generally less profound than SCID)**
     - DOCK2 deficiency
     - CD40 deficiency
     - CD40 ligand deficiency
     - ICOS deficiency, CD3γ deficiency, CD8 deficiency

2. **"Combined immunodeficiencies with associated or syndromic features" (selected sub-classifications and examples)**
   - Wiskott-Aldrich syndrome (WAS): Congenital thrombocytopenia-mutation in the WAS gene
   - Ataxia-telangiectasia: DNA repair defect-mutation in the ATM gene
   - DiGeorge syndrome: Thymic defect with more congenital anomalies-contiguous gene deletion in chromosome 22q11.2
   - Hyper-IgE syndromes: Job syndrome-STAT3 deficiency; Comel-Netherton syndrome-SPINK5 mutation
   - Cartilage hair hypoplasia: Immune-osseous dysplasias, mutations in RNAse MRP RNA (RMRP)
   - Anhidrotic ectodermodysplasia with immunodeficiency: Mutation in the NEMO (IKBKG) gene
   - Calcium channel defects: ORAI1 or STIM1 mutations

3. **"Predominantly antibody deficiencies" (selected examples)**
   - **Severe reduction in all serum immunoglobulin isotypes with profoundly decreased or absent B cell:** Bruton tyrosine kinase (BTK) deficiency, μ heavy chain, λ5, Igα, Igβ, BLNK deficiencies
   - **Severe reduction in at least 2 serum immunoglobulin isotypes with normal or low number of B cells:** Common variable immunodeficiency (CVID) disorders with no gene defect specified, CD19, CD81, CD20, CD21, TACI, BAFF receptor deficiencies
   - **Severe reduction in serum IgG and IgA with normal/elevated IgM and normal numbers of B cells:** Activation-induced cytidine deaminase (AID) deficiency, uracil N-glycosylase (UNG) deficiency
   - **Isotype or light chain deficiencies with generally normal numbers of B cells:** Specific antibody deficiency with normal Ig concentrations and normal numbers of B cells, selective IgA deficiency, isolated IgG subclass deficiency, transient hypogammaglobulinemia of infancy

4. **"Diseases of immune dysregulation" (selected examples)**
   - **Familial hemophagocytic lymphohistiocytosis (FHL) syndromes:** FHL syndromes without hypopigmentation such as perforin deficiency (FHL2); SH2D1A deficiency X-Linked lymphoproliferative syndrome type 1 (XLP1); XIAP deficiency (XLP2); and FHL syndromes with hypopigmentation such as Chediak-Higashi syndrome, Griscelli syndrome type 2, Hermansky-Pudlak syndrome
   - **T-regulatory cell genetic defects:** Immune dysregulation, polyendocrinopathy, enteropathy X-linked (IPEX) from mutation in FOXP3, CTLA4 deficiency, LRBA deficiency
   - **Autoimmunity with or without lymphoproliferation:** Autoimmune polyendocrinopathy with candidiasis and ectodermal dystrophy (APECED) mutation in the autoimmune regulator (AIRE) gene, autoimmune lymphoproliferative syndrome (ALPS)
   - **Immune dysregulation with colitis:** Interleukin (IL)-10 deficiency

- Susceptibility to Epstein-Barr virus (EBV) and lymphoproliferative conditions: e.g. SH2D1A deficiency (XLP1), XIAP deficiency (XLP2), CD27 deficiency, ITK deficiency, MAGT1 deficiency (XMEN)

5. **"Congenital defects of phagocyte number, function, or both" (selected examples)**
   - **Congenital neutropenias: Elastase deficiency (SCN1) from mutation in the ELANE gene**
   - **Defects of motility:** Leukocyte adhesion deficiency type 1 (LAD1), type 2 (LAD2), type 3 (LAD3), cystic fibrosis (CFTR gene)
   - **Defects of respiratory burst:** X-linked chronic granulomatous disease (CGD), autosomal recessive CGD
   - **Other non-lymphoid defects:** Congenital pulmonary alveolar proteinosis, GATA2 deficiency

6. **"Intrinsic and innate immunity defects" (selected examples)**
   - **Mendelian susceptibility to mycobacterial disease (MSMD):** IL-12 and IL-23 receptor β1 chain deficiency, IFN-γ receptor 1 deficiency, STAT1 deficiency (AD LOF), IRF8 deficiency
   - **Epidermodysplasia verruciformis:** Warts, hypogammaglobulinemia, infections, myelokathexis (WHIM) syndrome
   - **Predisposition to severe viral infection:** STAT1 deficiency (AR LOF)
   - **Herpes simplex encephalitis (HSE):** Toll-like receptor 3 (TLR3) deficiency
   - **Predisposition to invasive fungal diseases:** CARD9 deficiency
   - **Chronic mucocutaneous candidiasis (CMC):** IL-17RA deficiency, STAT1 GOF
   - **TLR signaling pathway deficiency:** IRAK-4 deficiency, MyD88 deficiency
   - **Isolated congenital asplenia (ICA)**

7. **"Autoinflammatory disorders" (selected examples)**
   - **Type 1 interferonopathies disease: Aicardi-Goutières syndrome, STING-associated vasculopathy**
   - **Defects affecting the inflammasome:** Familial Mediterranean fever (FMF)-mutations of the MEFV gene; patients present with recurrent fever, serositis and inflammation responsive to colchicine; predisposes them to vasculitis and inflammatory bowel disease; other examples: Muckle-Wells syndrome, familial cold autoinflammatory syndrome 1 (FCAS1), neonatal onset multisystem inflammatory disease (NOMID); all three have mutations in the NLRP3 gene. FCAS2 has a mutation in the NLRP12 gene. Mevalonate kinase (MVK) deficiency (Hyper IgD syndrome) with mutation in MVK
   - **Non-inflammasome-related conditions:** Tumor necrosis factor (TNF) receptor-associated periodic syndrome (TRAPS); patients present with recurrent fever, serositis, rash, and ocular or joint inflammation; another example is pyogenic sterile arthritis, pyoderma gangrenosum, acne (PAPA) syndrome

8. **"Complement deficiencies" (selected examples)**
   - **Integral complement cascade component deficiencies:** C1q deficiency (patient can have associated systemic lupus erythematosus [SLE] and infections from encapsulated organisms)' C5-C6-C7-C8-C9 deficiencies are all associated with *Neisseria* infections
   - **Complement regulatory defects:** C1 inhibitor deficiency (SERPING1 gene mutation) associated with hereditary angioedema (HAE); factor I and factor H deficiencies associated with disseminated neisserial infections, atypical hemolytic-uremic syndrome

9. **"Phenocopies of PID" (selected examples)**
   - Associated with autoantibodies: Chronic mucocutaneous candidiasis (isolated or with APECED syndrome), thymoma with hypogammaglobulinemia (Good syndrome)
   - Associated with somatic mutations: Autoimmune lymphoproliferative syndrome (ALPS–SFAS)

Making a diagnosis of PID requires a detailed history with a focus on severity, frequency and unusual complications of infections, autoimmunity, and malignancies. It is mandatory to obtain a detailed family history.

History

- Identification (age, sex): Male/female ratio of PID in children is approximately 5:1 but approaches 1:1 in adults (1).
- Past medical history/comorbidities.

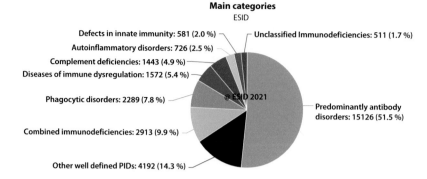

Figure 22.1 Distribution of the major PID groups: Percentage of diagnosed patients registered in the European Society for Immunodeficiencies (ESID) database. PIDs are classified according to the specific level of immune defect such as humoral (B-cell), cellular (T cell), combined (B and T cell), phagocytic, complement, or innate immune system. Autoimmune and autoinflammatory syndromes with genetic basis are also included. Humoral (antibody disorders) are the most commonly diagnosed PID. [Reproduced with permission from the European Society for Immunodeficiencies (ESID), 2021.]

- *Medications*: Determine whether any contribute and/or are a cause of immune deficiency, assess for presence of any that can cause secondary hypogammaglobulinemia (most commonly immunosuppressants such as glucocorticoids, rituximab, and antiepileptics).
- *Atopic disease (e.g. asthma, eczema, allergic rhinitis)*: Inhalant allergies may play a major role in contributing to upper airway infections.
- *Social history*: Having young children at home increases risk of upper airway infections and smoke exposure; teachers, nurses, and others in daily contact will the public often have recurrent respiratory infections (occupational).
- *Autoimmune disease*: Patients with PIDs may have concomitant autoimmune hemolytic anemia or Hashimoto thyroiditis. Patients with SLE, rheumatoid arthritis and other conditions undergo iatrogenic immunosuppression, making it difficult to evaluate the possibility of an underlying PID.
- *Recurrent infection history (viral, bacterial, fungal)*: During childhood and adulthood including (not limited to):
  - Otitis, sinusitis, bronchitis, pneumonia (documented).
  - Meningitis.
  - Oral ulcers.
  - Skin infections including skin abscesses, warts.
  - Other abscesses (e.g. intraabdominal).
  - Other infections: Osteomyelitis, septic arthritis, mastoiditis, parasitic infection, sepsis/bacteremia.
  - Previous hospitalization or complications from severe infection.
  - Treatments received including oral and intravenous (IV) antibiotics or other antimicrobial treatments (time, frequency, and duration of each treatment).
- *Malignancy*: Lymphoma, leukemia, other.
- Vaccination history including history of any disease following live vaccines, time from last vaccination is important, type of vaccine (e.g. polysaccharide or protein-conjugated) is also important.
- *Past surgical history*: Splenectomy, lung surgery, tonsillectomy, adenoidectomy, other.
- *Review of systems*: Ear, nose, and throat (ENT); cardiac; respiratory; gastrointestinal; musculoskeletal; neurological; genitourinary; skin; constitutional symptoms (e.g. fever, chills, night sweats, unexplained weight loss).
- *Family history*: Consanguinity, PID, genetic disease, early-unexplained childhood deaths, autoimmunity, hematological malignancies, recurrent spontaneous abortions, recurrent or severe infections.

Physical Examination

- General appearance, dysmorphic features
- Weight, height, vital signs
- Head and neck including oral cavity/ENT: Oral ulcers, oral thrush, teeth (including double row or conical teeth), nasal mucosa (pale or swollen), tympanic membrane, tonsils
- Sinuses

Table 22.2 Common Infectious Organisms and Sites According to Immune Defect

	Common infectious organisms	Infection sites
Humoral Immunity	• Pyogenic bacteria: *Streptococci, staphylococci, Haemophilus influenzae* • Enteroviruses: ECHO, polio • *Mycoplasma* species	Sinopulmonary, gastrointestinal, central nervous system, and joints
Cellular Immunity	• Viruses: CMV, adenovirus, measles, molluscum • Fungi: *Candida* and *Aspergillus* species, *Pneumocystis jiroveci* • Pyogenic bacteria • Protozoa: *Cryptosporidium* species	Lungs, sepsis, gastrointestinal tract, and skin
Complement System	• Pyogenic bacteria: *Streptococci, Haemophilus influenzae, Neisseria* species	Meningitis, systemic infections
Phagocytic System	• Bacteria: *Staphylococci, Serratia marcescens, Burkholderia cepacia, Klebsiella* species, *Escherichia coli, Salmonella* species, *Proteus* species • Fungi: *Candida, Aspergillus*, and *Nocardia* species	Skin infections, lymphadenitis, liver, lung, bone, GI tract, gingivitis/periodontitis

Note: Different immune defects predispose patients to specific pathogens and therefore identifying patterns of infectious organisms will help in diagnosis of specific PIDs.
Adapted from (4).

- Cardiac exam
- Respiratory exam
- Abdominal exam (including spleen and liver examination for hepatosplenomegaly)
- Skin and nails: For any skin infections, rash, onychomycosis
- Joints for signs of synovitis
- Neurological exam if indicated
- Lymph nodes: Head and neck, axillary, groin (presence or absence)
- Scoliosis, joint hyperlaxity

Differential Diagnosis of Hypogammaglobulinemia (Selected) [Adapted from "International Consensus Document (ICON): Common Variable Immunodeficiency Disorders" (7)]

- Infections: Human immunodeficiency virus (HIV), EBV
- Drugs: Glucocorticoids, phenytoin, carbamazepine, rituximab, sulfasalazine, antimalarials
- Malignancy: Non-Hodgkin lymphoma (NHL), chronic lymphocytic leukemia (CLL), multiple myeloma
- Systemic disease-causing protein (immunoglobulin) loss: Protein-losing enteropathy, nephrosis, lymphangiectasia, severe burns
- Hypercatabolic states

- PIDs: Hyper-IgM syndrome, X-linked agammaglobulinemia, CVID

Rule Out Causes of Secondary Immunodeficiency (Selected) [Adapted from (1)]

- See above—differential of hypogammaglobulinemia; in addition, consider:
  - Radiation
  - Malnutrition
  - Splenectomy
  - Any chronic illnesses including diabetes mellitus, cardiac, and respiratory diseases

Investigations in PID (Selected Investigations Including Quantitative and Functional Testing)

Tests for Suspected Antibody Deficiency (Selected Tests) [Adapted from (4)]

- Complete blood count (CBC) with differential for absolute lymphocyte counts
- Quantitative immunoglobulins: IgM, IgG, IgA, IgE, and IgG subclasses (only done in a very limited subset of patients and only if there is a particular indication)
- Specific antibody levels before and after vaccination: Tetanus, diphtheria, *Streptococcus pneumoniae* (protein and carbohydrate antigens)

- B-cell immunophenotyping/flow cytometry for percentage and total B cells (CD19, CD20) and memory B cells (CD27, surface IgM and IgD)
- In vitro functional studies (e.g. proliferation and cytokine production assays)
- Other tests to exclude secondary causes (selected tests):
  - Human Immunodeficiency Virus (HIV)
  - Stool alpha 1 antitrypsin, urinalysis (for proteinuria), serum albumin, total protein: To rule out gastrointestinal/urinary/lymphatic protein loss
  - Rule out complement deficiency: Classical pathway (CH50), alternative pathway (AH50), mannose-binding lectin (MBL)
  - Intracellular flow cytometry
  - Genetic evaluation
  - Karyotype or comparative genomic hybridization (CGH) microarray
  - Computed tomography (CT) of the chest to rule out thymoma, if clinically indicated

Tests for Suspected T-Cell and Combined (T- and B-Cell) Immunodeficiency (Selected) [Majority Adapted from (4)]

- CBC with differential (for absolute lymphocyte counts)
- Lymphocyte immunophenotyping: CD3+CD4+ (T helper), CD3+CD8+ (cytotoxic T cells), B cells as above, CD16-56, HLA DR, CD45RA+ (naïve T cells), CD45RO+ (memory T cells)
- Delayed type hypersensitivity skin testing
- HIV serology (and in certain cases viral load)
- Secondary tests (selected tests):
  - T-cell proliferation (mitogens, alloantigens, recall antigens)
  - Flow cytometry for surface or intracellular proteins (e.g. CD40 ligand, CD154 on activated T cells)
  - T-cell receptor excision circle (TREC) numbers (mostly in children)
  - Enzyme assays: Adenosine deaminase (mostly in children and also in adults with partial defects)
  - T-cell cytokine production
  - Fluorescence in situ hybridization (FISH) 22q11 deletion (mostly in children), CGH microarray
  - TCR V beta repertoire analysis
  - Panel sequencing of genes involved in combined immunodeficiencies

Tests for Suspected Complement Deficiency

- Classical complement pathway (CH50) by immune hemolysis
- Alternative complement pathway (AH50) by immune hemolysis
- MBL complement pathway by enzyme-linked immunosorbent assay (ELISA)

Tests for Suspected Defects in Phagocytes (Selected) [Adapted from (4)]

- Absolute neutrophil count and morphologic analysis (CBC with differential)
- Dihydrorhodamine 123 (DHR): To rule out CGD in children or in adults if suspected to have a milder form of the disease or to be a carrier
- Antineutrophil antibodies: Autoimmune neutropenia
- Bone marrow biopsy: Exclude defective myeloid production in neutropenia syndromes

Tests for Suspected Natural Killer (NK) Cell-Related Immunodeficiency (4)

- Flow cytometry (CD16CD56)
- Assaying cytotoxicity with standard in vitro assays (available in research labs)

Tests for Suspected Autoinflammatory Syndromes (Selected)

- Genetic testing (examples of mutations above): Is not a replacement for clinical diagnosis but should be done in cases that are highly suspected and for prognosis and genetic counseling.
- FMF: In acute attacks there can be leukocytosis on CBC, elevated erythrocyte sedimentation rate (ESR) and C-reactive protein (CRP) (5). Elevated levels of serum amyloid A (SAA) can be seen as a complication.
- TRAPS in acute attacks: Increased acute phase reactants, neutrophils, and anemia (5). TNF levels are low during acute flares and in between (6).

Management (General Aspects in Treatment) [Adapted from (1)]

- **Infection prophylaxis:** Prophylactic antimicrobials (antibiotics, antifungal)
- **Monitoring and management of associated conditions and complications:** Autoimmunity, malignancy, immune dysregulation, and atopic disease

- **Immunoglobulin replacement therapy:** Refer to Chapter 23
- **Avoid live vaccines:** e.g. in SCID, CID, MSMD, CGD
- **Isolation precautions when hospitalized:** In positive pressure rooms when indicated
- **Transplant:** Hematopoietic stem cell transplant (HSCT), bone marrow transplant in some cases
- **Gene therapy:** In some SCIDs, WAS, CGD
- **Others:** Biologics (e.g. abatacept), interferon gamma, JAK inhibitors

REFERENCES

1. Bonilla FA et al., J Allergy Clin Immunol. (2015), PMID: 26371839/DOI:10.1016/j.jaci.2015.04.049.
2. Jeffrey Modell Foundation. Primary Immunodeficiency Resource Centre. http://www.info4pi.org/library/educational-materials/10-warning-signs. Accessed on 08 June 2019.
3. Picard C et al., J Clin Immunol. (2018), PMID: 29226302/DOI: 10.1007/s10875-017-0464-9.
4. Oliveira JB et al., J Allergy Clin Immunol. (2010), PMID: 20042230/DOI:10.1016/j.jaci.2009.08.043.
5. Gattorno M et al., J Clin Immunol. (2008), PMID: 18368292/DOI:10.1007/s10875-008-9178-3.
6. Hull KM et al., Medicine (Baltimore). (2002), PMID: 12352631/DOI:10.1097/00005792-200209000-00002.
7. Bonilla FA et al., J Allergy Clin Immunol Pract. (2016), PMID: 26563668/DOI:10.1016/j.jaip.2015.07.025.

Immunoglobulin Replacement Therapy

ABEER FETEIH, FARIDA ALMARZOOQI, REZA ALIZADEHFAR, AND CHRISTOS TSOUKAS

GENERAL BACKGROUND

- Intravenous immunoglobulin (IVIg) is a sterile blood product prepared from pooled human plasma that usually consists of >95% unmodified IgG and trace amounts of IgA or IgM (1).
- Immunoglobulin replacement therapy (IRT) is indicated in a variety of primary and secondary immunodeficiencies (see Figure 23.2).

MECHANISMS OF ACTION OF IRT

- IRT is administered either in a low dose (e.g., 400–600 mg/kg/q 3–4 weeks) or a high dose (e.g., 1–2 g/kg/day) (14, 15):
  - *Low dose* is used in the context of low plasma IgG to replenish (substitute) the recipient IgG repertoire with protective antibodies against different infections, mainly bacterial.
  - *High dose* is used in autoimmune and autoinflammatory disorders (e.g. immune thrombocytopenia [ITP]) as an immuno-modulator therapy.
- The therapeutic impacts of IRT are attributed to its wide spectrum of actions, which involve the following mechanisms (see Figure 23.1):

1. **Immunoglobulin Fc (Fragment, crystallizable) region-mediated mechanism (14–16), through:**
   a. Preventing Fc gamma-receptor (FcγR) activation, which results in inhibition of FcγR-mediated cell functions including immune-complex binding, phagocytosis, antibody-dependent cellular toxicity, inflammatory cytokine release and antigen presentation.
   b. Increasing the expression of inhibitory FcγRIIb.

c. Blocking the complement cascade.
   d. Regulating immunoglobulin half-life and increasing catabolism of pathogenic antibodies by neonatal FcR (FcRn) saturation.
   e. Enhancing glucocorticoid receptor (GR) binding and response.

2. **Immunoglobulin fragment antigen-binding (Fab) region-mediated mechanisms, via (14–16):**
   a. Neutralizing pathogens and superantigens.
   b. Neutralizing cytokines, chemokines, apoptosis-inducing molecules (e.g. FasL) and adhesion molecules.
   c. Neutralizing autoantibodies by anti-idiotype antibodies (antibodies against the idiotype region of another immunoglobulin or T-cell receptor that consist of the antigen binding variable region).

3. **Antigen-presenting cells, in particular dendritic cells, regulation toward anti-inflammatory instead of pro-inflammatory response through (15, 16):**
   a. Decreasing surface molecule expression, such as HLA class II.
   b. Altering cytokine production, such as increase of IL-10 and reduction of IL-12.

4. **T-cell response regulation, by (15, 16):**
   a. T-regulatory (Treg) cells proliferating and response augmentation (17).
   b. Attenuating Th17 cells maturation and proliferation.

5. **B-cell response regulation, by enhancing anti-inflammatory response through (15, 16):**
   a. Upregulating the expression of inhibitory FcγRIIb.
   b. Alternating the TLR-9-dependent B-cell responses.

DOI: 10.1201/9781003174202-30

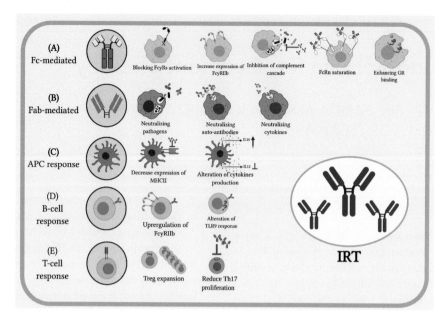

Figure 23.1 Mechanisms of action of immunoglobulin replacement therapy (IRT). The IRT therapeutic effects are illustrated through (A) the immunoglobulin Fc region-mediated mechanism; (B) Fab region-mediated mechanism; (C) APC response; (D) B-cells response control; and (E) T-cells response regulation. (Figure created with BioRender.com.) [Adapted from (14–17).] (*Abbreviations:* Fc: Fragment, crystallizable region; Fab: Fragment antigen-binding region; APC: Antigen presenting cells; MHCII: Major histocompatibility class II; GR: Glucocorticoid receptor.)

IVIG

Products Available in Canada

According to the 2016 Canadian Blood Services Professional Education (5):

- 5% or 10% [100 mg/mL] Gammagard˚ S/D [Solvent/Detergent-Treated (Lyophilized)].
- 5% or 10% Octagam˚.
- 10% Privigen˚.
- 10% IGIVnex˚.
- 10% GAMUNEX˚.
- 10% Panzyga˚.

Doses and Monitoring

- 400–600 mg/kg every 3–4 weeks used in most practices in Europe and the United states and Canada (6, 7).
- The goal of IRT is to achieve serum IgG trough levels that improve clinical results.
- IgG levels need to be monitored any time there is a major infection or when clinical response to treatment does not meet expectations (2).
- Periodic measurement of IgG trough levels may detect non-compliance in patients who are receiving treatment at home.

- Dose adjustments may be required due to patients' body weight change and/or the possibility of protein loss from other medical conditions (2).

Adverse Reactions (2)

Most reactions are related to the infusion rate, are mild, and occur in 5%–15% of infusions.

These reactions include:

- Headache
- Malaise
- Fever, chills
- Chest pain
- Rash
- Nausea
- Pruritus

Serious (Rare) Adverse Events

- Hemolysis
- Aseptic meningitis
- Thromboembolism (e.g. deep vein thrombosis, pulmonary embolism, stroke)
- Anaphylaxis
- Viral transmission
- Transfusion-related acute lung injury (TRALI)

Approved indications for use of IVIG*

Treatment of primary immunodeficiencies

Prevention of bacterial infections in patients with hypogammaglobulinemia and recurrent bacterial infection due to B-cell chronic lymphocytic leukemia

Prevention of coronary artery aneurysms in Kawasaki disease

Prevention of infections, pneumonitis, and acute graft-versus-host disease following bone marrow transplantation

Treatment of chronic inflammatory demyelinating polyneuropathy and multifocal motor neuropathy (3, 4)

Increasing platelet counts in idiopathic thrombocytopenic purpura to prevent or control bleeding

Reduction of serious bacterial infection in children infected with human immunodeficiency virus (HIV)

Figure 23.2 Approved indications for use of IVIG. (Figure created with BioRender.com.) [Adapted from (2).] *Indications listed are approved by the U.S. Food and Drug Administration (FDA). IVIG is used off-label in the treatment of numerous inflammatory, infectious, and immune-related diseases.

Management of Adverse Reactions and Pretreatment [Adapted from (2)]

- Decreasing the infusion rate or stopping it for 15–30 minutes will abort many of the reactions.
- One hour prior to infusion, pretreatment with nonsteroidal anti-inflammatory drugs (NSAIDs), acetaminophen, diphenhydramine (1 mg/kg per dose), or a non-sedating antihistamine and/or hydrocortisone (6 mg/kg per dose; maximum 100 mg) may prevent adverse reactions.
- Oral hydration before the infusion.

Note: In about 15%–18% of patients adverse reactions occur when switching between IVIg products (8).

SUBCUTANEOUS IMMUNOGLOBULIN (SCIG)

Indications

Primary immunodeficiency disease is the only licensed indication.

Products Available in Canada

- According to the 2016 Canadian Blood Services Professional Education (5):
  - 10% GAMUNEX®
  - 10% IGIVnex®
  - 20% Hizentra®
- 20% Cuvitru®

Dose

- *Initial dosing:* Usually 100–200 mg/kg per week (9).
- *Infusion rate:* 10–35 mL/h per site by pump, volumes of 15–40 mL per site (10, 11).
- To calculate the SCIg dose when switching from IVIg, the total monthly dose of IVIg being received is multiplied by a conversion factor (1.37 for the 16% preparations and 1.53 for the 20% preparation) and then divide it by the number of SCIg infusions to be given each month (12).

Site of Injections

- Abdomen, outer thigh, upper arm, and buttock

Adverse Reactions of SCIg

- Less serious adverse effects than IVIg.
- Most common: Local reaction at the infusion site (13).

REFERENCES

1. Rütter A et al., J Am Acad Dermatol. (2001), PMID: 11369915/DOI:10.1067/mjd.2001.112325.
2. Perez EE et al., J Allergy Clin Immunol. (2017), PMID: 28041678/DOI:10.1016/j.jaci.2016.09.023.
3. Hughes R, J Neurol. (2008), PMID: 18685920/ DOI:10.1007/s00415-008-3003-z.
4. Joint Task Force of the EFNS and the PNS. J Peripher Nerv Syst. (2010), PMID: 21199100/ DOI:10.1111/j.1529-8027.2010.00290.x.
5. Nahirniak S, Lazarus A. (2016) Chapter 4: Immune Globulin Products. In: Clinical Guide to Transfusion. Ottawa, Canada: Canadian Blood Services Professional Education. 2016. https://professional-education.blood.ca/en/transfusion/guide-clinique/ immune-globulin-products. Accessed 06-28-2019.
6. Yong PF et al., Clin Immunol. (2008), PMID: 18295543/DOI:10.1016/j.clim.2007.12.007.
7. Hernandez-Trujillo HS et al., Clin Exp Immunol. (2012), PMID:22670779/DOI:10.1111/j.1365-2249.2012.04588.x.
8. Ameratunga R et al., Clin Exp Immunol. (2004), PMID: 15030521/DOI:10.1111/j.1365-2249.2004.02412.x.
9. Stiehm ER et al., Adv Pediatr. (2010), PMID: 21056739/DOI:10.1016/j.yapd.2010.08.005.
10. Berger M, Immunol Allergy Clin North Am. (2008), PMID: 18940574/DOI:10.1016/j.iac.2008.07.002.
11. Moore ML et al., Ann Allergy Asthma Immunol. (2008), PMID: 18727465/DOI:10.1016/S1081-1206(10) 60197-4.
12. Wasserman RL et al., Clin Pharmacokinet. (2011), PMID: 21553933/DOI:10.2165/11587030-000000000-00000.
13. Ochs HD et al., J Clin Immunol. (2006), PMID: 16783465/DOI:10.1007/s10875-006-9021-7.
14. Nagelkerke SQ et al., Front Immunol. (2015), PMID: 25653650/DOI:10.3389/fimmu.2014.00674.
15. Gelfand EW, N Engl J Med. (2012), PMID: 23171098/ DOI:10.1056/NEJMra1009433.
16. Chaigne B et al., Transfus Apher Sci. (2017), PMID: 28161150/DOI:10.1016/j.transci.2016.12.017.
17. Maddur MS et al., J Clin Immunol. (2010), PMID: 20405183/DOI:10.1007/s10875-010-9394-5.

Index

Note: Locators in *italics* represent figures and **bold** indicate tables in the text.

A

AAAAI, *see* American Academy of Allergy, Asthma and Immunology
AAE, *see* Acquired angioedema
ABPA, *see* Allergic bronchopulmonary aspergillosis
ABRS, *see* Acute bacterial rhinosinusitis
AC, *see* Allergic conjunctivitis
ACAAI, *see* American College of Allergy, Asthma and Immunology
ACD, *see* Allergic contact dermatitis
ACE, *see* Angiotensin-converting enzyme-inhibitor cough
ACE inhibitor (ACE-I)-associated angioedema
    clinical, 97
    idiopathic, 97, **98**
    pathogenesis, 97
ACQ, *see* Asthma Control Questionnaire
Acquired angioedema (AAE)
    age and prevalence, 96
    associated underlying diseases, 96–97
    diagnosis, 97
    management, 97
    pathogenesis, 96
ACT, *see* Asthma Control Test
Acute attacks, 93
Acute bacterial rhinosinusitis (ABRS)
    antibiotics, 14–15
    defined, 14
    endocranial complications, 14
    immediate referral/hospitalization, 14
    orbital complications, 14
    osseous complications, 14
    physical examination, 14
    prevalence, 13
    symptoms, 14
Acute cough, 57
Acute facial eczema, *71*
Acute generalized exanthematous pustulosis (AGEP), 172, 180
Acute management, 119, 131

Acute rhinosinusitis (ARS), 13, 14
Acute severe asthma exacerbation, 44
Acute spontaneous urticaria (ASU), 81
Acute urticaria, 83, 145
Acute viral rhinosinusitis (AVRS), 13
AD, *see* Atopic dermatitis
Additives/residual components
    DNR latex, 184
    egg/chicken protein, 184
    gelatin, 184
    milk protein (casein), 184
    yeast protein, 184
Adverse drug reactions (ADRs), 167
AERD, *see* Aspirin-exacerbated respiratory disease
Aeroallergens, 45, 116
AFRS, *see* Allergic fungal rhinosinusitis
Aicardi-Goutières syndrome, 193
AIR, *see* Anti-inflammatory reliever
AIT, *see* Allergen immunotherapy
AKC, *see* Atopic keratoconjunctivitis
Alcohol-induced worsening, 15
Alemtuzumab, 140
Allergen immunotherapy (AIT), 12
    aeroallergen and venom desensitization, 31
    allergens and effective doses, **33**
    description, 31
    dosing, *36*
    indications and contraindications, **32**
    mechanism, 31, **32**
Allergic bronchopulmonary aspergillosis (ABPA), 48–49
Allergic conjunctivitis (AC), 23
Allergic contact dermatitis (ACD), 145
    differential diagnoses, 77
    non-pharmacologic, 78
    pharmacologic, 79
    physical examination, 77
Allergic disease, 109
Allergic facies, 5
Allergic fungal rhinosinusitis (AFRS), 18–19

Allergic proctocolitis, 149
Allergic rhinitis
   diagnosis, 6
   history taking, 5
   IgE-mediated inflammatory disease, 3
   non-pharmacologic, 6–7
   pharmacologic management, 7–11, **8–10**
   physical examination, 5
   pregnancy and lactation, 11
   symptoms, 4–5
Allergic Rhinitis and Its Impact on Asthma (ARIA),
   4
Allergic salute, 5
Allergic shiners, 5, *5*, 26
Allogeneic stem cell transplantation, 140
Allotussia, 58
American Academy of Allergy, Asthma and
   Immunology (AAAAI), 76, 167
American College of Allergy, Asthma and
   Immunology (ACAAI), 76, 167
Amoxicillin-clavulanate, 14
Anaphylaxis, 32, 146, 149, 174
   aeroallergens, 116
   allergy diagnostic tests/interventions, 115
   biphasic course, 116
   definition, 115
   diagnostic criteria, 117
   exercise and seminal fluid, 116
   fatality rate, 115
   food and medications, 115
   history of, 116
   idiopathic, 116
   insect stings and radiocontrast media, 115
   lifetime prevalence, 115
   pathogenesis, 115
   pathophysiology and clinical manifestations,
      115, *116*
   perioperative agents, 115
   severity grading, 118, **118**
   signs and symptoms, 116
   skin prick testing, 118
   uniphasic course, 116
Angioedema, 81, 83, 145; *see also* ACE inhibitor
   (ACE-I)-associated angioedema;
   Acquired angioedema (AAE); Hereditary
   angioedema (HAE)
Angiotensin-converting enzyme (ACE)-inhibitors,
   33, 44, 82
Angiotensin receptor blockers (ARBs), 97
Anthropomorphics, 43
Antifibrinolytics, 95

Antigen-presenting cells, 199
Anti-IgE (omalizumab), 87–88
Anti-inflammatory reliever (AIR), 46
Anti-leukotrienes, 112
ARBs, *see* Angiotensin receptor blockers
ARS, *see* Acute rhinosinusitis
Arthritis/arthralgia, 183
Aspirin challenge and desensitization, **179**
Aspirin desensitization, *180*
Aspirin-exacerbated respiratory disease (AERD),
   177–178
Associated biomarkers, 42
Associated HES, 138
Asthma
   asthma-related death, 45
   biologies and associated special features, *48*
   children and adults, 41
   clinical manifestations, 43
   comorbidities, *46*
   ICS-LABA combinations, 47
   initial controller treatment, *47*
   mild, moderate and severe, 41
   non-pharmacologic, 45–46
   non-type 2, 47
   pathophysiology endotypes and phenotypes,
      41–42, *43*
   pharmacologic, 46
   physical examination, 43–44
   symptoms, 41
Asthma and other lower airway diseases, 15
Asthma Control Questionnaire (ACQ), 43
Asthma Control Test (ACT), 43
Asthma inhaler therapies in Canada, **50–53**
ASU, *see* Acute spontaneous urticaria
Ataxia-telangiectasia, 192
Atopic dermatitis (AD), 145
   algorithm, *72*
   clinical manifestations, 67
   comorbidities, 68–69
   cytokine profiles, 67
   diagnosis and assessment, 67–68
   epidemiology, 67
   management approach, 69, **69–70**
   pathophysiology, *68*
   patient education and follow-up, 69, 72
   skin barrier defects, 67
Atopic eruption of pregnancy, 89
Atopic keratoconjunctivitis (AKC), 23
"Atypical" celiac sprue, 159
Autoinflammatory syndromes, 193, 196
AVRS, *see* Acute viral rhinosinusitis

B

Basal serum tryptase level, 84, 130, *131*
B-cell non-Hodgkin lymphoma (NHL), 159
B-cell response regulation, 199
Beta-lactam (BL) allergy, 174
Biologics, 18, 158
Biopsy indications, 161, **161**
Birch-apple syndrome, 148
Bird-egg syndrome, 148
Black fire ants *(S. richteri),* 128
Bone marrow-derived granulocytes, 135
Bone marrow evaluation, 109
Bradykinin-mediated angioedema, **98**
Bradykinin (B2) receptor antagonist, 91, 94
Bronchiectasis, 44
Budesonide (oral viscous), 157
Bumblebee *(Bombus* spp.), 127

C

Calcium channel defects, 192
Carbapenems, 174
Cardiovascular HES, 138–139
Cartilage hair hypoplasia, 192
Cat-pork syndrome, 148
CCAD, *see* Central compartment atopic disease
CD, *see* Contact dermatitis
CDC, *see* Contact dermatoconjunctivitis
Celiac disease (CD)
    adjunctive treatment of uncomplicated, 162–163
    autoimmune glutensensitive enteropathy, 159
    genotyping, 160
    pathogenesis and immunology, 159–160
    risk of malignancy, 159
    serological testing, 160, *161*
Celiac "iceberg," 159
Central compartment atopic disease (CCAD), 19, *20*
Central neuromodulators, 63
Chemokines, 135
CHF, *see* Congestive heart failure
Chronic cough
    CHS framework, 58–63
    description, 57
    diagnostic evaluation flowchart, **59**
    epidemiology, 58
    pathophysiologic components, *59*
    pathophysiology, 58
Chronic inducible urticaria (CIndU), 81, *82*, 84,
    85–86
Chronic mucocutaneous candidiasis (CMC), 193

Chronic obstructive pulmonary disease (COPD), 44
Chronic rhinosinusitis (CRS)
    asthma and other lower airway diseases, 15
    classification, 15
    CRSsNP, 15, **15**
    CRSwNP, 15, **15**
    description, 13
    differential diagnosis, 15–16
    environmental allergies, 15
    management, 17–18
    nasal inflammation, *17*
    N-ERD, 15
    normal and abnormal CT sinus imaging, *17*
    primary and secondary, 16
Chronic spontaneous urticaria (CSU), 81
Chronic urticaria (CU)
    defined, 81
    differential diagnosis, 83
    non-pharmacologic, 86
    pharmacologic, 86
    physical examination, 82–83
    prognosis, 88
    treatment algorithm, *87*
CHS, *see* Cough hypersensitivity syndrome
Cicatricial ectropion, 26
CIndU, *see* Chronic inducible urticaria
C1INH deficiency, *see* Acquired angioedema
C1INH replacement, 94
Circulation, airway, breathing (CAB), 119
Classic celiac sprue, 159
Combined immunodeficiencies, 192
"Complement deficiencies," 193
Complete blood count (CBC), 45
Component-resolved diagnosis (CRD), 147
Concurrent nutritional deficiencies, 162
C1 esterase inhibitor (C1INH) deficiency/
    impairment, 91
Congenital neutropenias, 193
Congestive heart failure (CHF), 44
Contact dermatitis (CD), 180
    aluminum, 185
    anatomic distribution, 75
    clinical manifestations, **76**
    eczematous skin disorder, 75
    elicitation phase, 75
    epidemiology, 75
    ICD, 75
    neomycin, 184
    sensitization phase, 75
    thimerosal, 184
Contact dermatoconjunctivitis (CDC), 23

Contact urticaria, 145
Contributing drugs, 170
COPD, *see* Chronic obstructive pulmonary disease
Corticosteroids, 139
Cough; *see also* Chronic cough
    classification, 57
    definition, 57
    hypersensitivity syndrome, *57*
Cough hypersensitivity syndrome (CHS), 44, 57
Cough/laryngeal hypersensitivity, 63
C-reactive protein (CRP), 84
Cross-reactivity, 145
CRS, *see* Chronic rhinosinusitis
CSU, *see* Chronic spontaneous urticaria
CU, *see* Chronic urticaria
Cutaneous HES, 138
Cutaneous systemic reactions, 129
Cyclosporine A, 88
Cytokines, 135
Cytotoxic therapies, 140

D

Delayed reactions, 174, 180
Delayed-type hypersensitivity reactions (DTHRs),
    see Contact dermatitis
Dennie-Morgan lines, 5, *5*
Dermatitis herpetiformis (DH), 159
DHRs, *see* Drug hypersensitivity reactions
Dietary protein-induced proctitis/proctocolitis,
    146
Differential diagnosis/syndromes, 149
Diffusing capacity for carbon monoxide (DLCO),
    45
DiGeorge syndrome, 192
DNR, *see* Dry natural rubber latex
Dose amoxicillin-clavulanate, 14
DRESS syndrome, 170
Drug allergies, 167
    classification, 167–168
    history, 169–170
    hypersensitivity reactions, 168
    physical examination, 170
Drug desensitization, 173–174
Drug hypersensitivity reactions (DHRs), 167
Drug provocation testing (DPT), 172–173
Drug rash with eosinophilia and systemic
    symptoms (DRESS), 180
Dry natural rubber (DNR) latex, 184
Dust mites, 6–7
Dysfunctional breathing/hyperventilation, 44

E

Ectopic ACD, 76
Eczema Area Severity Index, *71*
Eczema herpeticum (EH), 68
Egg/chicken protein, 184
EH, *see* Eczema herpeticum
EIMs management, 162
Elemental diet, 156–157
Empiric food elimination diet, 157
Encephalopathy, 185
Endocrine disorders, 109
End-organ involvement, 139
Endoscopic appearance, 161
Enteropathy, 149
Enteropathy-associated T-cell lymphoma (EATL),
    159
Environmental allergies, 15
Environmental control of indoor/outdoor allergens,
    6
EoE, *see* Eosinophilic esophagitis
Eosinophilia, *135*
    causes of, 136, *136*
    defined, 136
Eosinophilic bronchitis, 61
Eosinophilic esophagitis (EoE), 35, 146, 148
    definition, 153
    diagnosis, 154
    diet, 156–157
    differential diagnosis, 154
    epidemiology, 153
    history, 154
    management, 155–156
    and nutritional concerns, 154–155, *155*
    pathogenesis, 153, *153*
    signs and symptoms, 154
    systematic approach, *156*
Eosinophilic gastroenteritis, 146
Epidermodysplasia verruciformis, 193
Epinephrine auto-injector, 119–120
EPOS, see *European Position Paper on
    Rhinosinusitis and Nasal Polyps 2020*
Erythema marginatum, 92
Esophageal dilation therapy, 158
*European Position Paper on Rhinosinusitis and
    Nasal Polyps (EPOS) 2020*, 13
European Respiratory Society (ERS) Task Force, 57
European Society for the Study of Coeliac Disease
    (ESsCD), 160
Exacerbating factors, 82
Excited skin syndrome, 78

Exercise-induced anaphylaxis
    anaphylactic symptoms, 123
    clinical diagnoses, 123
    controlled exercise challenge, 123
    differential diagnoses, 125
    initial symptoms, 123
    life-threatening conditions, 123
    management, *124*
    prevalence, 123
    triggers, 123
    wheat-dependent, 125
Extra-intestinal manifestations (EIMs), 160, *160*

F

Familial hemophagocytic lymphohistiocytosis
        (FHL) syndromes, 192–193
Familial HES, 138
Family Apidae, 127
Family Vespidae (Vespid family), 127–128, *128*
FeNO, *see* Fractional excretion of nitric oxide
FFP, *see* Fresh frozen plasma
FIP1L1-PDGFR A mutation, 108
FIRE, *see* Food-induced immediate response of the
        esophagus
First-generation H1 antihistamines, 7
Fixed drug eruptions, 172, 180
Flushing syndromes, 118
Fluticasone propionate, 157
Food allergens, 145
Food allergy,
    defined, 145
    prevention, 150–151
Food-dependent exercise-induced anaphylaxis
        (FDEIA), 124, *124*, 148, 149; *see also*
        Exercise-induced anaphylaxis (EIA)
Food-induced immediate response of the esophagus
        (FIRE), 154
Food protein-induced enterocolitis syndrome
        (FPIES), 146, 148–149
Four-food elimination diet, 157
Fractional excretion of nitric oxide (FeNO), 42
Fresh frozen plasma (FFP), 94
Functional autoantibodies, 84

G

Gain-of-function *KIT* mutations, 104
Gastrointestinal HES, 139
GBS, *see* Guillain-Barré syndrome
GCD, *see* Gluten-containing diet

Gell and Coombs' Classification, 169, **169**
Gene therapy, 197
Gestational pemphigoid, 89
Giant papillary conjunctivitis (GPC), 23
GINA, *see* "Global Initiative for Asthma (GINA)
        2020 Update"
"Global Initiative for Asthma (GINA) 2020 Update,"
        41–43, 47
Gluten-containing diet (GCD), 160
Gluten-free diet (GFD), 162
GPC, *see* Giant papillary conjunctivitis
Graded intramuscular vaccine dosing, 186
Granule proteins, 135
Granulocyte-macrophage colony-stimulating factor
        (GM-CSF), 135
Guillain-Barré syndrome (GBS), 185

H

HAE, *see* Hereditary angioedema
H2 antihistamines, 87
HATS, *see* Hereditary alpha-tryptasemia syndrome
Health Canada approved sublingual
        immunotherapy tablets, 35, **35**
Hematologic HES, 138
Hereditary alpha-tryptasemia syndrome (HATS),
        103
Hereditary angioedema (HAE)
    characteristics of swelling, 92
    C1INH antigenic level, 93
    C4 level, 92
    diagnostic algorithm, *93*
    disease severity, 92
    morbidity and mortality, 92
    mutation, 91
    non-pharmacologic management, 93
    pharmacologic management, 93, *95*
    precipitating factors, 92
    prevalence, 91
    prodromal symptoms, 92
    types, 91, *92*
Herpes simplex encephalitis (HSE), 193
High-dose 17α-alkylated androgens, 94
Higher dose amoxicillin-clavulanate, 14
Histologic appearance, 162
HLA markers and disease associations, 173
Honeybee (*Apis mellifera* spp.), 127
Horner-Trantas dots, 26
Hornets: Yellow hornet (*Dolichovespula arenaria*),
        128
Human herpesvirus 6 (HHV-6) reactivation, 170

Hydroxyurea, 140
Hymenoptera
    cross-reactivity and cross-sensitization, 128
    family Apidae, 127
    family Formicidae, 128
    family Vespidae (Vespid family), 127–128, *128*
    subfamily Polistinae, 128
Hypereosinophilia, 136
Hypereosinophilic syndrome (HES), 136–137
Hyper-IgE syndromes, 192
Hypersensitivity reactions, 127
Hypertussia, 58

I

ICD, *see* Irritant contact dermatitis
ICS, *see* Inhaled corticosteroids
IDHRs, *see* Immediate drug hypersensitivity
        reactions
Idiopathic angioedema, 97
Idiopathic chronic cough (ICC), 57
Idiopathic MCASs (IMCASs), 105–106
ID test, 185–186
IFN-α, 140
IgE-mediated food allergy, 146–148
IgE-mediated reactions
    additives or residual vaccine components, 183
    anaphylaxis, 183
IMCASs, *see* Idiopathic MCASs
Immediate drug hypersensitivity reactions (IDHRs),
        168–169
Immediate GI hypersensitivity, 145
Immunodeficiencies affecting cellular and humoral
        immunity, 192
Immunodeficiency, 15
Immunoglobulin replacement therapy (IRT), 197
    antigen-presenting cells, 199
    B-cell response regulation, 199
    fragment antigen-binding (Fab) region, 199
    fragment, crystallizable region, 199
    primary and secondary immunodeficiencies,
        199
    T-cell response regulation, 199
Immunomodulators, 88
Immunosuppressants, 88
Impaired ciliary motility, 15
Imported fire ant (IFA), 132
INCS, *see* Intranasal corticosteroids
Infection prophylaxis, 196
Inhaled corticosteroids (ICS), 43
International Consensus Document (ICON), 195

"International Union of Immunological Societies:
        2017 Primary Immunodeficiency Diseases
        Committee Report on Inborn Errors of
        Immunity," 192
Intradermal (ID) tests, 11, 130, 147
Intrahepatic cholestasis of pregnancy, 89
Intranasal anticholinergics, 12
Intranasal antihistamine (INAH), 7
Intranasal corticosteroid (INCS), 7, 15
Intranasal cromolyn, 12
Intranasal decongestants, 12
Intranasal saline irrigation, 15
Intravenous (IV) crystalloid fluids, 119
Intravenous immunoglobulin (IVIg)
    adverse reactions, 200
    description, 199
    doses and monitoring, 200
    pretreatment, 201
    products in Canada, 200
    (rare) adverse events, 200
Immunoglobulin replacement therapy, 197
Intravenous plasma-derived C1INH, 94
Intrinsic and innate immunity defects, 193
Irritant contact dermatitis (ICD), 75
IRT, *see* Immunoglobulin replacement therapy
Isolated congenital asplenia (ICA), 193

J

Jeffrey Modell Foundation, **191**

K

Kallikrein inhibitor, 94
Keratoconjunctivitis, 23

L

Lagophthalmos, 26
Large local reactions (LLRs), 127
Laryngeal paresthesia, 58
Latent celiac sprue, 159
Latex-fruit syndrome, 148
Leukotriene inhibitors, 18
Leukotriene receptor antagonists (LTRAs), 11, 43,
        87
Lipid mediators, 136
5-Lipoxygenase inhibitors (zileuton), 11
Live and killed vaccines, *186*
Local reactions, 127
Local symptoms, 35

Long-term management, 119, 131
Long-term prophylaxis (LTP), 94
LTP, *see* Long-term prophylaxis
LTRA, *see* Leukotriene antagonist
Lung auscultation, 5

M

Macroscopic esophageal findings, 154
Maintenance immunotherapy, 11
Maintenance therapy, 157–158
Mast cell (MC), pathobiology, 103–104
Mast cell activation (MCA), 104
Mastocytosis, defined, 103
Material Safety Data Sheets (MSDS), 76
Mature activated eosinophils, 136
MC, *see* Mast cell
MCA, *see* Mast cell activation
MC activation syndromes (MCASs)
    bone marrow evaluation, 109
    clinical, 107
    defined, 103
    diagnostic criteria, 107, *108*
    FIP1L1-PDGFR A mutation, 108
    genetic test (buccal swab), *TPSAB1* gene, 108
    HAT, 106–107
    imaging, 109
    IMCASs, 105–106
    management, 109–110
    peripheral blood *KIT* D816V mutation, 107–108
    pharmacotherapy approach, 110
    primary, 105
    secondary, 105
    serum tryptase level, 107
MCASs, *see* MC activation syndromes
McGill University Health Centre Pre-Risk
        Assessment Protocol, 173
Mendelian susceptibility to mycobacterial disease
        (MSMD), 193
Mepolizumab (anti IL-5 monoclonal antibody),
        140
Methacholine provocation test, 45
Microscopic esophageal findings, 154
Milk protein (casein), 184
Mite-shrimp syndrome, 148
MMCAS, *see* Monoclonal MCAS
Monobactams, 174
Monoclonal MCAS (MMCAS), 105
MSDS, *see* Material Safety Data Sheets
Multiple NSAID-exacerbated urticaria/angioedema,
        178

Multiple NSAID-induced urticaria/angioedema,
        178–179
Myeloproliferative HES, 137

N

Nasal anatomic variations, 15
Nasal mucosa, 5
National Institute of Allergy and Infectious
        Diseases (NIAID) Sponsored Expert
        Panel, 145
Natural killer (NK) cell-related immunodeficiency,
        196
Neomycin, 184
Neuroendocrine disorders, 109
Neurologic HES, 139
NIDHRs, *see* Non-immediate drug hypersensitivity
        reactions
Non-celiac gluten sensitivity (NCGS), 163
Non-IgE-mediated food allergy, 150
Non-immediate drug hypersensitivity reactions
        (NIDHRs), 169
Non-inflammasome-related conditions, 193
Nonsteroidal anti-inflammatory drugs (NSAIDs)
    AERD, *see* Aspirin-exacerbated respiratory
            disease
    classification, **178**
    delayed reactions, 180
    description, 177
Non-type 2 endotype, 16
North American Contact Dermatitis Group
        (NACDG Research Group), 77
Novel peripheral neuronal treatments, 63
NSAID-exacerbated respiratory disease (N-ERD),
        15
NSAIDs, *see* Nonsteroidal anti-inflammatory drugs

O

OA, *see* Ocular allergies
Obstructive sleep apnea (OSA), 62
Occupational contact dermatitis (OCD), 75–76
Ocular allergies (OA)
    clinical presentations, 23, **24–25**
    diagnosis, 26–27, *27*
    management, 27
    pharmacotherapy, *28*
    treatment approach, *28*
    types of, 23, *23*
Ocular pruritus, 26
OFC, *see* Oral food challenge

Oral allergy syndrome (OAS), 145
Oral antibiotics, 18
Oral candidiasis, 157
Oral decongestants, 11
Oral food challenge (OFC), 147–149, 150, 151
Oral glucocorticoids, 17
Oral immunotherapy (OIT), 150
Oral steroids, 88
Osteoporosis, 109
Overlap disorders, 138
Oxidative products, 136

P

PAC, *see* Perennial allergic conjunctivitis
Patch testing (PT), 77, 78, *78*
Patch testing or delayed ID testing, 173
Patient-Oriented Eczema Measure (POEM), 72
Patient-Oriented SCORAD (PO-SCORAD), 72
Perennial allergic conjunctivitis (PAC), 23
Peripheral neuropathies, 139
PFAS/OAS, 148, 149
Phagocytes, 196
"Phenocopies of PID," 193
Pheochromocytoma, 118
Physical triggers, 82
Pittsburgh VCD Index, 44
Plasma-derived C1INH concentrate, 94
Polistes species (paper wasp), 128
Pollen-food allergy syndrome (PFAS), 145
Positive SPT, 147
Posterior pharynx, 5
Post-viral ARS, *see* Post-viral rhinosinusitis
Post-viral rhinosinusitis (Post-Viral ARS), 13
Predominantly antibody deficiencies, 192
Pregnancy, 19–20
    anesthesia, 111
    aspirin desensitization, 180–181
    breastfeeding, 111–112
    diagnosis, 95, 120
    epidemiology, 120
    first- and second-generation antihistamines, 111
    and lactation, 132–133, 140
    leukotriene antagonists, 111
    management, 120–121
    mastocytosis, 111
    MC stabilizer cromolyn, 111
    medical management, 96
    and postpartum, 96
    pre-conception, 95–96
Primary CRS, 16

Primary immunodeficiencies (PIDs)
    description, 191
    distribution, *194*
    history, 193–194
    physical examination, 194–195
Primary MCASs, 105
Progesterone hypersensitivity, 89
Prophylaxis, 94
Prurigo of pregnancy, 89
Pruritic urticarial papules and plaques of pregnancy (PUPPP), 89
PT reading, 77–78
Pulmonary involvement, 139
Pustular psoriasis of pregnancy, 89

R

Radiocontrast media (RCM) reactions, 174
RARS, *see* Recurrent acute rhinosinusitis
Recall dermatitis, 78
Recombinant human C1INH, 94
Recurrent acute rhinosinusitis (RARS), 13
Red fire ants (*Solenopsis invicta*), 128
Refractory chronic cough (RCC), 57
RegiSCAR scoring system, 170–171, **171**
Repeat open application test (ROAT), 78
Reslizumab (humanized anti-IL-5 monoclonal antibody), 140
Restaurant syndromes, 118
Rheumatologic HES, 139
Rhinitis
    atopic or non-atopic, 3
    causes of, 3, **4**
    classification of, *3*
    differential diagnosis, 5
    etiologies, 3
Rhinosinusitis, nasal cavities, 13

S

SAC, *see* Seasonal allergic conjunctivitis
SCF, *see* Stem cell factor
SCIg, *see* Subcutaneous immunoglobulin
SCIT, *see* Subcutaneous immunotherapy
Seasonal allergic conjunctivitis (SAC), 23
Seasonal allergic rhinitis (SAR), 3
Secondary CRS, 16
Secondary immunodeficiency, 195
Secondary MCASs, 105
Second-generation H1 antihistamines, 11
SERPIN peptidase inhibitor, 91

Serum tryptase, 103
17α-alkylated androgens, 94
Severe combined immunodeficiency (SCID), 192
SFED, *see* Six-food elimination diet
Shared decision-making process, 156
Short-course topical decongestant (oxymetazoline), 11
Short-term prophylaxis (STP), 94, 96
Silent celiac sprue, 159
Single inhaler maintenance and reliever therapy (SMART), 46
Single NSAID-induced anaphylactic reactions, 179–180, *180*
Six-food elimination diet (SFED), 157
Skin biopsy, 173
Skin examination, 5
Skin prick test (SPT), 11, 42, 130, 146, **147**, 172, 185
Skin testing and/or specific-IgE (sIgE) testing, 130
SLIT, *see* Sublingual immunotherapy
Slow-responders, 163
SMART, *see* Single inhaler maintenance and reliever therapy
Special patient populations
    immunocompromised patients, 185
    pregnant women, 185
Spontaneous and physical urticarias, *82*
SPT, *see* Skin prick test
Sputum eosinophils, 45
Stanozolol, 95
Stem cell factor (SCF), 103
Step-down approach, 157
Step-up approach, 157
Stevens-Johnson syndrome (SJS), 180
STING-associated vasculopathy, 193
Stinging Insect Venom Reaction Classifications and Management, **129**
STP, *see* Short-term prophylaxis
Subacute cough, 57
Subcutaneous immunoglobulin (SCIg), 201–202
Subcutaneous immunotherapy (SCIT)
    adverse effects, 31
    dose and scheduling, 31
    immunotherapy risks, 31
    vs. SLIT, *36*
Subcutaneous plasma-derived C1INH, 94
Sublingual immunotherapy (SLIT)
    adverse reactions, 33–34, **34**
    FDA, 35
    vs. SCIT, *36*
    side effects, 35
Sublingual (tablet) immunotherapy, 31

Supportive therapy, 119
Suspected antibody deficiency, 195–196
Symptomatic treatment, ISM, **110**
Systemic allergic reactions, 35
Systemic cutaneous reactions, 127, 129

T

T- and B-cell immunodeficiency, 196
Targeted elimination diet (allergy-testing directed), 157
T-cell response regulation, 199
TCS, *see* Topical corticosteroids
T2-high associated phenotypes, 42
T2-high endotype mechanism, 41–42
Thimerosal, 184
Thymic stromal lymphopoietin (TSLP), 42
Thyroid autoantibodies, 84
Thyroid function test, 84
T2-low associated phenotypes, 42
T2-low endotype mechanism, 42
TLR signaling pathway deficiency, 193
Topical calcineurin inhibitors, 79
Topical corticosteroids (TCS), *72*
Topical decongestants, 11
Topical swallowed steroids, 157
Toxic epidermal necrolysis (TEN), 171–172, 180
Trigger management, 63
TSLP, *see* Thymic stromal lymphopoietin
Tympanic membranes (TM), 5
Type 2 endotype, 16
Tyrosine kinase inhibitors, 140

U

UACS, *see* Upper airway cough syndrome
Undefined HEus, 137
Unexplained chronic cough (UCC), 57
Upper airway cough syndrome (UACS), 61
Urticaria
    cumulative lifetime prevalence, 81
    definition, 81
Urticaria Activity Score for Seven Days (UAS-7), 88
Urticarial lesions, 82

V

Vaccines; *see also* Additives/residual components; IgE-mediated reactions
    classification, *183*
    local injection site reactions, 183
    public health, 183

Vasoactive mediators, 103
Vasopressors, 119
VCD, *see* Vocal cord dysfunction
VCD/inducible laryngeal obstruction, 63
Venom hypersensitivity, 109, 127
Venom immunotherapy (VIT), 129, 131, 132
Vernal keratoconjunctivitis (VKC), 23
Vocal cord dysfunction (VCD), 44

W

White-faced hornet *(D. maculata),* 128
Wiskott-Aldrich syndrome (WAS), 192

Y

Yeast protein, 184
Yellow jacket (*Vespula* spp.), 127